Step-Up To The Bedside

SECOND EDITION

Step-Up To The Bedside

SECOND EDITION

WITHDRAWN

SAMIR MEHTA, MD
Administrative Chief Resident
Department of Orthopaedic Surgery
The Hospital of the University of Pennsylvania
University of Pennsylvania Health System
Philadelphia, Pennsylvania

LCDR EDMUND A. MILDER, MC USNR
Department of Pediatrics
Naval Medical Center
San Diego, California

ADAM J. MIRARCHI, MD
Chief Resident, Department of Orthopaedic Surgery
University Hospitals of Cleveland
Case Western Reserve University
Cleveland, Ohio

EUGENE MILDER, ENS MC USNR
Resident, Department of Ophthalmology
Naval Medical Center
San Diego, California

2nd Edition Editor

VERONICA SIKKA, MHA, MPH
Medical Student, School of Medicine
PhD Student, School of Allied Health Professions,
Department of Health Administration
Virginia Commonwealth University
Richmond, Virginia

. **Lippincott Williams & Wilkins**
a Wolters Kluwer business
Philadelphia · Baltimore · New York · London
Buenos Aires · Hong Kong · Sydney · Tokyo

Acquisitions Editor: Donna M. Balado
Managing Editor: Kelly Horvath
Marketing Manager: Emilie Linkins
Associate Production Manager: Kevin P. Johnson
Designer: Risa Clow
Compositor: International Typesetting and Composition
Printer: Data Reproductions

First Edition, 2001
Second Edition, 2006

Library of Congress Cataloging-in-Publication Data

Step-up to the bedside / [edited by] Samir Mehta . . . [et al.]. — 2nd ed.
   p. ; cm.
 "Preparatory text not only for the USMLE Step 1 (in conjunction with
Step-Up), but also for the Step 2 and CSA Examinations given the current
merging of formats underway by the NBME"—Pref.
 Includes bibliographical references and index.
 ISBN-13: 978-0-7817-7964-7 (alk. paper)
 ISBN-10: 0-7817-7964-2 (alk. paper)
 1. Differential diagnosis—Case studies. 2. Differential
diagnosis—Examinations, questions, etc. I. Mehta, Samir.
  [DNLM: 1. Diagnosis—Case Reports. 2. Diagnosis—Examination Questions.
3. Diagnostic Techniques and Procedures—Case Reports. 4. Diagnostic
Techniques and Procedures—Examination Questions.   WB 18.2 S8273 2007]
RC71.5.S74 2007
616.07'5076—dc22

2006015621

The publishers have made every effort to trace the copyright holders for borrowed material. If they have inadvertently overlooked any, they will be pleased to make the necessary arrangements at the first opportunity.

To my parents, Sudesh and Shobha, and to my sisters, Sonia and Sonul,

—Samir Mehta

To my parents James and Phyllis, and my siblings Eugene, Shannon, and Robert

—Edmund A. Milder

To my parents Anthony and Andrea, my brother Alan, and my wife Sharon

—Adam J. Mirarchi

To my parents James and Phyllis, and my siblings Edmund, Shannon, and Robert

—Eugene Milder

To my parents, Mahesh and Sunaina

—Veronica Sikka

To our teachers
To our friends
And to the physicians of the future

Preface

The transition from the basic science years to the clinical years is often marked by passing the United States Medical Licensing Exam (USMLE) Step 1 as administered by the National Board of Medical Examiners (NBME). In most medical school curricula, the basic science years consist of first learning "the normal state" followed by "what can go wrong." Diseases are first identified by name and subsequently expanded with information on signs, symptoms, histologic changes, diagnostic tests, and treatment methods. Despite the recent push toward problem-based learning and integration of principles, this approach still exists in many schools and curricula over the course of the first 2 years. During the clinical years, the approach to learning and teaching is quite different—essentially, students are provided with myriad facts and data about a patient and from that data are to make a conclusion about the patient's disease. Over the past few years, the NBME has utilized this latter approach in testing student knowledge of basic sciences. Each question administered by the NBME via its Computer Based Testing (CBT) is framed as a clinical case; however, the information needed to answer the clinical question is basic science in nature. Furthermore, the NBME has really blurred the line when it comes to questions for the Step 1 Examination and those geared toward the Step 2 Examination.

The first edition of *Step-Up to the Bedside* was created with the same concept in mind. It presented clinically oriented cases and provided basic science coverage of relevant material sufficient for USMLE Step 1 preparation, but also served as a springboard for Step 2 and the Step 2 CS. A significant effort was made to describe the "textbook" patient; however, it needs to be noted that very rarely do patients present with all the signs and symptoms typical of a certain disease. The second edition builds on the momentum of the first edition. The text has been re-tooled and multiple new educational features have been added including:

- Learning objectives for each case
- Medical workup sequence
- New, more comprehensive cases
- On-line learning tools and cases
- Case questions with annotated answers

The second edition has also been redesigned to serve as a preparatory text not only for the USMLE Step 1 (in conjunction with Step-Up), but also for the Step 2 and Step 2 CS Examinations given the current merging of formats under way by the NBME.

Each patient is introduced by a chief complaint followed by learning objectives and a brief history and physical. Based on the information given, students should attempt to determine the workup they would perform and a potential differential diagnosis should be offered. The differential here is listed alphabetically as a means of concealing the final diagnosis and allowing for the fact that different clinicians would derive their own rankings (most to least likely) for any given patient. Deriving a differential provides an excellent opportunity to synthesize all of the historical and physical data presented. It provides an opportunity to integrate various body systems and pool knowledge from various branches of medicine. Laboratory data are presented if they are pertinent; extraneous information was limited so as to maintain focus. Based on these data, a final diagnosis is then offered. An explanation of each differential is offered with pertinent positives and negatives. Making the final diagnosis is not the essential focus of this text—rather, it is the thought process that is used in determining the diagnosis that is most important. Finally, the case is completed with a refresher course on the basic science that one should know when dealing with such a patient and a USMLE-style vignette with an annotated answer. As with the USMLE itself, the patient in these cases simply serves as a springboard to access far-reaching basic science topics.

Step-Up to the Bedside 2e is designed to be used as both a self-study text and a self-test aid. After reviewing the history and physical examination findings, the student should generate a differential diagnosis list, then compare it to the list offered by the authors. The student should give thought to which diagnostic tests would be most appropriate and compare these to the tests listed. The reader should next attempt to determine the final diagnosis and the reasoning behind this diagnosis before reading the authors' explanation. The basic science section that follows should be used to review information related to the final diagnosis and other diseases mentioned within the case. Finally, a clinical vignette is offered to the students with a practice question and an annotated answer in the USMLE style (don't expect the annotated answers when you take the examination).

It would be hard to imagine a text that could summarize all of the important concepts students are expected to master over the course of medical school. We feel that

Step-Up to the Bedside 2e provides an excellent foundation for students to review this extensive body of knowledge in a practical way. The text also provides an opportunity to prepare students for the thought processes they must call upon during the clinical years of their medical education.

We were once in your situation—worried about passing the "boards" and not knowing where to begin. We authored this book with those concerns in mind, and now offer to you a resource that we wish had been available to us. This book will help you master your basic science knowledge and apply it to patient care. So, after you pass your Step 1 Exam, your Step 2 Exam, and your Step 2 CS Exam, you will be ready to STEP-UP to the bedside. Good luck!

Samir Mehta
Edmund A. Milder
Adam J. Mirarchi
Eugene Milder
Veronica Sikka

Acknowledgments

We extend our thanks to first edition contributors Oliver J. Wisco, Andrea Clark, Eiran Z. Gorodeski, Byron C. Leak, Marc S. Menkowitz, Melanie Schatz, and Kari Sproul and to first edition reviewers Alexandra Houck, MD; Fred William Markham, MD; Stuart Slavin, MD; Andrew Ulichney, MD; Michael M. White, PhD.; and Francine Wiest, MD.

Special thanks go to our editors and marketers at Lippincott Williams & Wilkins—Emilie Linkins, Kelly Horvath, Marette Smith, Donna Balado, Sharon Zinner and especially to Elizabeth Nieginski and Julie Scardiglia without whom the Step-Up series would not be possible— and to Holly Fischer for illustrations.

Contents

List of Cases by Diagnosis

● List of Cases by Diagnosis

● List of Cases by System

List of Cases by System

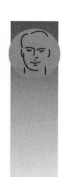

"I start to feel weak early into my exercise program or when I lift weights. Also, occasionally, my urine is red."

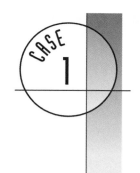

OBJECTIVES

1. Develop a differential diagnosis and an appropriate workup for weakness on exertion and change in urine color
2. Review glycogen metabolism
3. Compare and contrast the enzyme deficiencies and clinical manifestations of key glycogen storage and lysosomal storage diseases
4. Understand lactose, galactose, and fructose metabolism and the associated clinical manifestations with deficiencies in these three carbohydrates
5. Compare and contrast clinical features of phenylketonuria and albinism and the associated enzyme deficiencies

HISTORY AND PHYSICAL EXAMINATION

A 27-year-old man presents with muscle weakness on exertion. He describes **burning pain, cramping,** and exhaustion in his legs and arms whenever he attempts **strenuous exercise.** After a resting period, the symptoms resolve, then reappear when he resumes exercise. He also reports occasional **red urine.** He denies any skin rashes, progressive limb girdle weakness, or dysphagia. The patient is taking no medications except an occasional aspirin for pain. The neurologic exam reveals normal tone and strength bilaterally. The liver and spleen show no enlargement.

APPROPRIATE WORKUP

Blood chemistries, urinalysis, anaerobic exercise test, and muscle biopsy

DIFFERENTIAL DIAGNOSIS

Anemia, McArdle disease, muscular dystrophy, myasthenia gravis, polymyositis

DIAGNOSTIC LABORATORY TESTS AND STUDIES

Blood chemistry:
  CPK = 100 U/L (H)
  Hct = 45% (N)
  Hgb = 15.2 g/dL (N)
  BUN = 15 mg/dL (N)
Urinalysis:
  RBCs = 20–30 (H)
  Glucose = Elevated

Diagnostic anaerobic exercise test:
  Muscle cramping, pain, rapid
    exhaustion
  Substantial rise in CPK
  No rise in blood lactate
Muscle biopsy:
  Elevated **glycogen** content
  Reduced phosphorylase activity

DIAGNOSIS: MCARDLE DISEASE

McArdle disease is an **autosomal recessive** disorder involving **muscle glycogen phosphorylase** and characterized by pain, cramping, and muscle weakness upon exertion. It often does not present until the second or third decade of life. Strength returns following a rest period. Without **glycogen phosphorylase,** muscle tissue cannot use stored glycogen for energy during strenuous exercise. Patients also complain of **myoglobinuria,** which results from muscle breakdown in an attempt to liberate amino acids for conversion to glucose. If severe, the myoglobinuria can lead to renal failure. Treatment involves consuming a glucose load prior to exercise and avoiding excessively strenuous workouts.

EXPLANATION OF DIFFERENTIAL

Anemia must be considered because it is a common cause of weakness and presents with fatigue. Patients with anemia, however, typically complain of generalized fatigue and malaise rather than specific findings such as burning and cramping muscles. Intravascular hemolysis can cause hemoglobinuria, which would appear red, just as the myoglobinuria did in this patient. The normal Hgb and Hct levels in this patient are inconsistent with anemia.

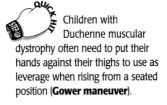

Children with Duchenne muscular dystrophy often need to put their hands against their thighs to use as leverage when rising from a seated position (**Gower maneuver**).

Duchenne muscular dystrophy is an **X-linked** disease and, as such, affects males almost exclusively. The **dystrophin** protein, which has an unknown function, is defective. Among the muscular dystrophies, it is the most common and most severe. Muscle weakness begins as early as 1 year of age. **Proximal muscles** are affected first, with compensatory hypertrophy of the distal muscles. Eventually the muscles undergo **pseudohypertrophy,** in which they become distended with deposits of fat and fibrous tissue. Death usually occurs during adolescence, often from pneumonia secondary to respiratory muscle weakness. Given the age and symptoms of this patient, Duchenne muscular dystrophy is not the likely diagnosis. A more mild form of muscular dystrophy (e.g., **Becker**) is a possibility. The muscle biopsy is diagnostic of McArdle disease, however, and rules out the other diseases.

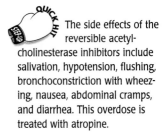

The side effects of the reversible acetyl-cholinesterase inhibitors include salivation, hypotension, flushing, bronchoconstriction with wheezing, nausea, abdominal cramps, and diarrhea. This overdose is treated with atropine.

Myasthenia gravis can present as muscle weakness exacerbated by exertion. The typical patient presents with **diplopia, ptosis,** and weakness of the muscles of speaking, chewing, and swallowing. These symptoms may worsen throughout the day. **Autoantibodies** directed against the **nicotinic acetylcholine receptor** of the neuromuscular junction cause this disease. It is associated with carcinoma or hyperplasia of the thymus. Reversible acetylcholinesterase inhibitors are used in the diagnosis (edrophonium) and treatment (pyridostigmine, neostigmine).

Polymyositis is a connective tissue disease that presents as progressive, **bilateral weakness** of the proximal limb muscles. It is more common in **women.** Typically levels of serum creatinine kinase and antinuclear antibodies are increased. **Dermatomyositis** is a related disease that involves the muscles and the skin. These patients develop a **lilac rash** and **periorbital edema.** The proximal, progressive limb girdle weakness typical of these connective tissue diseases does not resemble the symptoms in this patient.

Related Basic Science

Glycogen metabolism

Glycogen, a readily available source of glucose, can be stored in the liver or muscle. Breakdown of glycogen is one of the ways the body maintains blood levels of glucose (the others being dietary intake and gluconeogenesis). Working muscle can degrade glycogen to provide glucose during periods of strenuous exercise.

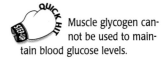

Muscle glycogen cannot be used to maintain blood glucose levels.

Genetic disorders leading to deficiencies in certain enzymes can lead to glycogen storage diseases (Figure 1-1 and Table 1-1).

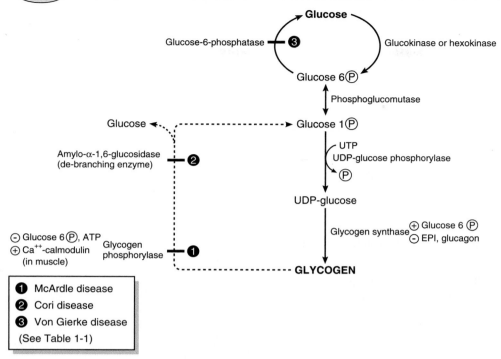

FIGURE 1-1 Glycogen metabolism (*EPI*=epinephrine; *UDP*=uridine diphosphate; *UTP*=uridine triphosphate)

❶ McArdle disease
❷ Cori disease
❸ Von Gierke disease
(See Table 1-1)

TABLE 1-1 Glycogen Storage Diseases

Disease	Enzyme Deficiency	Clinical Manifestations	Notes
McArdle disease (Type V)	Muscle glycogen phosphorylase	Cramping and weakness following exercise	Sugar load before exercise to prevent symptoms.
		Myoglobinuria CNS, liver, and blood glucose levels unaffected	
Cori disease (Type III)	Debranching enzyme (amylo-α-1,6-glucosidase)	Hepatomegaly	Frequent feedings are necessary.
		Hypoglycemia Failure-to-thrive	
Von Gierke disease (Type I)	Glucose-6-phosphatase	Severe hypoglycemia Fatty hepatomegaly Failure-to-thrive	Glucose-6-phosphatase is the final step in both glycogenolysis and gluconeogenesis; therefore, blood glucose levels cannot be maintained.
			Frequent feedings are necessary.

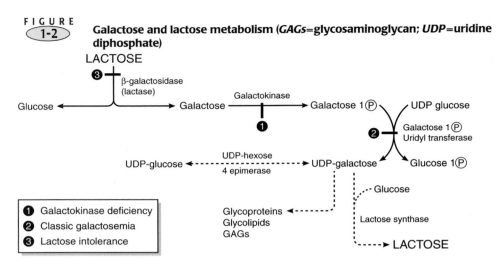

FIGURE **1-2** **Galactose and lactose metabolism (*GAGs*=glycosaminoglycan; *UDP*=uridine diphosphate)**

❶ Galactokinase deficiency
❷ Classic galactosemia
❸ Lactose intolerance

Carbohydrate metabolism and enzyme deficiencies

Galactose, the major source of which is lactose, is absorbed in the proximal portion of the small intestine via sodium-dependent glucose transporters. Galactosemias, which are inborn errors of galactose metabolism, can be classified as either classic galactosemia or galactokinase deficiency (Figure 1-2).

Classical galactosemia results from deficiency of **uridylyl transferase,** which in turn results in galactosemia and galactosuria and leads to accumulation of galactose-1-phosphate in the tissues (e.g., nerves, lens, liver, and kidney). Excessive accumulation can lead to **cataracts** and **mental retardation.** Cataracts, along with benign galactosemia and galactosuria, are the only clinical manifestation of **galactokinase deficiency.** When galactose is elevated (as in these deficiencies), aldose reductase reduces galactose to galactitol. Deposition of galactitol in the lens leads to the formation of cataracts.

Lactose is a disaccharide of galactose and glucose. Lactose synthase, composed of protein A (β-lactalbumin) and **protein B** (α-lactalbumin), forms lactose. It should be noted that protein B is found only in mature, lactating mammary glands. Protein B activates protein A by lowering its K_m and increasing its specificity substantially. Protein B levels are **downregulated by progesterone** during pregnancy. After pregnancy, progesterone levels decrease, prolactin levels increase, and protein B synthesis is stimulated.

Lactase deficiency (lactose intolerance) causes bloating, diarrhea, and dehydration following consumption of dairy products. Because lactose is not broken down or absorbed, intestinal bacteria metabolize it into by-products, leading to an **osmotic diarrhea.** Incidence of lactase deficiency increases with age and there is a higher incidence in **Blacks** and **Asians.**

Fructose, the major source of which is sucrose, is absorbed in the small intestine via facilitated diffusion. **Essential fructosuria** (Figure 1-3) is a benign, asymptomatic disorder resulting from a lack of **fructokinase. Hereditary fructose intolerance,** an absence of

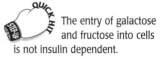

A small amount of glycogen is broken down by the lysosomal enzyme α-1,4-glucosidase. Deficiency in this enzyme results in Pompe disease, which is characterized by severe cardiomegaly (secondary to glycogen-filled vacuoles), normal blood glucose levels, and early death.

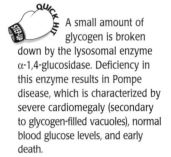

Excess fructose can overload aldolase B, which causes accumulation of fructose-1-phosphate and ADP, with depletion of inorganic phosphate. The excess ADP is catabolized, leading to hyperuricemia and gout.

The entry of galactose and fructose into cells is not insulin dependent.

FIGURE **1-3** **Fructose metabolism (*DHAP*=dihydroxyacetone phosphate)**

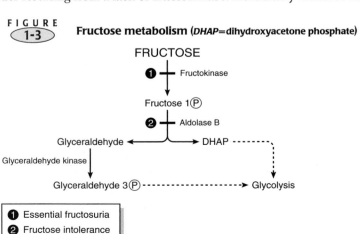

❶ Essential fructosuria
❷ Fructose intolerance

TABLE 1-2 Related Enzyme Deficiency Diseases

Disease	Defective Enzyme	Clinical Manifestations
Gaucher disease	Glucocerebrosidase	Hepatosplenomegaly Erosion of head of long bones **Wrinkled paper** appearance of cells in spleen, liver, and bone marrow
Niemann-Pick disease	Sphingomyelinase	**Foamy histiocytes** Hepatosplenomegaly Anemia Fever CNS deterioration Cherry-red macula (50%)
Tay-Sachs disease	Hexosaminidase A	**Ganglioside GM$_2$** accumulation CNS degeneration Blindness **Cherry-red macula (100%)**
Fabry disease	α-Galactosidase A	Skin lesions on trunk Fever Painful neuropathy Vascular involvement **Renal failure**
Hunter syndrome	Iduronate sulfatase	Hepatosplenomegaly Micrognathia Mental retardation Retinal degeneration

aldolase B, causes severe hypoglycemia, vomiting, jaundice, and hepatic failure if it is not diagnosed shortly after birth.

Lysosomal storage diseases also result from deficiencies in certain enzymes. This category of disease can be suspected on the basis of progressive neurologic dysfunction, enlarged viscera, and skeletal deformities (Table 1-2).

Phenylketonuria is another disease caused by deficiency of an enzyme (Figure 1-4). Because it is treatable and its manifestations are severe, a test for this disease is given at birth.

 Hurler syndrome is clinically similar to but more severe than Hunter syndrome. Both result from accumulation of heparan sulfate and dermatan sulfate. Hurler syndrome has the additional feature of **gargoyle facies.**

FIGURE 1-4 Phenylketonuria and albinism (*BH$_4$*=tetrahydrobiopterin; *DOPA*=dihydroxyphenylalanine; *I*=iodine; *PKU*=phenylketonuria)

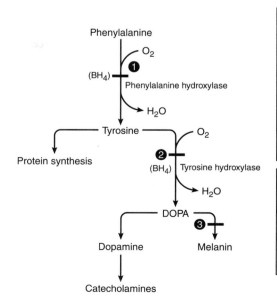

❶ Phenylketonuria
- Caused by deficiency of phenylalanine hydroxylase
- Can be due to deficiencies in enzymes. If related to BH$_4$ -must be treated with BH$_4$ supplementation
- CNS symptoms occur: mental retardation, microcephaly, tremor
- Hypopigmentation occurs
- Tyrosine becomes essential
- Treat by avoiding phenylalanine

❷ and ❸ Albinism
- Can be tyrosinase negative (2) or tyrosinase positive (3)
- Melanin defect leads to fair skin, fair hair, and red eyes
- Is most often autosomal recessive
- Increased incidence of actinic kerotosis and skin cancer

All the genetic enzyme deficiency diseases are autosomal recessive except for Fabry and Hunter, which are both X-linked.

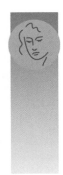

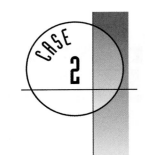

"Doctor, my vaginal area is very itchy."

OBJECTIVES

1. Develop a differential diagnosis and an appropriate workup for vaginal pruritus and discharge
2. Review the anatomy, innervation, and significance in parturition of the pudendal nerve
3. Understand the immunology and clinical presentation associated with toxic shock syndrome and the role of *Staphylococcus aureus*

HISTORY AND PHYSICAL EXAMINATION

A sexually active 22-year-old woman complains of vaginal itching and discharge. She has been taking her oral contraceptives regularly, and her menstrual cycle has been normal. Physical examination reveals small amounts of whitish vaginal discharge and slight vulvar erythema. Thrush-like white plaques are seen inside the vagina. The cervix appears normal.

APPROPRIATE WORKUP

KOH, wet mount, and "whiff" test of vaginal discharge

DIFFERENTIAL DIAGNOSIS

Bacterial vaginosis, vaginal candidiasis, trichomoniasis, vulvar dystrophy

DIAGNOSTIC LABORATORY TESTS AND STUDIES

KOH:
Yeast with pseudohyphae on discharge swab
Wet mount (saline):
No *Trichomonas vaginalis* or *Gardnerella vaginalis* "clue cells"
"Whiff" test:
Negative results

DIAGNOSIS: VAGINAL CANDIDIASIS

The yeast **Candida albicans** is the most common cause of **vaginal candidiasis.** *C. albicans* is part of the normal vaginal flora and rarely causes symptoms. Overgrowth usually stems from a change in vaginal pH, use of **broad-spectrum antibiotics,** or an **immunocompromised state.** The incidence of vaginal candidiasis is slightly increased in pregnant women,

FIGURE
2-1   (See also Color Plate 2-1). *C. albicans*

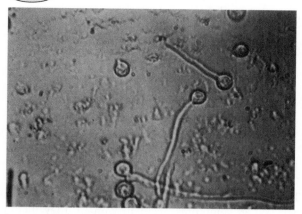

(From Mahon CR, Manuselis G: Textbook of Diagnostic Microbiology, 2nd Ed. Philadelphia: WB Saunders, 2000, p 751.)

patients with **Type 1 diabetes mellitus** or **HIV,** and women taking oral contraceptives. The most common presenting symptom is vulvar **pruritus,** which may be accompanied by **scant white discharge.** The pseudohyphae of *C. albicans* can be identified in a KOH preparation of a swab sample (Figure 2-1).

Treatment is intravaginal administrations of imidazole antifungal agents, which are available over the counter. Vaginal candidiasis also can be treated with a single dose of oral fluconazole.

EXPLANATION OF DIFFERENTIAL

Bacterial vaginosis, which usually is caused by **G. vaginalis,** is associated with risk factors for STDs, such as multiple partners; however, bacterial vaginosis itself has not been shown to be transmitted sexually. Other commonly implicated pathogens include **Mycoplasma hominis, Prevotella sp.,** and several anaerobes. All these organisms can be found as normal vaginal flora in healthy women. Many women with bacterial vaginosis have fewer H_2O_2-producing **lactobacilli** bacteria that may have a protective effect. Bacterial vaginosis usually presents with a **malodorous white-gray discharge.** Pruritus is not prominent. Diagnosis can be made by smelling the distinct fishy odor that results upon mixing KOH with the discharge (positive **"Whiff"** test), measuring an abnormally acidic pH in the vagina, or identifying **"clue cells"** (vaginal epithelial cells that appear granular because of adherent *G. vaginalis*) (Figure 2-2). This patient had none of the diagnostic findings of bacterial vaginosis.

QUICK HIT
Fluconazole is the drug of choice for infections with cryptococcus, candida, and coccidioides.

FIGURE
2-2   *G. vaginalis* **clue cell**

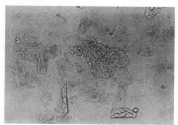

(From Beckmann CRB, Ling FW, Herbert WNP, Laube DW, Smith RP, and Barzansky BM. Obstetrics and Gynecology, 3rd Ed. Baltimore: Williams & Wilkins, 1998, p 329.)

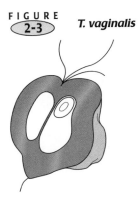

FIGURE
2-3

T. vaginalis

Trichomoniasis is a common STD caused by the parasite **T. vaginalis.** Many infections are **asymptomatic,** especially in men. When symptoms occur in women, they include vaginal **pruritus** and a copious **yellow, frothy discharge.** The epithelium of the vulva and the vagina are usually inflamed, and petechial lesions on the cervix can give the appearance of a **"strawberry cervix."** Identifying the parasite in a sample of discharge establishes the diagnosis (Figure 2-3). Both the patient and all sexual partners should be treated with metronidazole and tested for other STDs.

Vulvar dystrophies are disorders of epithelial proliferation that can present as **leukoplakia** (irregular white patch-like lesions) and **pruritus. Lichen sclerosis** and hyperplastic dystrophy are two benign forms. Conversely, **atypical hyperplastic dystrophy** is considered premalignant. If this patient's condition does not resolve with antifungal therapy, a biopsy should be obtained to rule out vulvar dystrophy.

Related Basic Science

The pudendal nerve

This nerve is derived from the ventral rami of S2–4. The nerve exits the pelvis via the greater sciatic foramen, passes near the ischial spine, and enters the gluteal region through the lesser sciatic foramen accompanied by the internal pudendal artery. The pudendal nerve branches into the inferior rectal nerve, which supplies the external anal sphincter, lower rectum, and perianal skin. Branches of the pudendal nerve also supply the skin of the scrotum/labia majora and the lower part of the vagina. Injection of local anesthetics from a needle passed through the wall of the vagina in the direction of the ischial spine and sacrospinous ligament can block the pudendal nerve. This procedure is used in obstetrics to ease the pain of parturition.

Toxic shock syndrome and *Staphylococcus aureus*

Toxic shock syndrome (TSS) is no longer common because superabsorbent tampons, whose misuse was the main cause, have been removed from the market. TSS can still occur, however, if a tampon is left in place for more than 24 hours or in wound infections. Certain strains of **S. aureus,** which can proliferate in the tampon or in unclean wounds, produce the **toxic shock syndrome toxin (TSST).** TSST enters the systemic circulation and acts as a **superantigen.** This means that TSST can activate many helper T cells by directly interacting with major histocompatibility complex (MHC) II, the β chain of the T-cell receptor (Figure 2-4). Subsequent widespread nonspecific T-cell activation ensues. Large amounts of **IL-1 and IL-2** cytokines are produced. These cytokines are responsible for symptoms including **fever,** diarrhea, **hypotension,** desquamating rash of the palms and soles, and an ascending rash in the lower extremities. Tampon removal or wound debridement and fluid resuscitation are the first line of treatment.

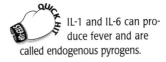

Like all the azole antifungals, fluconazole inhibits the production of ergosterol, an essential component of the cell membrane of fungi, and antagonizes the action of amphotericin.

Patients taking metronidazole should avoid alcohol because it can cause a disulfiram-like reaction. When taken with alcohol, disulfiram inhibits aldehyde dehydrogenase, increasing levels of acetylaldehyde. High levels of acetylaldehyde lead to nausea, flushing, thirst, palpitations, chest pain, and vertigo.

IL-1 and IL-6 can produce fever and are called endogenous pyrogens.

Other diseases caused by *S. aureus* include osteomyelitis, food poisoning (onset often 6 hours after ingestion as a result of preformed toxin), impetigo and other skin infections, scalded skin syndrome, and endocarditis.

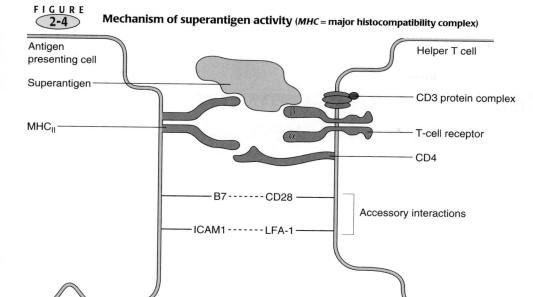

FIGURE 2-4   **Mechanism of superantigen activity** (*MHC* = major histocompatibility complex)

Antigen presenting cell

Superantigen

MHC$_{II}$

Helper T cell

CD3 protein complex

T-cell receptor

CD4

B7 ------ CD28

ICAM1 ------ LFA-1

Accessory interactions

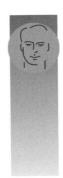

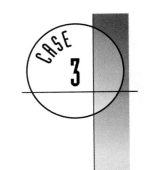

"My hands and arms are getting weaker and weaker."

OBJECTIVES

1. Develop a differential diagnosis and an appropriate workup for progressive weakness in extremities
2. Understand the physiology associated with neurons
3. Review the associated physiology of the skeletal muscle action potential
4. Discuss the neuromuscular junction and key neurotransmitters
5. Compare and contrast classic lesions of the spinal cord
6. Review the corticospinal tract and the result of lesions above and below the pyramids

HISTORY AND PHYSICAL EXAMINATION

A 45-year-old male presents with marked, progressive weakness in his hands and arms. His wife has noticed slurred speech with **involuntary muscle contractions** around his mouth. The patient reports no history of sensory loss, bladder or bowel dysfunction, fever, or spinal or cranial trauma. On physical exam, **bilateral wasting of hands** is evident with stiffness and spasticity of the upper limbs. **Deep tendon reflexes are absent** in the upper limbs with a positive Babinski sign. The funduscopic exam is normal with all cranial nerves intact. Sensation is intact to all modalities in all areas tested. A mental status exam is within normal limits with some difficulty in articulation.

APPROPRIATE WORKUP

Blood chemistries, cerebrospinal fluid analysis, electromyogram (EMG), CT of the brain and cervical spine

DIFFERENTIAL DIAGNOSIS

Multiple sclerosis, amyotrophic lateral sclerosis (ALS), Guillain-Barré syndrome, and myasthenia gravis

DIAGNOSTIC LABORATORY TESTS AND STUDIES

Blood chemistry:
  TSH = 2.5 μU/mL (N)
  Triiodothyronine (T_3) = 150 ng/mL (N)
  Thyroxine (T_4) = 10 μg/mL (N)
  Total
Cerebrospinal fluid (CSF):
  Cell count = 2 cells/mm³ (N)
  Glucose = 54 mg/dL (N)
  Protein = 22 mg/dL (N)

Electromyogram (EMG):
  Fibrillations (abnormal spontaneous activity in resting muscle)
CT, brain and cervical spine:
  Normal; some degeneration in the lateral spinal cord; no disc herniations or cord impingement noted

FIGURE
3-1
Neuromuscular diseases

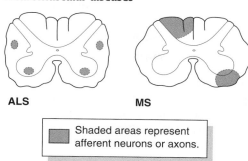

ALS   MS

Shaded areas represent
afferent neurons or axons.

DIAGNOSIS: AMYOTROPHIC LATERAL SCLEROSIS (ALS)

Amyotrophic lateral sclerosis (ALS, Lou Gehrig disease) (Figure 3-1) is the most common motor neuron disease. It is characterized by **degeneration of both the upper motor neurons (UMN) and the lower motor neurons (LMN),** including the **lateral corticospinal tracts** and the anterior motor neurons of the spinal cord. It results in a denervation atrophy of the muscles. Clinical manifestations include symmetric atrophy and fasciculation, hyperreflexia, and spasticity. Onset is **early adulthood to middle age.** The disease has a **rapid course leading to death,** usually from respiratory failure. In most cases, ALS does not impair a patient's cognitive functions, personality, intelligence, or memory, nor does it affect sensory functions.

ALS is more commonly acquired (80%) as opposed to inherited (20%). Mutations are believed to occur in the zinc/copper superoxide dismutase gene which is key to scavenging free radicals in metabolically active cells, such as neurons.

The cause of ALS is unknown with no cure to date. However, the FDA has approved the first drug treatment for the disease—riluzole. **Riluzole** is believed to reduce damage to motor neurons and prolongs survival by several months, mainly in those with difficulty swallowing. Other treatments are designed to relieve symptoms and improve the quality of life for people with ALS. Drugs also are available to help individuals with pain, depression, sleep disturbances, and constipation. Individuals with ALS may eventually consider forms of mechanical ventilation (respirators).

QUICK HIT
Amyotrophic lateral sclerosis presents with both LMN *and* UMN symptoms while polio usually only presents with LMN signs.

EXPLANATION OF DIFFERENTIAL

Multiple sclerosis (MS) (see Figure 3-1) is the **most common demyelinating disease** with relative preservation of axons. The first symptoms of MS usually appear between **20 to 30 years of age** and occur more commonly in **women** than men. Increased incidence is associated with specific HLA types and birth in the Northern Hemisphere. Generally, the etiology of MS is unknown, although immune and viral factors have been proposed. Both environmental and genetic factors seem to play a role in the development of MS. MS is characterized by multiple focal areas of demyelination called **plaques** that are most typically in the paraventricular areas, optic nerve, and brainstem. A reactive gliosis can occur later. Frequently with MS, **multiple oligoclonal bands appear on electrophoresis of the CSF.** The absence of these findings makes the diagnosis of MS improbable. Another key distinguishing feature between ALS and MS is that MS affects both motor and sensory neurons, whereas ALS only affects the motor system.

MS follows a variable clinical course, depending on the location of plaques. Many affected patients have a relapsing, remitting course. Early manifestations include weakness of the lower extremities, visual and sensory disturbances, and possible loss of bladder control. The classic **charcot triad** of MS is **nystagmus, intention tremor,** and **scanning speech.**

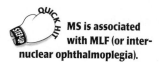
QUICK HIT
MS is associated with MLF (or internuclear ophthalmoplegia).

Guillain-Barré syndrome is an acute, **inflammatory demyelinating disease,** usually involving the peripheral nerves, with highest incidence in **young adults.** The etiology is thought to be autoimmune, and the syndrome commonly follows a viral infection, immunization, or allergic reaction. Manifestations are **ascending muscle weakness** and paralysis, beginning in the distal lower extremities. The CSF often reveals increased protein levels but normal cell counts.

Myasthenia gravis can present as muscle weakness exacerbated with exertion. The typical patient presents with **diplopia, ptosis,** and weakness of the muscles associated with speaking, chewing, and swallowing. These symptoms may worsen throughout the day. This patient exhibited none of these symptoms. **Autoantibodies** directed against the **nicotinic acetylcholine receptor** of the neuromuscular junction in skeletal muscle cause this disease. It is associated with carcinoma or hyperplasia of the thymus. Reversible acetylcholinesterase inhibitors are used in the diagnosis (edrophonium) and treatment (pyridostigmine, neostigmine).

In Guillain-Barré syndrome, elevated CSF protein with normal cell counts is referred to as "albumino-cytologic dissociation."

Related Basic Sciences

Neurons

A synapse is the functional membrane-to-membrane contact between neuronal and neuromuscular cells. Synapses can be either **excitatory or inhibitory signals.** One-to-one synapses, such as those found at the neuromuscular junction, are characterized by an action potential in the presynaptic element, producing an action potential in the postsynaptic element. Many-to-one synapse arrangements, spinal motor neurons for example, require that multiple synapses fire simultaneously on one postsynaptic cell for it to depolarize. When the input brings the membrane potential of the postsynaptic cell to threshold, an action potential is fired. **Excitatory postsynaptic potentials (EPSPs)** drive the postsynaptic cell toward threshold by opening **sodium and potassium channels,** resulting in a release of neurotransmitters such as **acetylcholine** (excitatory), or **GABA** (inhibitory). **Inhibitory postsynaptic potentials (IPSPs)** hyperpolarize the postsynaptic cell by opening **chloride channels,** which inhibits the release of any neurotransmitter.

Myelin serves as an insulator to the electrical signal that is conducted down the axon as a neuron fires. Myelination in the CNS is accomplished by **oligodendrocytes** that wrap around **several axons at once.** In the PNS, **Schwann cells** serve this function and wrap around a **single axon.** In demyelinating diseases, the myelin sheath around axons is targeted. After patches of myelin are damaged, oligodendrocytes attempt to repair the damage but in the process cause scar tissue (gliotic plaques). These hard plaques then begin to interfere with the flow of electrical impulses that move through the axon.

An example of a schwannoma is an acoustic neuroma which is associated with the internal acoustic meatus through which cranial nerves VII and VIII pass.

Skeletal action potential

Action potentials are properties of excitable cells (i.e., nerves and muscle). An action potential consists of a rapid depolarization (upstroke) followed by repolarization of the membrane potential. Key features of action potentials are their stereotypical size and shape, propagating nature, and an all-or-none firing. In the upstroke of the action potential (depolarization), there is an influx of Na^+ current. Nicotinic acetylcholine (ACh) receptors are ligand-gated sodium channels, and the binding of ACh to nicotinic receptors produces an endplate potential in skeletal muscle cells. If above a certain threshold value for activation of fast voltage-gated sodium channels, there will be a muscle contraction by triggering the release of calcium from the sacroplasmic reticulum. In myasthenia gravis, the number of ACh receptors to respond to the synaptic ACh and depolarize the cell to reach threshold are decreased.

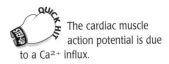

The cardiac muscle action potential is due to a Ca^{2+} influx.

Neuromuscular junction

The **neuromuscular junction** is a **synapse** between **axons of motor neurons and skeletal muscle.** When an action potential reaches the presynaptic terminal of the motor neuron, depolarization opens calcium channels and releases acetylcholine from the presynaptic terminal into the synaptic cleft. Acetylcholine binds to the **nicotinic** receptor on the post-synaptic terminal, which ultimately stimulates muscle contraction. Two types of drugs can block the neuromuscular junction. **Succinylcholine** is the prototypical **depolarizing** neuromuscular blocker, while the **curare drugs (e.g., vecuronium, pancuronium)** are **nondepolarizing.**

QUICK HIT

Reversal of a blockade with nondepolarizing drugs can be achieved with edrophonium, neostigmine, and other acetylcholinesterase inhibitors.

Classic lesions of the spinal cord (Figure 3-2)

Corticospinal tract

The corticospinal tract is the descending pathway that originates in the cerebral cortex (areas 6, 4, 3, 1, 2) and mediates voluntary movement of striated muscle. First-order neurons project to the posterior limb of the internal capsule and descend through the middle three-fifths of the midbrain's crus cerebri and base of the pons, decussating in the pyramids of the medulla. These axons continue down the spinal cord as the corticospinal tract. Corticospinal fibers synapse on second-order neurons of the ventral horn via interneurons.

F I G U R E 3-2 **Classic lesions of the spinal cord**

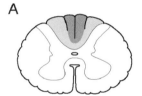

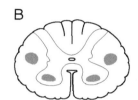

Tabes dorsalis

- Seen in tertiary syphilis
- Bilateral loss of touch, vibration and tactile sense from lower limbs due to lesion of fasciculus gracilis

Amyotrophic lateral sclerosis

- Combined UMN and LMN lesion of corticospinal tract
- Spastic paresis (UMN sign)
- Flaccid paralysis with fasciculations (LMN)

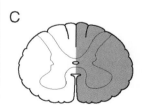

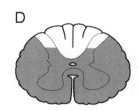

Brown-Séquard syndrome

- Ipsilateral loss of touch and vibration, and tactile sense below lesion due to posterior white column lesion
- Contralateral loss of pain and touch due to loss of spinothalamic tract
- Ipsilateral spastic paresis below lesion due to lesion of corticospinal tract
- Ipsilateral flaccid paralysis at level of lesion due to loss of LMN
- If lesion occurs above T1, Horner syndrome on side of lesion will result

Spinal artery infarct

- Bilateral loss of pain and temperature one level below lesion due to loss of spinothalamic tract
- Bilateral spastic paresis below lesion due to lesion of corticospinal tract
- Bilateral flaccid paralysis at level of lesion due to loss of LMN
- Loss of bladder control due to lesion of corticospinal tract innervation of S2–S4 parasympathetics
- Bilateral Horner syndrome if above T2

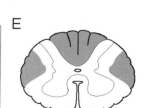

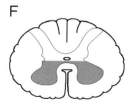

Subacute combined degeneration (Vitamin B12 deficiency)

- Bilateral loss of touch, vibration and tactile sense due to posterior white column lesion
- Bilateral spastic paresis below lesion due to lesion of corticospinal tracts

Syringomyelia

- Bilateral loss of pain and temperature one level below due to lesion of ventral white commissure (spinothalamic tract)
- Bilateral flaccid paralysis of level of lesion due to loss of LMN

Any lesions above the pyramids, UMN lesions, produce contralateral spastic paresis and a positive Babinski sign. Lesions below the pyramids, also referred to as UMN lesions, produce ipsilateral spastic paresis (the muscles have an increased resistance to passive movement or manipulation) and a positive Babinski sign. The most widely accepted theory of hyperreflexia and spastic paresis with UMN lesions is the tonically inhibitory effect UMNs have on LMNs. When UMNs are disrupted, they disinhibit or activate LMNs, making DTRs more active and increasing baseline muscle tone. This increases resistance to passive movement. Muscle atrophy with UMN lesions may occur secondary to muscle disuse but is not a direct result of muscle denervation. Lesions of the second-order neurons, (LMN lesions), produce flaccid paralysis and fasciculations.

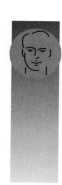

"Over the past 2 weeks, I've had really bad back pains, especially when I walk or bend over. I've also been feeling tired."

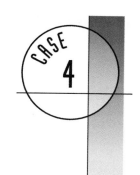

CASE
4

OBJECTIVES

1. Develop a differential diagnosis and an appropriate workup for recent onset of back pain and fatigue
2. Review key principles of humoral immunity
3. Compare and contrast four major plasma cell disorders besides multiple myeloma: Waldenstrom macroglobulinemia, AL amyloidosis, monoclonal gammopathy of undetermined significance
4. Learn major geriatric behavioral and medical issues
5. Understand the role of parathyroid hormone (PTH), phosphorus, and alkaline phosphatase levels in differentiating among common causes of hypercalcemia

HISTORY AND PHYSICAL EXAMINATION

A 68-year-old African American man complains of **back pain** and **fatigue.** He recalls recent bouts of **confusion, weakness, polyuria,** and **constipation.** He reports no history of trauma. Physical examination reveals **tenderness to palpation in the thoracic and lumbar spine** and a **limited range of motion** because of pain. Auscultation reveals **a systolic flow murmur** over the left sternal border. The neurologic examination is normal.

APPROPRIATE WORKUP

Blood chemistries, bone marrow aspirate, urinalysis, and skull radiograph

DIFFERENTIAL DIAGNOSIS

Fibromyalgia, herniated disk (nerve root impingement), metastatic bone lesions, multiple myeloma, osteoarthritis (OA)

DIAGNOSTIC LABORATORY TESTS AND STUDIES

Blood chemistry:
Pancytopenia
RBC rouleaux formation
Monoclonal "M" spike on electrophoresis (Figure 4-1)
Ca^{2+} 15 mg/dL (H)
ESR 50 mm/h (H)
Radiograph:
Diffuse **lytic lesions** of the skull, vertebrae, and long bones (Figure 4-2)

Bone marrow:
Infiltrate of **plasma cells** with morphologic atypia (Figure 4-3)
Urinalysis:
Marked **proteinuria** despite a finding of only mild proteinuria (1+) on dipstick examination
Bence-Jones proteins

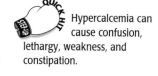
Hypercalcemia can cause confusion, lethargy, weakness, and constipation.

The RBCs in a peripheral smear can form stacks called **rouleaux.** This phenomenon, which is secondary to hyperglobulinemia, is seen in multiple myeloma and Waldenstrom macroglobulinemia.

FIGURE 4-1   Serum protein electrophoretic patterns in multiple myeloma

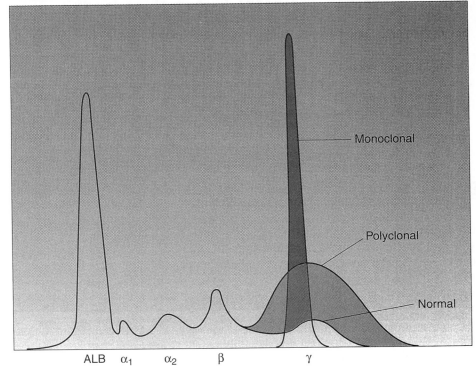

Monoclonal

Polyclonal

Normal

ALB α_1 α_2 β γ

(From Mehta S, Milder EA, Mirarchi AJ. Step-Up: A High-Yield, Systems-Based Review for the USMLE Step 1. Philadelphia: Lippincott Williams & Wilkins, 2000, p 354.)

FIGURE 4-2   Multiple myeloma—a radiograph of the skull

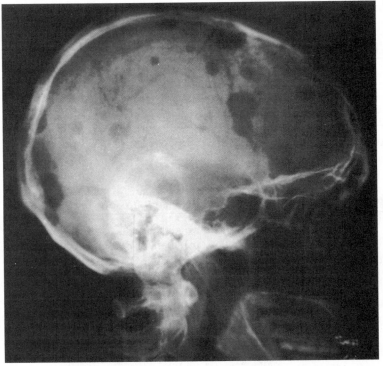

(From Mehta S, Milder EA, Mirarchi AJ. Step-Up: A High-Yield, Systems-Based Review for the USMLE Step 1. Philadelphia: Lippincott Williams & Wilkins, 2000, p 354.)

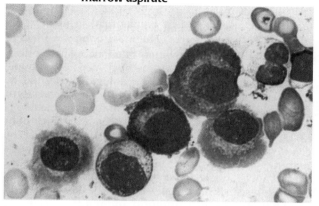

FIGURE 4-3   Multiple myeloma—a smear of bone marrow aspirate

(From Mehta S, Milder EA, Mirarchi AJ. Step-Up: A High-Yield, Systems-Based Review for the USMLE Step 1. Philadelphia: Lippincott Williams & Wilkins, 2000, p 354.)

DIAGNOSIS: MULTIPLE MYELOMA

Multiple myeloma, a disease of unknown etiology, usually presents in the seventh decade of life. It occurs most commonly in patients with an earlier disorder of the plasma cells, such as monoclonal gammopathy of undetermined significance (MGUS). Multiple myeloma is a disorder in which **monoclonal malignant plasma cells** proliferate in the bone marrow and produce immunoglobulins, usually IgG or IgA. The proliferation of these cells causes a space-occupying lesion in the marrow, resulting in a myelophthisic anemia and **pancytopenia.** The most common clinical features of multiple myeloma include **osteolytic lesions,** pathologic fractures, **anemia, renal insufficiency,** and **recurrent bacterial infections.** The osteolytic lesions, which lead to **hypercalcemia,** are thought to be secondary to osteoclast activation by cytokines produced by the neoplastic cells. Renal involvement occurs in approximately 70% of cases and includes interstitial infiltrates of plasma cells, tubular protein casts, calcifications, and a predisposition to pyelonephritis. Suppression of normal antibody production predisposes patients to infection, especially with encapsulated bacteria such as pneumococci. The most common presenting symptom is bone pain, usually in the back and ribs, with movement. Patients sometimes also suffer from the symptoms of hyperviscosity (see Waldenstrom macroglobulinemia below) or primary (AL) amyloidosis (cardiomyopathy, macroglossia, neuropathy). Multiple myeloma is responsible for about 1% of all cancer-related deaths in Western countries. The incidence of multiple myeloma increases with advancing age, male gender, or African American race.

EXPLANATION OF DIFFERENTIAL

Fibromyalgia, a disorder of unknown etiology, is characterized by widespread musculoskeletal pain, including back pain, stiffness, and paresthesia. Sleep problems, fatigue, and multiple tender points that are widely and symmetrically distributed are also common. Fibromyalgia affects predominantly women. This patient's symptoms are much more specific, and the combination of the radiographic and bone marrow findings is diagnostic of multiple myeloma.

A **herniated intervertebral disk** can **impinge nerves** exiting the intervertebral foramina. The pain caused by a herniated disk tends to be sharp, localized to a **specific dermatome,** and associated with paresthesia, motor weakness, and reflex loss. This patient's pain was localized to the bone, with no signs of nerve impingement.

Metastatic bone lesions are much more common than primary bone cancers. **Prostate, breast,** and **lung** metastases account for 80% of all bone metastases. The vertebrae are the sites most often involved, and the most common presenting symptom is gradual localized

QUICK HIT   A herniated disk typically causes impingement of the nerve corresponding to the second number in the designation of the disk. For instance, herniation of the C3-C4 disk is most likely to impinge on the C4 nerve.

back pain. In this patient, the bone marrow studies showed the plasma cell infiltrate typical of multiple myeloma and no infiltration of metastatic cancer.

Osteoarthritis (OA) is most often a primary disease resulting from genetic and environmental factors. This noninflammatory disease caused by **mechanical injury** ("wear-and-tear") most often develops in the weight-bearing joints. The **most common form of arthritis,** OA has the highest incidence in older women. Clinical manifestations are deterioration of the articular cartilage and **osteophyte formation.** In the hands, OA usually affects the **interphalangeal joints** and can be **asymmetric,** while rheumatoid arthritis tends to show symmetric involvement of the metacarpophalangeal joints.

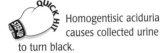
Homogentisic aciduria causes collected urine to turn black.

Related Basic Science

Humoral immunity

Plasma cells (Figure 4-4) are derived from B cells, and their sole purpose is to manufacture antibodies (Ig). Antibody-mediated immunity is called **humoral immunity.** B cells are found in the germinal centers of lymph nodes, the white pulp of the spleen, and the Peyer patches of the small intestine. B cells have IgM monomers as surface receptors and can recognize free antigen. This recognition activates B cells to proliferate into a clone of plasma cells, each making the antibodies that the B cell was genetically preprogrammed to produce.

Along with macrophages and Langerhans cells, B cells have **major histocompatibility complex (MHC)** II receptors and act as antigen-presenting cells to CD4+ T helper cells. An activated T cell then produces IL-4 and IL-5, which are required for **B-cell class switching** by alternate RNA splicing. Without these cytokines, only IgM antibodies are produced. Help from the T cell allows the plasma cell to produce other classes of Ig, such as IgG and IgA. These Igs have the same specificity but different heavy chains. Only peptide antigens can be presented in association with MHC II. Therefore, polysaccharide antigens are capable of activating B cells but not T cells. The Ig produced to polysaccharide antigens, such as the ABO blood group antigens and some bacterial capsule antigens, can only be of the IgM class.

FIGURE 4-4 **(See also Color Plate 4-4.) Plasma cells and multiple myeloma**

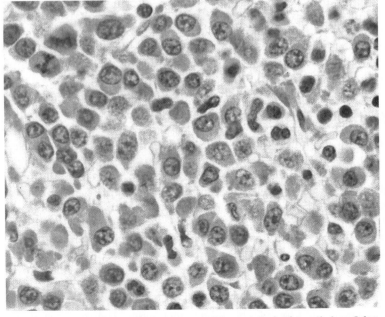

(From Burkitt HG, Stevens A, Lowe JS, Young B. Wheater's Basic Histopathology Color Atlas and Text, 3rd Ed. Churchill Livingstone, 1996, p 193.)

TABLE 4-1 Properties of Antibody Classes

Class	Structure	Major Functions
IgM	Pentamer	Complement fixation, B-cell receptor (monomer)
IgG	Monomer	Complement fixation, opsonization, crosses placenta
IgA	Dimer	Present in secretions
IgD	Monomer	Unknown, possible b-cell receptor
IgE	Monomer	Receptor on mast cells and basophils, mediates type I hypersensitivity and immunity against certain parasites

The different **heavy chains** of the different Ig classes are responsible for conferring unique properties to each class. Table 4-1 summarizes these properties, while Figure 4-5 outlines the basic structure of an antibody protein. Among the most important functions of antibodies are toxin neutralization and **opsonization.** Both IgG and the complement component C3b can opsonize, which means that their presence on the surface of a pathogen facilitates their phagocytosis by macrophages. IgG can opsonize directly, and both IgG and IgM can opsonize indirectly by fixing complement, leading to the generation of C3b.

An important distinction can be drawn between primary and secondary humoral responses (Figure 4-6). This difference results from the **memory B cells** that are produced during the first exposure and rapidly activated during the second. Also, with each successive exposure to the same antigen, the Ig produced binds more avidly because of two processes called **somatic mutation** and **affinity maturation.** Mutations occur in the hypervariable region of the DNA of the antibody (somatic mutation). Some of these mutations lead to higher affinity to the antigen; some do not. In a Darwinian selection process, the next exposure to the antigen leads to selective activation of those B cells bearing Ig with increased affinity (affinity maturation). For this reason, as well as generation of more memory cells, booster shots enhance the effectiveness of active immunization.

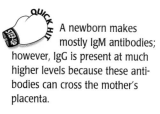 A newborn makes mostly IgM antibodies; however, IgG is present at much higher levels because these antibodies can cross the mother's placenta.

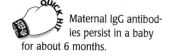 Maternal IgG antibodies persist in a baby for about 6 months.

Other plasma cell disorders

The plasma cell disorders include multiple myeloma, Waldenstrom macroglobulinemia, AL amyloidosis, monoclonal gammopathy of undetermined significance (MGUS), and heavy chain disease. All result from the proliferation of plasma cells. Multiple myeloma has been described above; heavy chain disease is extremely rare and will not be covered. The others will be briefly outlined here.

FIGURE 4-5 Antibody structure

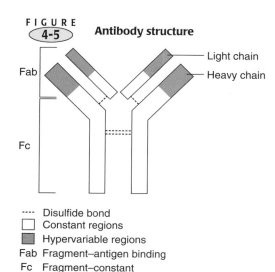

Light chain
Heavy chain
Fab
Fc

```
----  Disulfide bond
[ ]   Constant regions
[▓]   Hypervariable regions
Fab   Fragment–antigen binding
Fc    Fragment–constant
```

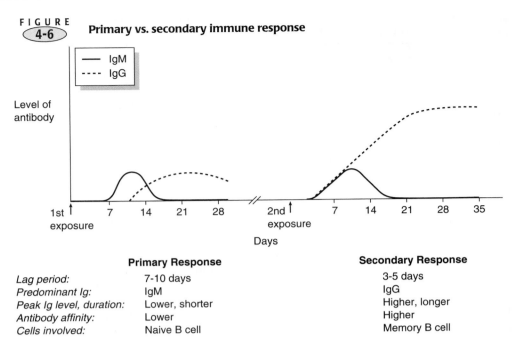

FIGURE 4-6

Primary vs. secondary immune response

	Primary Response	Secondary Response
Lag period:	7-10 days	3-5 days
Predominant Ig:	IgM	IgG
Peak Ig level, duration:	Lower, shorter	Higher, longer
Antibody affinity:	Lower	Higher
Cells involved:	Naive B cell	Memory B cell

Waldenstrom macroglobulinemia results from **IgM**-producing cells that are of intermediate differentiation between B cells and plasma cells. It occurs most frequently in men older than 50 years and presents with generalized lymphadenopathy, weakness, weight loss, mild anemia, hepatosplenomegaly, and hyperviscosity syndrome. The **hyperviscosity syndrome** results from the high levels of IgM and can cause retinal vascular dilation, CNS symptoms, and Raynaud phenomenon. Sometimes emergency plasmapheresis is necessary to prevent blindness.

AL amyloidosis results from deposition of amyloid fibrils of Ig light chain. It can be secondary to multiple myeloma but most cases are not caused by a B-cell neoplasm. AL amyloidosis typically affects the **heart**, GI tract, **peripheral nerves**, and tongue, with **macroglossia** as a classic feature.

MGUS is present in 1 to 3% of healthy individuals older than 50 years and is characterized by a monoclonal **M spike** on plasma electrophoresis but **no Bence-Jones proteinuria.** Bence-Jones proteins are the monoclonal immunoglobulin light chains produced by B-cell neoplasms. These proteins have a low molecular weight and are therefore freely filtered across the glomerulus and largely reabsorbed in the proximal tubule. Those proteins not reabsorbed appear in the urine. When the tubular reabsorptive capacity is surpassed, **intratubular casts** of precipitated proteins can appear in the distal segments of the nephron. These casts obstruct flow and induce tubular injury, which can lead to **renal failure.**

> **QUICK HIT**
> Amyloid is birefringent, β-pleated sheets and stains with Corgo red dye. Secondary amyloidosis (AA) complicates chronic inflammatory diseases (e.g., rheumatoid arthritis). A4 amyloid is seen in Alzheimer disease. Transthyretin is the protein that composes the amyloid of senile amyloidosis.

Prominent behavioral and medical issues of older adults

In the United States, 80% of people reach 60 years of age. While age does not affect intelligence, strength and health gradually decline. Included in this decline are visual and hearing impairment, decreased muscle mass, increased fat deposits, osteoporosis, and impaired immune responses. Older individuals generate a weaker response to immunizations than young people. Older patients are subject to reactivation of latent infections such as tuberculosis (TB) and herpes zoster. **Depression** is the most common psychiatric disorder in older adults, but it is not a natural result of aging. Many older people also report changes in sleep patterns resulting in poor sleep.

Hypercalcemia

> **QUICK HIT**
> The macrophages involved in granulomatous inflammation can convert vitamin D to its active form, leading to excess vitamin D and hypercalcemia.

Table 4-2 shows some common causes of hypercalcemia. Levels of parathyroid hormone (PTH), phosphorus, and alkaline phosphatase can help differentiate between these diseases.

TABLE 4-2 Hypercalcemia

Disease State	Common Causes	Ca^{2+}	P	PTH	Alkaline Phosphatase	25-Vit D	1,25-Vit
Multiple myeloma		↑	↑	↓	↑		
Primary hyper-parathyroidism	Parathyroid adenoma	↑	↓	↑	↑	N	↑
Granulomatous inflammation	Sarcoidosis, TB	↑	↓	↓	↑	N	↑
PTH producing tumor	Squamous cell carcinoma of the lung	↑	↓	↑ (PTH related peptide)	↑		
Skeletal metastasis	Prostate, breast, lung cancer	↑	↑	↓	↑		

PTH, parathyroid hormone; TB, tuberculosis.

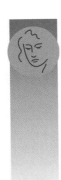

"I've had a high fever for a few days and have been coughing up a lot of greenish red mucus. Now my chest hurts."

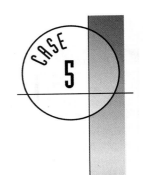

OBJECTIVES

1. Develop a differential diagnosis and an appropriate workup for a common respiratory infection
2. Differentiate among common causative agents of pneumonia by age
3. Describe in detail the bacterial, viral, and fungal causes of pneumonia in terms of presentation, acquisition, pathogenesis, and diagnosis
4. Review the inflammatory response and regulation
5. Know the specific functions and origins of inflammatory mediators

HISTORY AND PHYSICAL EXAMINATION

A 45-year-old white woman comes to the office, complaining of **chills, fever,** dyspnea, and a **cough** that is bringing up **rust-colored sputum.** These signs and symptoms began a few days ago after she had finished shoveling her driveway. She states that **right-sided chest pain** has been increasing since last night. She denies any history of smoking, drinking, injecting drugs, or recently traveling. On physical examination, she is tachypneic with **rhonchi,** and percussion reveals consolidation in her right lower lung base.

APPROPRIATE WORKUP

Blood chemistries, chest X-ray, and sputum culture

DIFFERENTIAL DIAGNOSIS

Bronchitis, foreign body aspiration, hospital-acquired pneumonia, community-acquired pneumonia, upper respiratory tract infection (URI)

DIAGNOSTIC LABORATORY TESTS AND STUDIES

Blood chemistry:
  WBCs = 18,000/mm^3 (H)
  Neutrophils = 78% (H)
Chest radiograph:
  Pulmonary infiltrate with consolidation of right lower lobe (Figure 5-1)

Sputum culture:
  Gram-positive, lancet-shaped, diplococci catalase-negative α-hemolytic colonies inhabited by optochin

DIAGNOSIS: COMMUNITY-ACQUIRED PNEUMONIA

In individuals between 40 and 60 years of age (Table 5-1), *Streptococcus pneumoniae* and *Haemophilus influenza* are the most common causative agents of **community-acquired pneumonia.** The most common mechanism for acquiring pneumonia is aspiration of

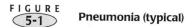

FIGURE 5-1 Pneumonia (typical)

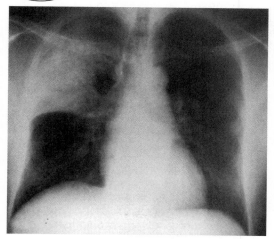

(From Brant WE and Helms CA. **Fundamentals of Diagnostic Radiology,** 2nd Ed. Philadelphia: Lippincott Williams & Wilkins, 1999, p 402.)

organisms from the oropharynx. Typically, the patient presents with an **acute fever,** chills, and **purulent sputum** (often rust-colored or blood-tinged). Physical examination reveals evidence of extra fluid in the lungs, consistent with the findings of **rales** or consolidation upon auscultation. Chest radiograph often demonstrates an **infiltrate** localized to one or many lobes. In this case, if *Haemophilus influenza* were the causative agent, then the Gram stain would have revealed Gram-negative coccobacilli.

EXPLANATION OF DIFFERENTIAL (TABLES 5-2, 5-3, 5-4)

Bronchitis is an inflammation of the airways that causes a cough with abundant, thick sputum, fever, chest pain, and wheezing. Chronic bronchitis is characterized by **cough with expectoration for at least 3 months for 2 consecutive years.** Smokers are predisposed to developing bronchitis. Often, the chest radiograph is normal, and auscultation fails to reveal rales or consolidation.

Foreign body aspiration may lead to airway obstruction and present as acute respiratory distress or hypoxemia with stridor. Chest radiograph may show evidence of pulmonary infiltrate or lobar collapse.

In **hospital-acquired pneumonia,** common causative organisms include *Mycoplasma pneumoniae, Legionella pneumophila,* oral anaerobes, and *Pneumocystis carinii.* Hospital-acquired pneumonia also can present with fever and cough; however, the **fever is usually low-grade,** and the onset of symptoms is **gradual.** Often, the cough is **nonproductive.** The infection is associated with many extrapulmonary manifestations such as headache,

QUICK HIT

Rare pathogens causing atypical pneumonia include *Chlamydia psittaci, Coxiella burnetii, Francisella tularensis, Histoplasma capsulatum,* and *Coccidioides immitis.*

TABLE 5-1 Most Common Causative Agents of Pneumonia by Age			
Children (Birth to 20 Years)	**Young Adults (20 to 40 Years)**	**Adults (40 to 60 Years)**	**Older Adults (Older than 60 Years)**
RSV	*M. pneumoniae*	*S. pneumoniae*	*S. pneumoniae*
Mycoplasma pneumoniae	*S. pneumoniae*	*M. pneumoniae*	Anaerobes
Chlamydia pneumoniae		*H. influenzae*	*H. influenzae*
Streptococcus pneumoniae			RSV

RSV, respiratory syncytial virus.

TABLE 5-2 Bacterial Causes of Pneumonia

Bacterial Agent	Streptococcus pneumoniae	Klebsiella pneumoniae	Legionella pneumophila	Mycoplasma pneumoniae
Typical vs. atypical presentation	Typical	Atypical	Atypical	Atypical
Community vs. hospital acquired	Community	Hospital	Community	Community
Disease	• Pneumonia • Meningitis	• Pneumonia • Urinary tract infections • Sepsis	**Legionnaires disease**	Atypical pneumonia
Characteristics	• Gram-positive cocci • **"Lancet" shaped** • In pairs or short chains • **α-hemolytic on blood agar** • **Catalase negative**	• Gram-negative rod • Facultative • Polysaccharide capsule • **Currant-jelly** sputum • Seen in patients with **alcoholism**	• Gram-negative rod • Requires cysteine and iron for growth	• Smallest free-living organism • No cell wall (Gram stain not effective) • B-hemolytic on blood agar • Cholesterol in membrane • Colonies take on **"fried-egg" appearance**
Pathogenesis	• Induces inflammatory response • Often secondary to a viral infection, which damages cilia of mucosal membranes • **Polysaccharide capsule inhibits phagocytosis** and is the major virulence factor.	• **Endotoxin** resulting in fever and shock • Capsule retards phagocytosis. • Chronic pulmonary disease and catheterization predispose to infection.	• **Endotoxin** • Intracellular replication in macrophages • Predisposing factors include age (>55 years), smoking, high alcohol consumption, and immunosuppression.	• Hydrogen peroxide and cytolytic enzymes that damage respiratory tract
Laboratory diagnosis	• Gram stain and culture • α-hemolytic colonies • Bile and Optochin (P disk) inhibit growth. • **Positive Quellung reaction**	• Gram stain and culture • Mucoid colonies (as a result of the capsule) • **Lactose fermenting** on MacConkey agar • Positive Quellung reaction	• **Silver stain** • Fluorescent antibody • Culture on charcoal yeast extract agar with increased cysteine and iron	• Can be cultured, but requires 10 days to grow • Diagnosis via **cold agglutinins** in serum • Complement fixation test for antibodies more specific

TABLE 5-3 Fungal Infections Causing Pneumonia

Fungal Agent	Histoplasma capsulatum	Blastomyces dermatitidis	Coccidioides immitis	Pneumocystis carinii
Typical vs. atypical presentation	Atypical	Atypical	Atypical	Atypical
Community vs. hospital acquired	Community	Community	Community	Community
Characteristics	• Thermally dimorphic (yeast at body temperature, mold at ambient temperature) • Mold form produces asexual spores (**micro-conidia**) and is associated with bird or bat feces.	• Thermally dimorphic • Yeast form has single broad-based bud and thick wall.	Thermally dimorphic (spherule at body temperature, mold at 25°C)	• Respiratory pathogen • Some consider it to be a protozoan.
Habitat	**Ohio** and **Mississippi River valleys**	Rich soil (near beaver dams)	**Southwestern United States**	Human reservoir occurring world-wide
Pathogenesis	• Microconidia enter lung, become yeast cells, and are engulfed by macrophages. • Multiply in macrophages • **Caseous granulomas form.** • Suppression of cell-mediated immunity can lead to widespread disease.	Inhaled conidia differentiate into yeast, resulting in abscess and granuloma formation.	• Arthrospores differentiate into spherules in the lungs, which rupture resulting in new spherules throughout the lungs. • High risk of dissemination in immunocompromised patients	• Usually asymptomatic • Results in alveolar inflammation • Immunosuppressed patients are predisposed to disease. • Most common opportunistic infection in patients with **AIDS** in North America and Europe
Laboratory diagnosis	Culture on Sabouraud's agar	Sputum or skin lesions examined for yeast buds	• Sputum or tissue examined for spherules • Increased IgM antibodies indicate recent infection. • Increased IgG indicates dissemination.	• **Silver stain of lung tissue** or lavage fluid • Increased LDH

TABLE 5-4 **Viral Causes of Pneumonia**

Viral Agent	Influenza (Orthomyxovirus)	Respiratory Syncytial Virus (Paramyxovirus)
Typical vs. atypical presentation	Atypical	Atypical
Community vs. hospital acquired	Community	Community
Disease	Influenza	• Bronchiolitis • Pneumonia in infants
Characteristics	• Single-stranded (−) RNA • Segmented • Enveloped • Three antigenic types (A,B,C) determined by nucleocapsid ribonucleoprotein • **Hemagglutinin** (HA) and **neuraminidase** (NA) are antigens on the envelope.	• Single-stranded (−) RNA • Nonsegmented • Enveloped • One antigenic type • One type of protein spike on envelope (unlike other paramyxoviruses) • Fusion (F) protein
Pathogenesis	• Colonizes respiratory tract • Occurs most often from **December to March** in the United States • 1–4 day incubation period • Self-limited	• Involves lower respiratory tract • Immune response may contribute to pathogenesis
Laboratory diagnosis	• Grows in cell culture and embryonated eggs • Hemagglutination inhibition and complement fixation can be used to identify virus.	• Cell culture • Multinucleated giant cells

QUICK HIT Aerobic Gram-negative bacilli (e.g., **Pseudomonas aeruginosa**) colonize the oropharynx and stomach more frequently in hospitalized and institutionalized patients than in other individuals. *P. aeruginosa* is a common cause of **nosocomial pneumonia.**

S. pneumoniae is among the leading causes of otitis media and sinusitis in children.

Pneumovax vaccine for *S. pneumoniae* is a polysaccharide vaccine against 23 of the most prevalent capsular antigens. The vaccine prevents bacteremia, not pneumonia, and has been shown to decrease mortality.

L. pneumophila is spread via aerosol droplets and should be suspected when patients have a history of working on or near **air conditioners** or **water towers.**

malaise, sore throat, and GI distress. Chest radiograph reveals a **patchy, diffuse pattern** (Figure 5-2); radiograph findings are often more serious than physical findings and symptoms indicate.

URIs can present with rhinorrhea, coryza, cough, sore throat, and low-grade fever. When influenza is the causative **virus,** other symptoms such as headache, myalgia, and high fevers may be seen. Rhinovirus is the most common cause of a "cold." URIs are **self-limited,** and the characteristic patterns seen on chest radiograph with pneumonia do not appear.

FIGURE 5-2 **Pneumonia (atypical)**

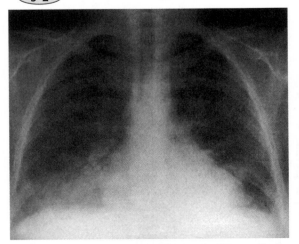

(From Brant WE and Helms CA. Fundamentals of Diagnostic Radiology, 2nd Ed. Philadelphia: Lippincott Williams & Wilkins, 1999, p 404.)

Related Basic Sciences

Inflammatory response and regulation

Recurrent pneumonia or chest colds may be signs of **bronchiectasis,** an irreversible dilatation of the bronchi caused by a suppurative infection in an obstructed bronchus. Bronchiectasis is characterized by inflammation and damage to the bronchial wall. **Pyogenic bacteria** (either Gram-positive cocci or Gram-negative rods) usually cause the initial suppurative infection. The resulting inflammation is secondary to the increased vascular permeability and leukotaxis of neutrophils attracted to the infection. Along with recurrent infections, chronic cough with purulent sputum, intermittent hemoptysis, and pleuritic pain characterize bronchiectasis. Chest radiograph can reveal peribronchial fibrosis in the involved segment.

Cytokines are low-molecular weight hormones involved in **cell-to-cell communication.** Various inflammatory cells release cytokines to mediate the immunologic response. Cytokines have specific functions based on their ability to interact with other cells and membranes (Figure 5-3, Table 5-5, Table 5-6, Table 5-7).

Immunodeficiency syndromes resulting in respiratory tract infections

Selective IgA deficiency, the **most common congenital B cell deficiency,** affects nearly 1:700 children. The inherited form (as opposed to the sporadic form) involves genes on chromosome 14 that code for the heavy chain of IgA. Because of this defect, maturation of cells bearing IgA is arrested. Reduced secretion of IgA from the respiratory and GI tracts increases the chances of infections developing in these body systems.

Chronic granulomatous disease (CGD) results from deficiency in nicotinamide adenine dinucleotide phosphate **(NADPH) oxidase** in neutrophils. NADPH oxidase creates an **oxidative burst** in neutrophils, which helps kill phagocytized bacteria. This **X-linked** disease makes patients susceptible to infections by Aspergillus, Gram-negative rods, and catalase-producing organisms (e.g., *Staphylococcus aureus*). Severe, recurrent infections begin early in life.

 Antigenic shift and drift (change in antigenicity) of the HA and NA antigens on the influenza envelope cause viral evasion of host immunity and allow for annual worldwide epidemics.

The fusion protein of RSV causes cell fusion (syncytia) and allows the virus to escape detection by the immune system. Treatment is via aerosolized **ribavirin,** a deoxyguanosine analog that interferes with guanosine triphosphate (GTP) that is required for capping of messenger RNA.

The bindings of TCR and CD4 from the T helper cell to the major histocompatibility complex (MHC) II-antigen complex of the antigen-presenting cell (APC) and of B7 to CD28 are required for T-cell activation.

Cyclosporine A, an immunosuppressant used to prevent transplant rejection, inhibits T helper cell activity by blocking the activity to **calcineurin.**

Slow reacting substance of anaphylaxis (SRS-A) is a combination of leukotrienes C4 and D4. In the treatment of asthma, **zileuton** blocks the production of leukotrienes by inhibiting the lipoxygenase enzyme, while **zafirlukast** blocks leukotriene receptors.

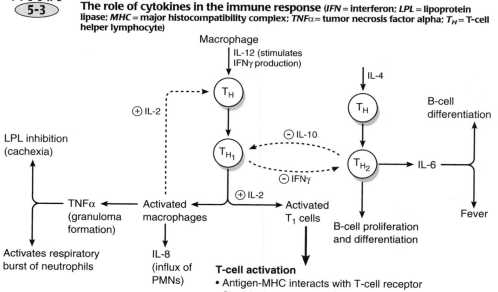

FIGURE 5-3

The role of cytokines in the immune response (*IFN* = interferon; *LPL* = lipoprotein lipase; *MHC* = major histocompatibility complex; *TNFα* = tumor necrosis factor alpha; T_H = T-cell helper lymphocyte)

TABLE 5-5 Function of Inflammatory Mediators

Substance	Released by	Function
Histamine, serotonin	Mast cells, platelets, basophils	↑ vascular permeability
Bradykinin	Plasma substrate	↑ vascular permeability, pain
C3b, C5a	Plasma substrate	↑ vascular permeability, **chemotaxis** (C5a), **opsonization** (C3b), leukocyte adhesion and activation
Prostaglandins	Mast cells, membrane phospholipids	↑ vascular permeability, pain, vasodilatation, fever
Leukotriene B4	Leukocytes	Chemotaxis, leukocyte adhesion and activation
Leukotrienes C4, D4, E4	Leukocytes, mast cells	↑ vascular permeability, **bronchoconstriction,** vasoconstriction
Oxygen metabolites (O_2^-, H_2O_2, $C10^-$)	Leukocytes	↑ vascular permeability, **endothelial and vascular damage,** microbicidal
PAF	Leukocytes, mast cells	↑ vascular permeability, chemotaxis, bronchoconstriction
IL-1 and tumor necrosis factor-β	Macrophages	Chemotaxis, endothelial activation, **fever** (IL-1)
IL-8	Macrophages, endothelium	Chemotaxis, leukocyte activation
NO	Macrophages, endothelium	**Vasodilatation, cytotoxicity**

NO, nitric oxide; *PAF,* platelet-activating factor.

TABLE 5-6 Mediators in Acute Inflammation

Mediators Increasing Vascular Permeability		Mediators Involved with Chemotaxis	
Substance	*Released by*	*Substance*	*Released by*
Histamine	Mast cells, platelets, basophils	C5a	Plasma substrate
Serotonin	Mast cells, platelets, basophils	Leukotriene B4	Leukocytes
C3a, C5a	Plasma substrate	Oxygen metabolites	Leukocytes
Bradykinin	Plasma substrate	PAF	Leukocytes, mast cells
Leukotriene C4, D4, E4	Leukocytes, mast cells	IL-1	Macrophages
Oxygen metabolites	Leukocytes	TNF	Macrophages
PAF	Leukocytes	IL-8	Macrophages, endothelium

PAF, platelet-activating factor; TNF, tumor necrosis factor.

TABLE 5-7 Inflammatory Mediators Released by Cells of the Immune System

Cell	Substance Released
Mast cells	Histamine Serotonin Prostaglandins Leukotrienes C4, D4, E4 PAF
Macrophages	IL-1 TNF IL-8 NO MIF
Leukocytes	Leukotrienes Oxygen metabolites PAF
Endothelium	NO IL-8
Basophil	Histamine Eosinophil chemotactic factor Neutral proteases PAF Leukotrienes Prostaglandins

MIF, müllerian inhibiting factor; PAF, platelet-activating factor; TNF, tumor necrosis factor.

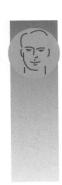

"Over the past few months, I've been feeling increasingly tired and out of breath. Recently, I've been walking stiffly and falling down a lot."

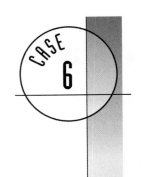

OBJECTIVES

1. Develop a differential diagnosis and an appropriate workup for increasing fatigue, dyspnea, and difficulty walking
2. Review the anatomy, function, and effects of lesions of the lateral corticospinal, tract, dorsal column/medial lemniscus, and lateral spinothalamic tract
3. Understand the biochemistry of vitamin B_{12}
4. Learn the effects of deficiencies in vitamin B_{12} and appropriate treatment

HISTORY AND PHYSICAL EXAMINATION

A 62-year-old man complains of gradually increasing **fatigue,** weakness, dyspnea, and "pins and needles" in his feet and lower legs. The patient is taking no medications other than captopril to control his hypertension. He denies a history of renal disease, melena, or alcohol abuse. Physical examination reveals that his conjunctivae and nailbeds are pale and his **skin is lemon yellow.** The patient also points out that his tongue has become glazed and "beefy" **(atrophic glossitis).** No alcohol odor is on his breath and he shows no evidence of asterixis, hepatosplenomegaly, or ascites. Auscultation reveals a 2/6 systolic flow murmur over the left sternal border. Neurologic examination reveals a stiff, unsteady gait, **hyperreflexia,** and **loss of position and vibratory sense** in the lower limbs. The mental status examination is normal.

APPROPRIATE WORKUP

Blood chemistries, peripheral smear, and Schilling test

DIFFERENTIAL DIAGNOSIS

Beri beri, diabetes mellitus, folate deficiency (alcoholism, poor diet, pregnancy), lead poisoning, uremia, vitamin B_{12} deficiency (bacterial overgrowth, disease of the terminal ileum, infection with *Diphyllobothrium latum* tapeworm, pernicious anemia, vegan diet)

DIAGNOSTIC LABORATORY TESTS AND STUDIES

Blood chemistry:
Hgb = 10.5 μg/L (L)
Mean corpuscular volume
(MCV) = 120 fL (H)
Leukocyte count = 3,500/mm³ (L)
Platelet count = 80,000/mm³ (L)
B_{12} = 89 pg/mL (L)
Methylmalonic acid = (H) (also in urine)
Creatinine = 1.1 mg/dL (N)

BUN = 15 mg/dL (N)
Antiparietal cell antibodies = (H)
Peripheral smear: (Figure 6-1)
Megaloblastic anemia with hyper-
segmented granulocytes
Schilling test:
Positive
Marked reticulocytosis (3.5%) follow-
ing B_{12} injection

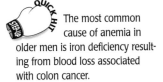

QUICK HIT The most common cause of anemia in older men is iron deficiency resulting from blood loss associated with colon cancer.

Megaloblastic anemia–smear of peripheral blood cells

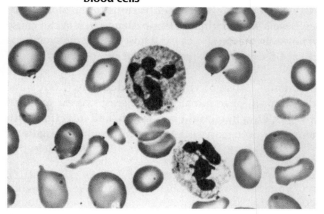

(From Mehta S, Milder EA, Mirarchi AJ. Step-Up: A High-Yield, Systems-Based Review for the USMLE Step 1. Philadelphia: Lippincott Williams & Wilkins, 2000, p 357.)

DIAGNOSIS: PERNICIOUS ANEMIA

Pernicious anemia, an autoimmune disease, usually occurs in the fifth or sixth decade of life and is associated with a **predisposition to other autoimmune disorders,** especially of the adrenal and thyroid glands. Antiparietal cell antibodies develop, leading to **chronic fundal (type A) gastritis.** With the destruction of parietal cells, acid and intrinsic factor production are diminished. Goblet cells replace the damaged gastric mucosa. This process is called "**intestinalization**" and is an example of metaplasia. Lack of intrinsic factor, which is required for B_{12} (extrinsic factor) absorption, results in B_{12} **deficiency.** This deficiency leads to the insidious onset of **megaloblastic anemia** and **subacute combined degeneration** of the posterior and lateral spinal tracts. Patients with pernicious anemia are at **increased risk for gastric carcinoma,** even when they receive treatment with regular injections of B_{12}.

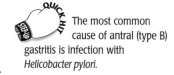 The most common cause of antral (type B) gastritis is infection with *Helicobacter pylori.*

EXPLANATION OF DIFFERENTIAL

Beri beri is a disease caused by **thiamine deficiency,** often secondary to **alcoholism.** The first stage, called dry beri beri, is characterized by **peripheral neuropathy** with muscle atrophy. Wet beri beri is the next stage; its most prominent feature is high output **heart failure.** The final stage, **Wernicke-Korsakoff syndrome,** involves the brainstem and diencephalon, often with hemorrhage in the mamillary bodies. **Confusion, ataxia, ophthalmoplegia,** and **confabulation** are classic manifestations of this stage of the disease. Some other typical manifestations of chronic alcoholism include cirrhosis, hepatosplenomegaly, ascites, gynecomastia, dilated cardiomyopathy, and chronic relapsing pancreatitis. Although this patient has neuropathy (as in dry beri beri), he shows no other signs of alcoholism.

Diabetic neuropathy often affects the autonomic nerves, leading to **gastroparesis** and an inability to regulate heart rate. This patient has neither these symptoms nor any sign of retinopathy or nephropathy, both of which are complications of diabetes.

Folate deficiency causes megaloblastic anemia but not subacute combined degeneration of the posterior spinal column. Deficiency of this vitamin can result from poor intake (e.g., patients with alcoholism, people on specific diets) or increased demand (e.g., pregnancy). Other causes of folate deficiency include celiac sprue, giardiasis, and certain drugs (e.g., phenytoin, oral contraceptives, antifolate chemotherapeutic agents).

Lead poisoning can cause motor neuropathy, often leading to **wrist drop** or foot drop. Other signs of lead poisoning are microcytic, hypochromic anemia, basophilic stippling of erythrocytes, encephalopathy, Fanconi syndrome, and a lead line deposit in the gums. This patient has both motor and sensory neuropathies but no other signs of lead poisoning.

Uremia is defined as **elevated BUN and creatinine concentrations** in the blood, usually secondary to renal failure. These levels were normal in this patient. Uremia can cause anemia and **peripheral neuropathy;** however, uremia also causes a host of systemic symptoms including **bleeding,** heart failure, **pericarditis,** esophagitis, pruritus, and encephalopathy, none of which the patient had.

Pernicious anemia is the most common cause of **vitamin B$_{12}$ deficiency,** but some rarer causes include resection of the stomach or terminal ileum, diseases of the terminal ileum (e.g., **Crohn disease**), **strict vegan diet, bacterial overgrowth,** and **infection with D. latum.** None of these conditions, however, is associated with atrophic glossitis or antiparietal cell antibodies.

Related Basic Science

Spinal tracts (Figure 6-2)

Lateral corticospinal tract

Anatomy:
- The first neuron is in the motor strip (anterior to central sulcus) in the frontal cortex of the brain.
- Axons pass through the posterior limb of the internal capsule, medial two-thirds of the crus cerebri, and base of the pons.
- Axons of this tract terminate on ventral horn lower motor neurons.
Function:
- Motor signals are carried by this tract to muscles involved with skilled motor movements, especially those of the upper limbs.
- Ninety percent of the fibers cross in the pyramidal decussation and become the lateral spinothalamic tracts. The uncrossed fibers become the anterior spinothalamic tract.
Lesions:
- Lesions can occur anywhere from the cortex (Figure 6-3) to the peripheral nerves.
- Lesions above the decussation result in contralateral deficits. Lesions below the decussation result in ipsilateral deficits.
- Lesions within the CNS (e.g., stroke, demyelination of the spinal tract) result in upper motor neuron damage, while lesions of the peripheral nerves (trauma) result in lower motor neuron damage (Table 6-1).

Dorsal column/medial lemniscus

Anatomy:
- Receptors are Pacinian and Meissner corpuscles, joint receptors, muscle spindles, and Golgi tendon organs.
- First-order neurons are in the dorsal root ganglion. Axons from the dorsal root ganglions below T6 form the fasciculus gracilis, while the fibers above T6 form the fasciculus cuneatus.
- Second-order neurons are in the gracile and cuneate nuclei of the caudal medulla. These project axons that form the internal arcuate fibers and decussate to form the medial lemniscus.

TABLE 6-1 **Upper Motor Neuron Lesions vs. Lower Motor Neuron Lesions**

Upper Motor Neuron Lesion	Lower Motor Neuron Lesion
Spastic paralysis	Flaccid paralysis
Exaggerated muscle stretch reflexes	Loss of muscle stretch reflexes
Muscle hypertonia	Muscle fasciculations and atrophy

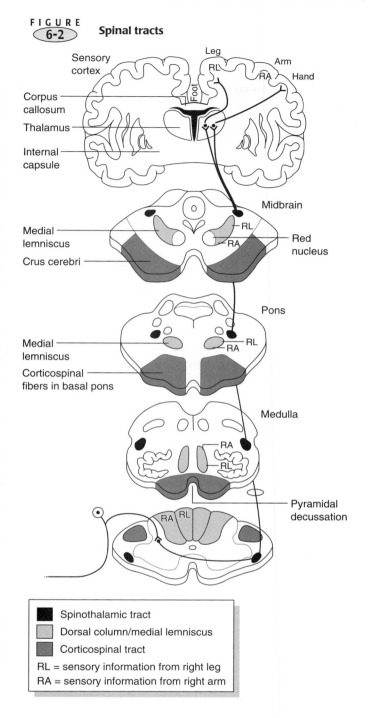

FIGURE 6-2   Spinal tracts

Sensory cortex
Leg — RL
Arm — RA
Hand
Foot
Corpus callosum
Thalamus
Internal capsule
Midbrain
Medial lemniscus — RL
Crus cerebri — RA
Red nucleus
Pons
Medial lemniscus — RL
Corticospinal fibers in basal pons — RA
Medulla
RA
RL
Pyramidal decussation
RA RL

Legend:
■ Spinothalamic tract
▨ Dorsal column/medial lemniscus
▦ Corticospinal tract
RL = sensory information from right leg
RA = sensory information from right arm

- Third-order neurons are in the ventral posterior lateral (VPL) nucleus of the thalamus. They project axons that pass through the posterior limb of the internal capsule and terminate in the primary somatosensory cortex (area 3,1,2).

Function:

- The fasciculus gracilis and fasciculus cuneatus carry the following sensory information: tactile discrimination, vibratory sense, and form recognition.

Lesions:

- Cord level lesions of the dorsal column result in ipsilateral loss of vibratory sense, joint position sense, tactile discrimination, and form recognition. Lesions of the sensory cortex (see Figure 6-3) result in localized contralateral sensory losses.

FIGURE
6-3   **The homunculus**

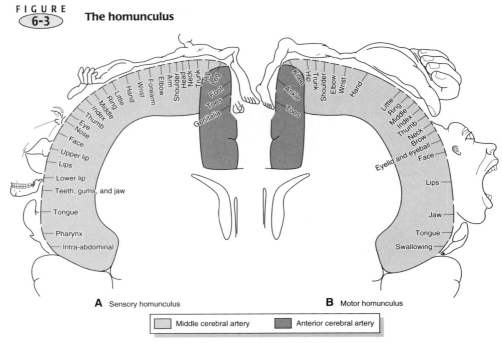

(Modified from Fix JB. BRS Neuroanatomy, 2nd Ed. Philadelphia, Lippincott Williams & Wilkins, 1997, p 348.)

Lateral spinothalamic tract

Anatomy:
- Receptors are free nerve endings.
- First-order neurons are in the dorsal root ganglion. They project a very short distance to the dorsal horn of the same cord level.
- Second-order neurons are in the dorsal horn and project axons that ascend a few cord levels before they decussate in the ventral white commissure and form the lateral spinothalamic tract.
- Third-order neurons are in the VPL nucleus of the thalamus. These project via the posterior limb of the internal capsule to the primary sensory cortex (area 3, 1, 2).

Function:
- This tract carries pain and temperature information.

Lesions:
- Cord level lesions of the lateral spinothalamic tract result in contralateral loss of pain and temperature sensation beginning a few levels below the lesion.
- Syringomyelia is dilatation of the central canal of the spinal cord. This disease of unknown etiology normally occurs in the cervical region. The ventral white commissure at cervical levels is often destroyed, interrupting the decussating spinothalamic fibers. The result is bilateral loss of pain and temperature in the upper limbs and trunk.

Vitamin B$_{12}$

Vitamin B$_{12}$ (also called cobalamin and extrinsic factor) contains cobalt coordinated in a corrin ring. Intrinsic factor, a glycoprotein secreted by parietal cells, binds B$_{12}$ in the stomach. Without intrinsic factor, B$_{12}$ cannot be effectively absorbed. Together, B$_{12}$ and intrinsic factor are absorbed in the terminal ileum. Transcobalamin carries B$_{12}$ in the blood.

B$_{12}$ is involved in two reactions. The first involves a common final step in the metabolism of odd-chain fatty acids (FA) and branched-chain amino acids (bc-aa) (Figure 6-4). In a fasting state, falling glucose levels lead to decreased insulin and increased epinephrine levels. This combination activates hormone sensitive lipase (HSL) in adipocytes,

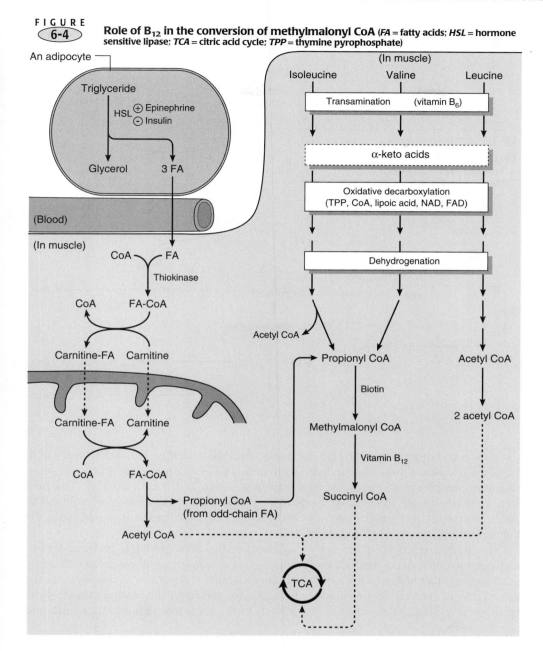

FIGURE 6-4 Role of B$_{12}$ in the conversion of methylmalonyl CoA (*FA* = fatty acids; *HSL* = hormone sensitive lipase; *TCA* = citric acid cycle; *TPP* = thymine pyrophosphate)

which breaks down triglycerides, releasing free FA and glycerol. Tissues such as skeletal muscle can take up the free FA, which albumin carries in the serum. The **carnitine shuttle** transports FA into the mitochondria. Once here, the reactions of β-oxidation remove two carbons at a time, releasing acetyl coenzyme A (CoA). Acetyl CoA can then enter the TCA cycle and provide the energy needed during starvation.

B$_{12}$ is involved only when an odd-chain FA is broken down. In this case, as two-carbon acetyl CoA units are removed, a three-carbon propionyl CoA remains. Two reactions, the second of which requires B$_{12}$, convert propionyl CoA to succinyl CoA. Succinyl CoA then enters the TCA cycle.

The metabolism of two of the bc-aa (valine and isoleucine) also produces propionyl CoA. Valine, isoleucine, and leucine are all essential and metabolized primarily in muscle, not the liver. The first step is transamination to α-ketoacids, which requires vitamin B$_6$. Deficiencies of the α-ketoacid dehydrogenases involved in this step result in **maple syrup urine disease.** This disease is characterized by elevated levels of bc-aa and α-ketoacids in

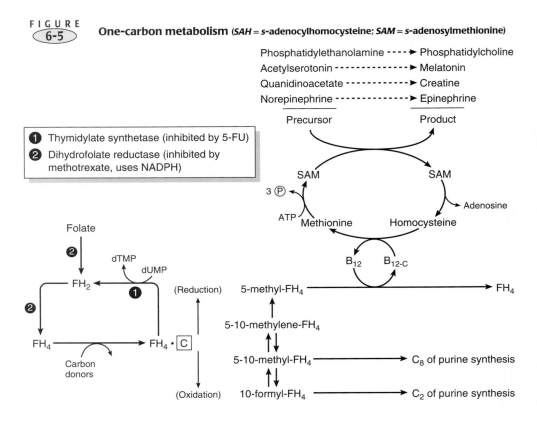

FIGURE 6-5 One-carbon metabolism (*SAH* = *s-adenocylhomocysteine; SAM* = *s-adenosylmethionine*)

the plasma and urine, neurologic deterioration, and high mortality. The second reaction in bc-aa metabolism is an oxidative decarboxylation. This reaction requires five coenzymes: thiamine pyrophosphate, lipoic acid, coenzyme A, FAD, and NAD (TLCFN). The final step common to all three bc-aa is dehydrogenation. The metabolism of valine and isoleucine yields propionyl CoA, which the same enzymes involved in odd-chain FA metabolism must convert to succinyl CoA.

The second reaction in the body that requires B_{12} involves folate and one-carbon metabolism. One-carbon metabolism (Figure 6-5) is a complex set of reactions that partly produces many important substances, including thymine and purines. A deficiency in the production of these DNA precursors affects rapidly dividing cells, such as those of the bone marrow. Thus, a deficiency of either folate or B_{12} leads to megaloblastic anemia and pancytopenia.

Tetrahydrofolate (FH4) can receive carbon units from many sources. Once such carbon units are attached to FH4, they become part of the "one-carbon pool" and can be oxidized or reduced. These carbons, at different levels of oxidation or reduction, are donated to certain recipients, such as B_{12} and purine precursors.

Vitamin B_{12} receives carbon from folate only in the methyl form. The methylated B_{12} then participates in the production of s-adenosylmethionine (SAM). In states of B_{12} deficiency, folate accumulates in its methylated form (5-methyl-FH4), which cannot be reoxidized. Therefore, in the absence of B_{12}, folate is unavailable to participate in reactions such as purine synthesis.

Administrations of sufficient amounts of folate will correct the anemia of B_{12} deficiency by providing enough folate to overcome the trapping phenomenon. Administration of folate, however, will not correct the neurologic deterioration associated with B_{12} deficiency that results from elevated levels of methylmalonyl CoA.

Two chemotherapeutic agents, **5-fluorouracil (5-FU)** and **methotrexate,** act on folate one-carbon metabolism. These drugs can halt the two-step regeneration of folate that occurs as part of thymine synthesis. The bone marrow toxicity of these agents is useful in the treatment of certain neoplasms.

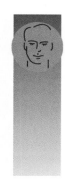

"I get this weird chest pain every time I work."

OBJECTIVES

1. Develop a differential diagnosis and an appropriate workup for chest pain on exertion
2. Compare and contrast aortic versus mitral regurgitation and stenosis
3. Learn the associated pathologies with systolic and diastolic murmurs
4. Carefully dissect the seven phases of the cardiac cycle
5. Understand the physiology of the baroreceptor reflex and its response to a decrease in blood pressure

HISTORY AND PHYSICAL EXAMINATION

A 40-year-old male complains of increasing angina that is getting worse even with minimal physical activity. He reports several recent episodes of dizziness while playing golf. Last week, he fainted while working in the garden. Physical exam reveals a **narrow pulse pressure** with a **delayed and weak carotid pulse** (*pulsus parvus et tardus*). Auscultation reveals a **crescendo-decrescendo systolic ejection murmur** heard in the second right interspace.

APPROPRIATE WORKUP

EKG, chest X-ray, and echocardiograph

DIFFERENTIAL DIAGNOSIS

Mitral stenosis, aortic stenosis, mitral regurgitation, aortic regurgitation

DIAGNOSTIC LABORATORY TESTS AND STUDIES

EKG:
 left ventricular hypertrophy
Chest radiograph:
 Enlarged cardiac shadow with
 calcifications on valve leaflets
 (Figure 7-1)

Echocardiograph:
 Decrease in the maximal aortic cusp
 separation; bicuspid aortic valve

DIAGNOSIS: AORTIC STENOSIS

Aortic stenosis (AS) is due to the narrowing or obstruction of the aortic valve which prevents it from opening properly and hence, blocking the flow of blood from the left ventricle to the aorta. Based on this patient's chest X-ray, the most likely cause of his condition is

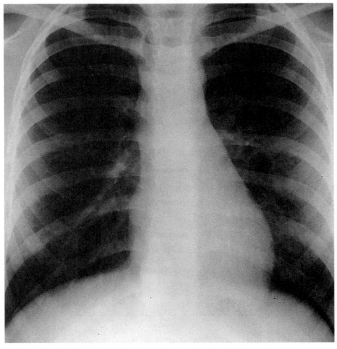

FIGURE 7-1 **Chest radiograph** This chest X-ray shows features of aortic stenosis: prominent ascending aorta, normal pulmonary vasculature, and normal heart size with well-rounded left cardiac border

(LifeART image, 2006. Lippincott Williams & Wilkins.)

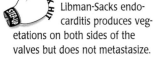

Acute bacterial endocarditis results in large vegetations on valves. The most common causative agent is *S. aureus.* The vegetations can embolize to the brain, producing ring-enhancing lesions on CT.

Libman-Sacks endocarditis produces vegetations on both sides of the valves but does not metastasize.

calcium buildup on his aortic valve. With age, valves can accumulate deposits of calcium, which is a mineral found in blood. As blood repeatedly flows over the aortic valve, deposits of calcium can accumulate on valve leaflets (**senile calcific aortic stenosis**). These deposits can be asymptomatic but a patient with congenital bicuspid valve may be predisposed to developing calcification and stenosis much earlier.

A **narrow pulse pressure** (systolic–diastolic BP) suggests a severe aortic valve stenosis. Physiologically, this is due to the fact that during AS, a significant portion of cardiac energy is devoted to generating sufficient force to overcome the aortic valve resistance. As a result, a smaller portion of energy is available for cardiac output, causing a lower stroke volume and pulse pressure. In addition, the left ventricular hypertrophy can impair diastolic filling.

On physical exam, AS may also present with a delayed pulse, carotid thrill, and a **crescendo-decrescendo systolic ejection murmur** following an **ejection click.** Other indicators of severe aortic stenosis are **left ventricular hypertrophy or failure,** which is a compensatory mechanism to overcome the resistance to flow presented by the stenotic valve.

Since the left ventricular mass requires more oxygen to overcome the outflow resistance, **its myocardial oxygen demand (MVO_2) increases.** The time spent in systole to eject the blood also increases the MVO_2. However, this increased demand is not met by equal supply. Since more time is spent in systole, less time is spent in diastole where coronary perfusion occurs. In addition, reduced ventricular compliance increases left ventricular pressure, further reducing perfusion. Finally, since aortic pressure is reduced, coronary blood flow also decreases. Figure 7-2 summarizes the long-term consequences of this **mismatch between myocardial oxygen supply and demand.**

EXPLANATION OF DIFFERENTIAL

Table 7-1 compares and contrasts the differential diagnosis in terms of key differences in etiology, physical exam, and clinical manifestation.

FIGURE
7-2

Mismatch between myocardial oxygen supply and demand in aortic stenosis

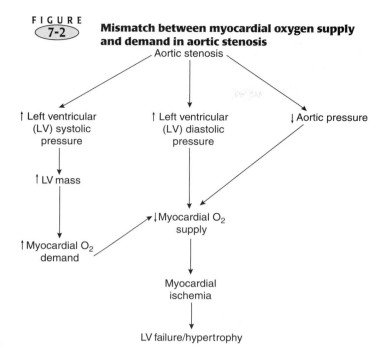

Murmurs are caused by **turbulent flow at elevated velocities.** With aortic stenosis, for instance, the calcified aortic valve forces the heart to contract more forcefully, generating a high pressure gradient between the left ventricle and aorta and resulting in high flow velocities across the aortic valve. Table 7-2 compares and contrasts the systolic and diastolic murmurs.

Marfan syndrome is due to a **fibrillin gene mutation.** Besides skeletal abnormalities (i.e., tall with long extremities), cardiovascular complications include cystic medial necrosis of the aorta with aortic incompetence and dissecting aortic aneurysms. The mitral valve is often floppy, resulting in a late-systolic murmur.

PDA is associated with a **left-to-right shunt** resulting in late cyanosis/"**blue kids**" versus **right-to-left shunts** (i.e., tetralogy of Fallot and transposition of great vessels) which causes early cyanosis/"**blue babies.**"

Eisenmenger syndrome: an uncorrected PDA (or VSD, ASD) can result in the reversal of a left-to-right shunt to a right-to-left shunt as pulmonary resistance increases.

TABLE 7-1 Valvular Heart Diseases

Valvular Disease	Etiology	Physical Examination	Clinical Manifestations
Mitral stenosis	Usually **rheumatic heart disease**	Cyanosis; **opening snap;** diastolic rumbling murmur	Dyspnea; orthopnea; left atrial enlargement; mid- to late diastolic murmur
Mitral regurgitation	**Rheumatic heart disease** (50% of cases); mitral valve prolapse; hypertrophic cardiomyopathy; papillary muscle dysfunction (secondary to myocardial infarction)	Splitting of S_2; S_3; systolic murmur	Arrhythmias; infective endocarditis; dilated left atrium; holosystolic murmur
Aortic regurgitation	**Rheumatic heart disease;** syphilitic aortitis; nondissecting aortic aneurysm; **Marfan syndrome**	Wide pulse pressure; water-hammer pulse; S_3 **blowing, decrescendo diastolic murmur**	Left ventricular enlargement; dyspnea; early diastolic murmur

TABLE 7-2 Murmurs

Systolic			Diastolic		
Ejection	**Holosystolic**	**Late-Systolic**	**Early**	**Mid-to-Late**	**Continuous**
• Aortic valve stenosis • Hypertrophic cardiomyopathy • Pulmonic valve stenosis	• Mitral regurgitation • Tricuspid regurgitation • Ventricular septal defect	• Mitral valve prolapse	• Aortic valve regurgitation • Pulmonic valve regurgitation	• Mitral stenosis	• Patent ductus arteriosus

Related Basic Sciences

Cardiac Cycle

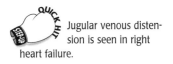 Jugular venous distension is seen in right heart failure.

Table 7-3 corresponds to Figure 7-3 above and explains the mechanical and electrical events that occur in each of the seven phases (vertically).

FIGURE
7-3   **The cardiac cycle**

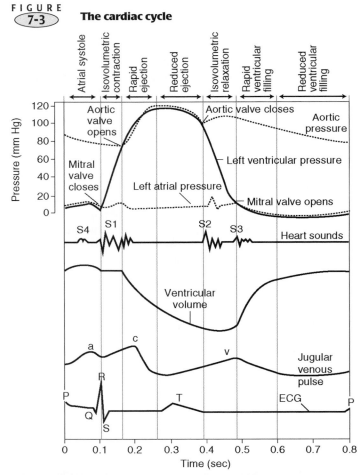

(Reprinted with permission from Mehta S, Milder EA, Mirarchi AJ. Step-Up: A High-Yield, Systems-Based Review for the USMLE Step 1 Examination, 2nd Ed. Philadelphia: Lippincott Williams & Wilkins, 2003, p 75.)

TABLE 7-3 Cardiac Cycle

	Left Ventricular Pressure	Heart Sounds	Ventricular Volume	Jugular Venous Pulse	ECG
Atrial systole: Prior to this phase, blood was flowing passively from the atrium into the ventricle through the open AV valves; during this phase, the atrium contracts and ejects any residual volume of blood into the ventricle	Relatively low; mitral valve closes at end of this phase	**4th heart sound** with filling of the ventricle by atrial systole; not audible in normal adults	Increases due to ventricular filling from atria	"A" wave represents the increase in atrial pressure caused by atrial systole; blood arriving at the heart cannot enter the atrium so it flows back up the jugular vein, causing the first discernible wave in the jugular venous pulse	Preceded by the P wave which signifies electrical activation of atria
Isovolumetric contraction: AV valves close at the beginning of this phase and the ventricles contract against closed valves	Ventricular pressure increases significantly with ventricular isovolumetric contraction	**1st heart sound** when the ventricular pressure becomes greater than the atrial pressure resulting in the AV valves to close (may be split as the mitral valve closes before the tricuspid valve)	No volume change since the aortic valve is closed	—	Begins **after the onset of the QRS wave** which signifies electrical activation of the ventricles
Rapid ejection: Aortic valves open at the beginning of this phase when ventricular pressure becomes greater than the aortic pressures	Reaches its maximum	—	Decreases significantly as most of the stroke volume is ejected	"C" wave of atrial pressure occurs when the right ventricular contraction pushes the tricuspid valve into the atrium and increases atrial pressure, creating a small wave into the jugular vein	—

(continued)

TABLE 7-3 Cardiac Cycle (Continued)

	Left Ventricular Pressure	Heart Sounds	Ventricular Volume	Jugular Venous Pulse	ECG
Reduced ejection: Continued but slower ejection of blood from the ventricle; at end of phase, aortic valve closes	—	—	Continues to decrease	—	"T" wave signifies repolarization of the ventricles at the end of ventricular contraction and ejection
Isovolumetric relaxation: AV valves are closed at the beginning of this phase	Decreases rapidly since ventricles are relaxed. The dicrotic notch in the left atrial pressure tracing occurs after the aortic valve closes	**2nd heart sound** when aortic valve closes; inspiration causes splitting of this heart sound with the aortic valve closing first followed by the pulmonic valve	Remains constant because all valves are closed	"V" wave is due to the backflow of blood after it hits a closed AV valve	—
Rapid ventricular filling: AV valves open and blood rushes from the atria to ventricles	Remains constant	**3rd heart sound** is abnormal in adults and is due to rapid passive ventricular filling; occurs in **dilated congestive heart failure,** severe hypertension, myocardial infarction, or mitral incompetence; in **children, a S3 is normal**	Increases as blood flows from the atria to ventricles	—	—
Reduced ventricular filling: Remaining blood in the atria flows slowly into the ventricles	Remains constant	—	Increases more slowly	—	—

FIGURE 7-4 **Baroreceptor reflex**

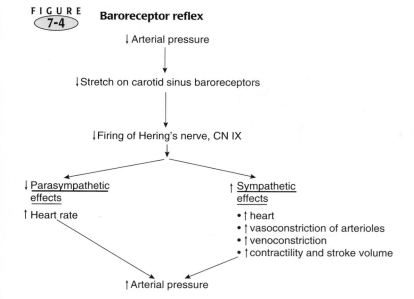

↓ Arterial pressure

↓ Stretch on carotid sinus baroreceptors

↓ Firing of Hering's nerve, CN IX

↓ Parasympathetic effects
↑ Heart rate

↑ Sympathetic effects
- ↑ heart
- ↑ vasoconstriction of arterioles
- ↑ venoconstriction
- ↑ contractility and stroke volume

↑ Arterial pressure

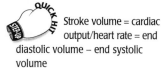 The renin–angiotensin–aldosterone system is a slow hormonal mechanism that is effective in the long-term regulation of blood pressure by altering blood volume.

Stroke volume = cardiac output/heart rate = end diastolic volume – end systolic volume

Contractility can also increase with catecholamines that increase the activity of the calcium pump in the sarcoplasmic reticulum, digitalis which increases sodium and hence calcium, increased intracellular calcium, and decreased extracellular sodium.

Baroreceptor Reflex

The baroreceptor reflex (Figure 7-4) is a fast, neural mechanism involved in the **minute-to-minute regulation of the arterial blood pressure.** Baroreceptors are located in the walls of the **carotid sinus** near the bifurcation of the common carotid arteries. They transmit signals via the **glossopharyngeal nerve** to the medulla. The aortic arch also contains baroreceptors that respond only to an increase in blood pressure via the vagus nerve to the medulla. The figure below details the reflex response to a decrease in arterial pressure. This reflex would be particularly helpful in cases of **acute hemorrhage,** where there is significant blood loss that decreases arterial pressure, or going from a seated or lying down position to standing quickly.

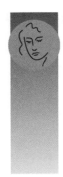

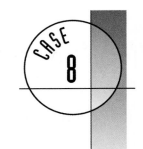

"I have this hard bump on the side of my face."

OBJECTIVES

1. Develop a differential diagnosis and an appropriate workup for unilateral mandibular swelling
2. Compare and contrast the pathophysiologies and clinical features of key environmental lung diseases
3. Understand properties of acid fast bacilli and be able to list a few examples
4. Review the anatomy, function, pathology, and common tests for the 12 cranial nerves
5. Understand the synthesis and flow of cerebrospinal fluid

HISTORY AND PHYSICAL EXAMINATION

A 29-year-old female medical student presents to her primary care physician with a red, **indurated swelling** over her right **mandible.** She reports no pain associated with the swelling but earlier that morning noticed that it had begun to **drain pus.** She is currently on no medications. She is concerned this is contagious and does not want to spread it to her roommates. The only major surgery she recalls is a **recent molar extraction.**

Physical exam revealed no abnormal findings with all cranial nerves in tact. A chest and lung exam was unremarkable.

APPROPRIATE WORKUP

Culture of exudate and radiograph of mandible

DIFFERENTIAL DIAGNOSIS

Asbestosis, nocardiosis, actinomycosis

DIAGNOSTIC LABORATORY TESTS AND STUDIES

Culture of exudate:
Branching Gram-positive filaments with **sulfur granules;** anaerobic and non-acid fast (Figure 8-1)
Radiograph, mandible:
No bony destruction

DIAGNOSIS: ACTINOMYCOSIS

Actinomyces israeli is part of the **normal flora of the mouth.** Patients who develop actinomycosis usually have some history of trauma or oral surgery. The swellings may soften and discharge pus that contains small, round, **yellowish granules.** Because of their resemblance

FIGURE
8-1   (See also Color Plate 8-1.) Culture of exudate color sulfur
granules of *Actinomyces israeli*

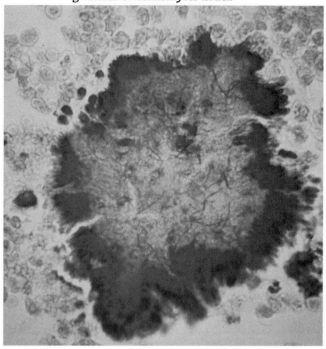

(From Sweet RL, Gibbs RS. *Atlas of Infectious Diseases of the Female
Genital Tract.* Philadelphia: Lippincott Williams & Wilkins, 2005.)

to sulfur, these granules are sometimes called **sulfur granules.** They do not, however, contain sulfur. The infection may extend to the **cheek, tongue, throat, salivary glands, skull, facial bones,** brain, or the tissues covering the brain (meninges). There is no person-to-person spread. Actinomycosis is a chronic, suppurative infection that can involve the abdomen or lungs such as with trauma to the chest (i.e., bullet wound) or following gastrointestinal surgery. The most appropriate treatment would be **ampicillin** followed with **amoxicillin or penicillin G** and finally, **oral penicillin V.** The necrotic tissue could be surgically drained and/or removed.

There is a **thoracic form** of *Actinomyces* which presents with **chest pain, fever, and a productive cough.** These symptoms, however, may not appear until the lungs are severely infected. If an abscess develops in the chest, pus may drain through the skin by way of channels connecting the abscess to the chest wall. *Actinomyces* can also be found in the female genital tract and are often isolated on intrauterine devices.

QUICK HIT If a patient has penicillin allergies, aztreonam can be administered instead.

EXPLANATION OF DIFFERENTIAL

Asbestosis is diffuse pulmonary interstitial fibrosis caused by inhaling asbestos fibers. Common occupations with exposure to asbestos are **plumbers** and **shipbuilders.** Asbestosis increases the risk for **malignant mesothelioma** and **bronchogenic carcinoma.** On microscopic examination, **ferruginous bodies,** which are asbestos fibers coated with hemosiderin, are evident. Chest X-ray can reveal ivory-white pleural plaques.

QUICK HIT Asbestosis and smoking are two common risk factors associated with bronchogenic cancer.

Nocardiosis is also caused by a Gram-positive rod with long, branching filaments resembling fungi. However, *Nocardia asteroides* is a weakly acid-fast aerobe that causes pulmonary infection in patients with diabetes, leukemia, and lymphoma. Nocardiosis can involve the lungs and spread to the brain, subcutaneous tissue, liver, and kidney. Sputum is often **foul smelling, thick, and greenish.** A gross examination of a lesion would reveal necrotic centers with regions of consolidation and abscess formation. Microscopically, the alveoli will be consolidated with exudate of polymorphonuclear leukocytes and fibrin. Treatment consists of a 6-month course of **TMP-SMX.**

QUICK HIT Key side effects of sulfa drugs include hypersensitivity reactions, kernicterus in infants, hemolysis if G6PD deficient, and nephrotoxicity.

TABLE 8-1 Environmental Lung Diseases (Pneumoconiosis)

Disease	Pathophysiology	Clinical Features
Anthracosis	Carbon dust ingested by alveolar macrophages; visible **black deposits**	Usually asymptomatic
Asbestosis	Asbestos fibers ingested by alveolar macrophages; fibroblast proliferation; interstitial fibrosis (lower lobes); **asbestos bodies and ferruginous bodies;** pleural plaques and effusions	Increased risk of bronchogenic carcinoma and **malignant mesothelioma;** synergistic effect of asbestos and tobacco
Coal worker's pneumoconiosis	Carbon dust ingested by alveolar macrophages forms bronchiolar **macules;** may progress to fibrosis	Plaques as asymptomatic; often benign, may progress to fibrosis; may be fatal due to pulmonary hypertension and **cor pulmonale**
Silicosis	Silica dust ingested by alveolar macrophages causing release of harmful enzymes; **silicotic nodules**	Nodules may obstruct air or blood flow; concurrent tuberculosis common (**silicotuberculosis**)
Berylliosis	Induction of cell-mediated immunity leads to noncaseating granulomas; several organ systems affected; histologically identical to sarcoidosis	Increased lung cancer

Reprinted with permission from Mehta S, Milder EA, Mirarchi AJ: *Step-Up: A High-Yield, Systems-Based Review for the USMLE Step 1 Examination.* Philadelphia, Lippincott Williams & Wilkins, 2000, p 75.

Kallmann syndrome is hypogonadotropic hypogonadism associated with deficits in the sense of smell.

Naegleria fowleri is a fatal disease that crosses the cribriform plate through the olfactory bulbs and gains access to the meninges. Patients often report a recent history of swimming, fever, headache, stiff neck, nausea, and vomiting. CSF analysis reveals a neutrophil count, low glucose, and high protein.

Weber syndrome occurs with medial midbrain injury, resulting in ipsilateral CN III paralysis and contralateral spastic hemiparesis.

Injury to CN III: 1) ptosis because of loss of innervation to the levator palpebrae, 2) lateral deviation of the eye because of unopposed pull of the lateral rectus, 3) dilation of the pupil because of unopposed action of the dilator pupillae muscle, and 4) impairment of near vision with loss of accommodation of the ciliary muscle

The medial inferior pontine syndrome results in ipsilateral lateral rectus paralysis with contralateral spastic hemiparesis and loss of sensation of pain and temperature.

Noncommunicating hydrocephalus occurs when the aqueduct of Sylvius is blocked resulting in dilation of the lateral and 3rd ventricles.

Related Basic Sciences

Environmental lung diseases

Environmental lung diseases (Table 8-1) are often caused by workplace exposure to various organic and chemical irritants. A careful history and pulmonary function testing are often important for diagnosis.

Acid-fast bacilli

Acid-fast bacilli are a group of bacteria that can retain carbolfuchsin stain despite treatment with ethanol hydrochloric acid (EtOH-HCl) washings. The **high lipid content of their cell walls** is responsible for this characteristic. **Mycobacteria, actinomyces,** and **nocardia** are examples of acid-fast bacilli.

Cranial Nerves

It is important to recognize the anatomy, function, common lesions, and tests of the 12 cranial nerves. Table 8-2 outlines these features and Figure 8-2 displays the 12 cranial nerves as they arise from various nuclei within the brain stem and cortex.

Cerebrospinal fluid (CSF) production and flow

CSF is produced by an active secretory process of the **choroid plexus** in the lateral, third, and fourth ventricles. CSF flows from the lateral ventricles into the third ventricle via the foramen of Monroe and from the third ventricle through the cerebral aqueduct, or the aqueduct of Sylvius, to the fourth ventricle. From the fourth ventricle, CSF flows into the subarachnoid space through the medial foramen of Magendie and the lateral foramen of Luschka (Figure 8-3).

TABLE 8-2 Cranial Nerves

Nerve	Site of Exit From Skull	Function	Fiber Types	Common Lesions	Test
I-Olfactory	Cribriform	Smell	SVA	Cribriform plate fracture; Kallmann syndrome	Smell
II-Optic	Optic canal	Sight	SSA	See Figure 8-2	Snellen chart; peripheral vision
III-Oculomotor	Superior orbital fissure	**Parasympathetic** to **ciliary** and **sphincter muscles;** medial rectus, superior rectus, inferior rectus, inferior oblique	GVE, GSE	Transtentorial (uncal) herniation; **diabetes;** Weber syndrome	"H" in space; pupillary light reflexes; convergence
IV-Trochlear	Superior orbital fissure	Superior oblique muscle	GSE	Head trauma	"H" in space
V-Trigeminal V1-Ophthalmic	Superior orbital fissure	Sensory from medial nose, forehead	SVE, GSA	Tic douloureux (trigeminal neuralgia)	Facial sensation; open jaw **(deviates toward lesion)**
V2-Maxillary	Foramen rotundum	Sensory from lateral nose, upper lip, superior buccal area			
V3-Mandibular	Foramen ovale	**Muscles of mastication,** tensor tympani, tensor veli palantini; sensory from lower lip, lateral face to lower border of mandible			
VI-Abducens	Superior orbital fissure	Lateral rectus muscle	GSE	**Medial inferior pontine syndrome**	"H" in space
VII-Facial	Internal acoustic meatus	Parasympathetic to lacrimal, submandibular, and sublingual glands; **muscles of facial expression and stapedius, stylohyoid muscle, posterior belly of digastric muscle;** sensory from anterior 2/3 of tongue (including taste **via chorda tympani**)	GVE, SVE, GSA, SVA	**Bell's palsy**	Wrinkle forehead; show teeth; puff out cheeks; close eyes tightly
VIII-Vestibulocochlear	Internal acoustic meatus	Equilibrium; hearing	SSA	**Acoustic schwannoma**	Hearing; nystagmus (slow phase toward lesion)

(*continued*)

TABLE 8-2 Cranial Nerves (Continued)

Nerve	Site of Exit From Skull	Function	Fiber Types	Common Lesions	Test
IX-Glossopharyngeal	Jugular foramen	Parasympathetic to parotid gland; stylopharyngeus muscle; sensory from pharynx, middle ear, auditory tube, carotid body and sinus, external ear, posterior third of tongue (including taste)	GVE, SVE, GSA, GVA, SVA	Posterior inferior cerebellar artery (**PICA**) infarct	Gag reflex (no response ipsilateral to lesion)
X-Vagus	Jugular foramen	Parasympathetic to body viscera; laryngeal and pharyngeal muscles; sensory from trachea, esophagus, viscera, external ear, epiglottis (including taste)	GVE, SVE, GSA, GVA, SVA	Thyroidectomy, **PICA** infarct	Gag reflex (**uvula deviates away from lesion**)
XI-Accessory	Jugular foramen	Sternocleidal-mastoid and trapezius muscles	SVE	**PICA** infarct	Turning head (weakness turning away from lesion); raising shoulder against resistance (ipsilateral)
XII-Hypoglossal	Hypoglossal canal	Intrinsic tongue muscles	GSE	Anterior spinal artery infarct	Tongue protrusion (deviates toward lesion)

GSA, general somatic afferent; GSE, general somatic efferent; GVA, general visceral afferent; GVE, general visceral efferent; SSA, special somatic afferent; SVA, special visceral afferent; SVE, special visceral efferent.
Reprinted with permission from Mehta S, Milder EA, Mirarchi AJ: *Step-Up: A High-Yield, Systems-Based Review for the USMLE Step 1 Examination*, 2nd Ed. Philadelphia, Lippincott Williams & Wilkins, 2000, p 75.

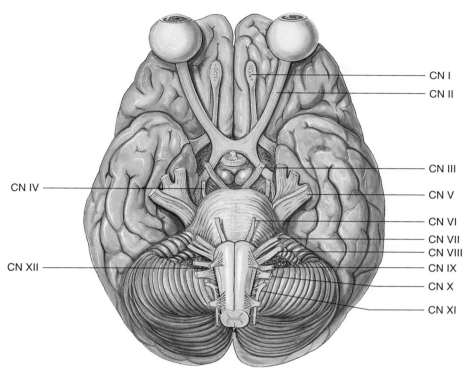

FIGURE 8-2 Cranial nerves

CN I
CN II
CN III
CN IV
CN V
CN VI
CN VII
CN VIII
CN IX
CN X
CN XI
CN XII

(From Anatomical Chart Company.)

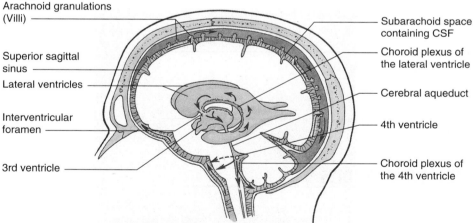

FIGURE 8-3 Cerebral spinal fluid flow

Arachnoid granulations (Villi)
Superior sagittal sinus
Lateral ventricles
Interventricular foramen
3rd ventricle

Subarachoid space containing CSF
Choroid plexus of the lateral ventricle
Cerebral aqueduct
4th ventricle
Choroid plexus of the 4th ventricle

(From Moore KL, Agur A. Essential Clinical Anatomy, 2nd Ed. Philadelphia: Lippincott Williams & Wilkins, 2002.)

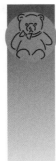

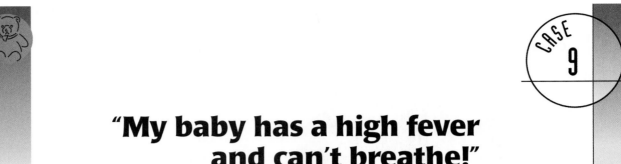

"My baby has a high fever and can't breathe!"

OBJECTIVES

1. Develop a differential diagnosis and an appropriate workup for high fever and wheezing in an infant
2. Understand the physical findings on a chest exam and their clinical significance
3. Review the synthesis and function of surfactant and its associated pathology
4. Learn Laplace's law and its clinical significance
5. Discuss the direction of the FEV_1/FVC ratio in obstructive and restrictive pulmonary diseases

HISTORY AND PHYSICAL EXAMINATION

A 7-month-old female is brought to the pediatric ER with **wheezing and labored breathing** for 5 hours. Her mother reports that she has had a **runny nose and fever of 38°C (101°F)** for 3 days. She refuses to eat and is "fussy." The mother recalls several children at the daycare center having colds. Family history includes an older **asthmatic sister.** On physical exam, the infant is tachypneic with nasal flaring and mild central cyanosis. On auscultation, **expiratory and inspiratory wheezes** are heard over both lung fields.

APPROPRIATE WORKUP

Blood chemistries, nasal swab and culture, and chest X-ray

DIFFERENTIAL DIAGNOSIS

RSV, asthma, influenza, common cold

DIAGNOSTIC LABORATORY TESTS AND STUDIES

Blood chemistry:
　WBCs = 6,000/ μL (N)
Nasal swab and culture:
　Positive for a virus with multinucleated giant cells (Figure 9-1)
Chest Radiograph:
　Slightly hyperinflated lung fields with marked peribronchial cuffing

DIAGNOSIS: RESPIRATORY SYNCYTIAL VIRUS (RSV)

Respiratory syncytial virus (RSV) is the **most common respiratory virus** in infants and young children and can cause lower respiratory tract disease such as **bronchiolitis and pneumonia.** Nonspecific clinical symptoms include cough, coryza, wheezing and rales,

FIGURE
9-1

(See also Color Plate 9-1.) Nasal swab
and culture

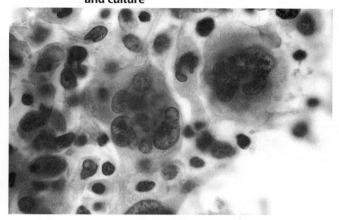

(From Cagle PT. Color Atlas and Text of Pulmonary Pathology. Philadelphia:
Lippincott Williams & Wilkins, 2005.)

low-grade fever (<101°F), and decreased oral intake. Most children recover from this infection in 8 to 15 days. **Premature infants** are at particularly high risk because the final stages of **normal lung development are interrupted.** These vulnerable premature infants have developed neither a normal immune response nor the lung capacity of full-term children. This makes it difficult for these infants to fight infections.

RSV is **spread from person to person.** This patient probably contracted the virus from **daycare.** Inoculation of the virus occurs in the **upper respiratory tract** in respiratory epithelial cells. Spread of the virus down the respiratory tract occurs by cell-to-cell transfer of the virus along syncytia from the upper to lower respiratory tract.

RSV is a **negative-sense, single-stranded, enveloped RNA virus.** The surface spikes are fusion proteins that fuse to form **multinucleated giant cells or syncytia.** The virion is variable in shape and size (average diameter of between 120 and 300 nm), is unstable in the environment (surviving only a few hours on environmental surfaces), and is readily inactivated with soap and water disinfectants.

The chest radiograph and blood chemistries are nonspecific and do not help in confirming RSV but they do support the diagnosis.

A medication called **ribavirin** is effective against RSV if begun in the first few days after symptoms appear. There is also a medication called **palivizumab** that is indicated for the prevention of serious lower respiratory tract disease caused by RSV in pediatric patients. **Synagis** is a humanized monoclonal antibody. Adverse events with synagis may include upper respiratory tract infection, ear infection, fever, and runny nose.

EXPLANATION OF DIFFERENTIAL

Influenza results from infection with one of three basic types of virus, A, B, or C, which are classified within the family ***Orthomyxoviridae.*** These viruses share structural and biological similarities, but vary antigenically. The RNA core consists of 8 gene segments surrounded by a coat of 10 (influenza A) or 11 (influenza B) proteins. The most significant surface glycoprotein antigens that allow for virus entry and infection are **hemagglutinin** and **neuraminidase.** This patient most likely does not have the flu because fevers are usually higher and children are not wheezing. Treatment for influenza includes **amantadine** and **rimantadine** prophylactically for influenza A. **Zanamivir** and **oseltamivir** is used as a neuraminidase inhibitor in influenza A and B.

The **common cold** is most often caused by the nonenveloped RNA virus, the ***Rhinovirus,*** which can be transmitted by aerosol or direct contact. The symptoms of a cold are **limited to the head and neck** with coryza, sneezing, sore throat, cough, and headache. This is because the *Rhinovirus* is acid-labile, meaning it is unstable in the highly acidic environment of the gastrointestinal tract.

QUICK HIT RSV rarely causes pneumonia, leaving the alveoli intact with no purulent exudate. Small airways are inflamed with distal collapse, causing atelectasis.

QUICK HIT **Genetic shift** is due to a reassortment of segments of the RNA genome while **genetic drift** is a random mutation that is a minor change in the genome sequence. Both occur in the influenza virus which makes it difficult to establish one vaccine to administer every year.

QUICK HIT Reye's syndrome occurs when children are given aspirin to reduce fever in viral infections such as influenza or chicken pox. Life-threatening complications such as liver degeneration and encephalopathy can occur.

FIGURE
9-2

(See also Color Plate 9-2.) Curschmann spiral
Corkscrew-shaped mucinous cast with radiating
filaments in an exfoliative cytology specimen
from a patient with asthma

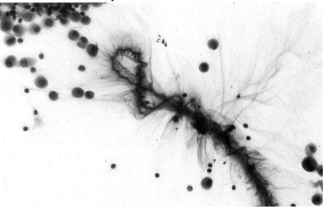

(From Cagle PT. Color Atlas and Text of Pulmonary Pathology. Philadelphia:
Lippincott Williams & Wilkins, 2005.)

The diagnosis of **asthma** is harder to rule out given the clinical presentation but the lab tests are helpful. On nasal swab, a virus would not be isolated with asthma. However, one of the most powerful triggers of an asthma exacerbation is a **viral URI.** Therefore many of the asthma exacerbation patients will present with rhinorrhea and fever. Asthma is regarded as a **chronic, obstructive but reversible bronchoconstriction.** Wheezing points toward intrathoracic obstruction but only pulmonary function testing can truly confirm. Often patients are given **albuterol** to help differentiate. If the wheezing and respiratory distress are reversible, then there must be some component of asthma-like disease. The wheezing associated with RSV usually does not respond well to albuterol. The **inspiration to expiration (I/E) ratio** (indicating airway narrowing) **is reduced** with **pulsus paradoxus.** Curschmann spirals are noted on microscopy of the mucus (Figure 9-2).

Eosinophilia would also be helpful in diagnosing acute asthma. The eosinophil count tends to be elevated in parasitic diseases (particularly those caused by nematodes) and hypersensitivity diseases, such as asthma and serum sickness. Arterial blood gas measurement provides important information in acute asthma. This test may reveal dangerous levels of **hypoxemia or hypercarbia secondary to hypoventilation;** typically, results are consistent with **respiratory alkalosis.** Chest X-ray of patients with acute asthma rarely reveals clinically significant findings, although it may show streaky infiltrates or hyperinflation of the lung fields.

Related Basic Sciences

Physical Findings on Chest Exam and Clinical Significance

Fremitus refers to the palpable vibrations that are transmitted through the bronchopulmonary tree to the chest wall when the patient speaks. It is decreased or completely absent when transmission of vibration to the surface of the chest is impeded in conditions such as an obstructed bronchus, COPD, pleural effusion, fibrosis, or pneumothorax.

Normal lungs are **resonant. Dullness** replaces resonance when fluid or solid is present in the lungs such as with lobar pneumonia or pleural accumulation of serous fluid (pleural effusion), blood (hemothorax), pus (empyema), or tumor. **Hyperresonance** is heard if the lungs are hyperinflated as in emphysema or asthma. Unilateral hyperresonance suggests **pneumothorax.** Table 9-1 summarizes physical exam findings for key lung diseases.

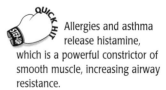 Asthma is considered a type I hypersensitivity reaction with elevated IgE levels.

The major human *Rhinovirus* receptor is intercellular adhesion molecule-1 (ICAM-1), which aids the binding between endothelial cells and leukocytes. The virus takes advantage of the ICAM-1 by using it as a receptor for attachment. Some virus serotypes can upregulate the ICAM-1 expression on human epithelial cells to increase infection susceptibility.

Allergies and asthma release histamine, which is a powerful constrictor of smooth muscle, increasing airway resistance.

The trachea deviates away from the side of the lesion in cases of tension pneumothorax and toward the lesion with bronchial obstruction.

TABLE 9-1 Physical Exam Findings

Disease	Fremitus	Resonance
Pleural effusion	↓	Dullness
Lobar pneumonia	↑	Dullness
Pneumothorax, emphysema	Absent	Hyperresonant
Bronchial obstruction	↓	↓

Surfactant

Surfactant plays a key role in **reducing surface tension** and **increasing lung compliance.** The alveoli have a tendency to collapse. However, surfactant increases alveoli compliance, allowing it to remain open, reducing pressure to collapse by removing intermolecular forces between liquid molecules lining the alveoli. Surfactant is produced by **type II pneumocytes** and consists primarily of the **phospholipids dipalmitoyl phosphatidylcholine.** It is made most abundantly after the **35th week of gestation.** The **lecithin-to-sphingomyelin ratio** in the amniotic fluid is a good measure of fetal lung maturity.

In **neonatal respiratory distress syndrome,** which occurs in premature infants, type II pneumocytes are not fully developed and fail to produce sufficient surfactant, resulting in atelectasis or collapse of the alveoli. Treatment includes **steroids** to the mother before birth and **artificial surfactant** to the infant after birth.

Laplace's law states that an alveolus with a small radius has more collapsing pressure than an alveolus with a large radius according to the following relationship:

$$P \propto T/r$$

P = collapsing pressure on the alveolus
T = surface tension
r = alveolar radius

Therefore, with large alveoli (↑ r) there is a tendency for the alveoli to remain open with low collapsing pressures (↓ P) while small alveoli (↓ r) collapse and are more difficult to keep open (↑ P). In the absence of surfactant, small alveoli then have an increased tendency toward atelectasis.

OBSTRUCTIVE VERSUS RESTRICTIVE PULMONARY DISEASES

Forced vital capacity (FVC) is the volume of air that can be forcibly expired after maximal inspiration. Forced expiratory volume (FEV_1) is the volume of air that can be expired in the first second of forced expiration. Normally, FEV_1 is 80% of FVC.

In **obstructive diseases,** such as asthma, emphysema, and COPD, airways are narrowed or completely blocked. Therefore, the amount of air that can be exhaled from the lungs is reduced, **decreasing FEV_1/FVC.** In **restrictive diseases,** such as with fibrosis or sarcoidosis, the lungs become "stiff" and there is a decrease in the lung capacity owing to an inability to expand on inhalation. Therefore, both the forced expiratory volume and vital capacity are reduced resulting in a **FEV_1/FVC ratio that is normal or increased.**

QUICK HIT It is important *not* to give oxygen at birth because it can cause blindness and retinopathy of prematurity.

QUICK HIT Poiseuille's law describes that there is an inverse fourth-power relationship between resistance (R) and airway size (r), $R = 1/r^4$.

QUICK HIT On inspiration, the diaphragm is considered the most important muscle while on expiration it is passive.

QUICK HIT In the bronchopulmonary tree, the site of greatest airway resistance is the medium-sized bronchi. The smallest airways actually have decreased resistance because of their parallel arrangement.

"My child has been drinking a lot and now can't keep anything down. She's also complaining that her stomach hurts."

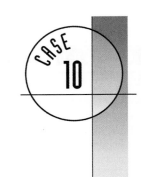

CASE
10

OBJECTIVES

1. Develop a differential diagnosis and an appropriate workup for polydipsia, upset stomach, and labored breathing
2. Review insulin and glucagon regulation in diabetic ketoacidosis (DKA)
3. Compare and contrast acid-base balance in tissue, RBCs, lungs, and kidneys
4. Understand the endocrine function of the pancreas
5. Review the body's response to fasting and starvation
6. Differentiate between the DKA and nonketotic hyperglycemic hyperosmolar (NHHK) states
7. Understand the body's synthesis and use of ketones
8. Compare and contrast Types 1 and 2 diabetes mellitus
9. Learn the chronic symptoms of diabetes
10. Review the pharmacologic management of diabetes

HISTORY AND PHYSICAL EXAMINATION

An **11-year-old** girl presents to the ED with her mother. The mother states that her daughter has not been acting "normal" and has been complaining of excessive **thirst** for more than 1 week. The child has been **unable to eat** or drink today because of **nausea and vomiting** but continues to urinate more than usual and reports being very hungry. The mother has not given the child any medications recently but reports that her child had a high-grade fever 3 weeks ago, for which she brought her to the ER. On examination, the patient is breathing rapidly and deeply **(Kussmaul respirations),** and a sweet smell is noticed on her breath. Her **skin and oral mucosa are dry.**

APPROPRIATE WORKUP

Blood chemistries and urinalysis

DIFFERENTIAL DIAGNOSIS

Diabetic ketoacidosis (DKA), gastroenteritis, hypoglycemic coma, metabolic acidosis, nonketotic hyperglycemic hyperosmolar coma (NHHK)

DIAGNOSTIC LABORATORY TESTS AND STUDIES

Metabolic acidosis results in Kussmaul respirations in response to the fall in serum pH. **Cheyne-Stokes** breathing, associated with hypoxia [i.e., congestive heart failure (CHF)] and CNS depression (i.e., opioid overdose), manifests as variably increasing and decreasing tidal volumes with periods of **apnea.**

Blood chemistry:
  Glucose = 485 mg/dL (H)
  Ketone bodies = ___ (H)
  Na^+ = 131 mEq/L (L)
  K^+ = 5.8 mEq/L (H)
  HCO_3^- = 10 mEq/L (L)
  pH = 7.18 (L)
  Anion gap = 22 (H)

Osmolality = 320 mOsm/kg (H)
BUN = 23 mg/dL (H)
Creatinine = 1.0 mg/dL (N)
Lactate = (N)
Urinalysis:
  Ketones = >80 (H)
  Glucose = >1000 mg/d (H)

DIAGNOSIS: DIABETIC KETOACIDOSIS

In patients with **Type 1 diabetes mellitus** (who **lack circulating insulin**), **DKA** may occur secondary to infection or lack of insulin therapy. Insulin normally suppresses the breakdown of adipose tissue into fatty acids (FAs). Therefore, without insulin, **FA formation increases,** which is the substrate for hepatic ketone body synthesis. The lack of insulin also prompts counterregulatory hormones such as glucagon, epinephrine, cortisol, and growth hormone to rise. These factors result in increased glycogen breakdown, increased gluconeogenesis in the liver, inhibition of glycolysis, and decreased peripheral use of glucose—leading to hyperglycemia (Figure 10-1). The increased glucose and ketones in the urinary filtrate (as a result of reaching a transport maximum for the resorption of glucose) causes **osmotic diuresis,** provoking hypovolemia, dehydration, and loss of electrolytes in the urine. **Hyperkalemia** results from the movement of potassium out of cells in exchange for the hydrogen ions that are prevalent in the serum from the metabolic acidosis (Figure 10-2). An **increased anion gap acidosis** results from both the production of excess organic acids (particularly ketone bodies) and the body's inability to neutralize the excess acid (Figure 10-3).

EXPLANATION OF DIFFERENTIAL

Gastroenteritis refers to an infection (usually viral or bacterial) of the stomach and small bowel. Although a viral or bacterial infection of the GI tract could explain some of the symptoms in the patient (i.e., nausea and vomiting), the laboratory values are inconsistent with a diagnosis of gastroenteritis. Furthermore, profuse vomiting causes a **metabolic alkalosis** as a result of the loss of hydrogen and chloride ions from the stomach.

The mental status changes of **hypoglycemic coma** can mimic those of DKA; however, glucose levels in hypoglycemic coma are low. The symptoms of hypoglycemia, including pallor, sweating, hunger, tremors, increased heart rate, increased blood pressure, and angina, are **the results of increased levels of epinephrine.** Hypoglycemia in patients known to have diabetes can result from excessive insulin administration, skipped meals, or increased physical activity. Hypoglycemia can also result from an insulinoma or consumption of ethanol.

Metabolic acidosis can present with nausea, vomiting, and Kussmaul respirations. There are several other causes of metabolic acidosis besides DKA. Low pH and serum bicarbonate levels are indicative of metabolic acidosis (Table 10-1). Either a **normal** or an **elevated anion gap,** as is the case with this patient, can accompany metabolic acidosis. Normal anion gap acidoses include diarrhea, renal tubular acidosis, or acetazolamide overdose. Anion gap can be elevated in chronic renal failure, lactic acidosis, **DKA,** uremia, salicylate overdose, methanol ingestion, and ethylene glycol consumption. Normal creatinine

> **QUICK HIT**
> The **anion gap** reflects the concentrations of anions that are present in the serum but not normally measured. It is calculated by the equation $[Na^+] - ([Cl^-] + [HCO_3^-])$, with normal values ranging from 8 to 14. An increased anion gap represents a metabolic acidosis with excess anions in the serum (usually owing to organic acids like ketones).

> **QUICK HIT**
> Dehydration activates the renin–angiotensin–aldosterone axis. **Aldosterone** stimulates the **principal cells** of the distal collecting tubule to increase potassium secretion into the urine.

> **QUICK HIT**
> **Transport maximum** (T_m) is the concentration of a substance within the glomerulus at which all transporters are saturated. Concentrations above T_m result in excretion of the excess. The T_m for glucose is approximately **300 mg/dL.** Higher concentrations result in osmotic diuresis.

> **QUICK HIT**
> The administration of β-blockers is discouraged in patients with diabetes. These drugs can mask the symptoms of hypoglycemia by blocking the effect of epinephrine, causing **"hypoglycemic unawareness."**

FIGURE 10-1 **Metabolic events regulated by insulin and glucagon in diabetic ketoacidosis**

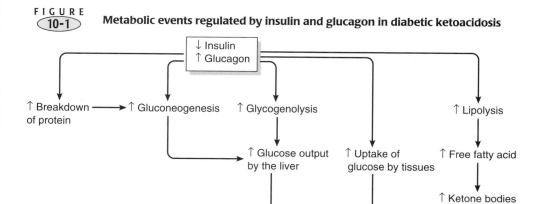

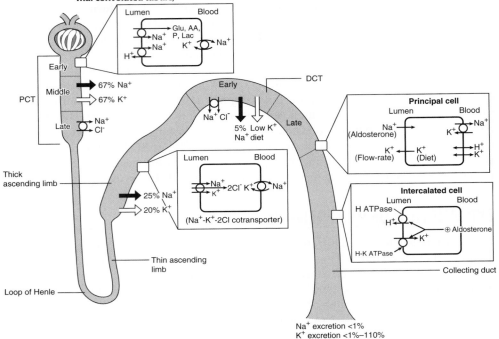

FIGURE **10-2** Renal sodium and potassium balance. Lungs regulate the rate of alveolar ventilation and retain or excrete CO_2 to regulate acid component of HCO_3^- buffer system (*AA* = amino acid; *DCT* = distal convoluted tubule; *glu* = glucose; *Lac*=lactose; *PCT* = proximal convoluted tubule)

TABLE 10-1	Diabetic Ketoacidosis (DKA) and Nonketotic Hyperglycemic Hyperosmolar (NHHK) State	
	DKA	**NHHK**
Pathology	Increased serum **ketone bodies** (>2 mMol/L) Anion gap metabolic acidosis (pH <7.2) **Hyperglycemia** (glucose 300 mg/dL owing to increased production and decreased uptake)	**Hyperglycemia** (>800 mg/dL) **Hyperosmolarity** (>350 mg/dL) > pH > 7.3
Patient	Type 1 diabetes mellitus	Older, with Type 2 diabetes mellitus
Precipitating event	50% **infection** (look for fever), 25% insufficient insulin	**Decreased ability to sense thirst or obtain enough water** Infection Vascular event (e.g., CVA, MI)
Fluid loss	5–7 L	8–9 L
Clinical presentation	Nausea and vomiting **Kussmaul respiration** Osmotic diuresis Shock Coma	Usually **coma** if serum osmolarity is greater than 350 mg/dL
Mortality	10%	17%
Treatment	Saline (essential) Insulin (essential) Potassium replacement	Saline (essential) Insulin
Complications	**Cerebral edema** Hyperchloremic (nongap) metabolic acidosis	More severe dehydration (older patients have decreased body water stores)

CVA, cerebrovascular accident; MI, myocardial infarction.

FIGURE 10-3 Acid-base balance (*CA* = carbonic anhydrase; *TCA* = the citric acid cycle)

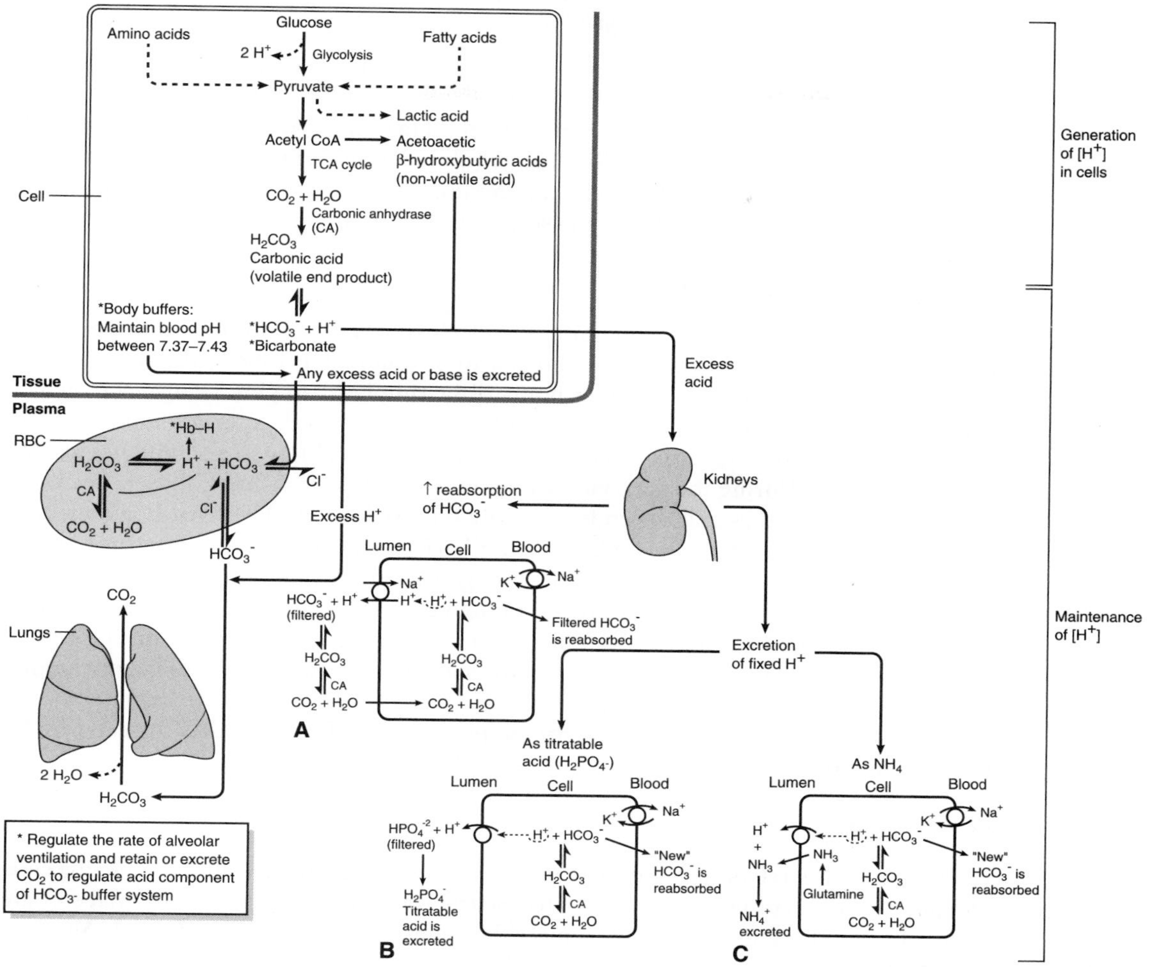

levels rule out chronic renal failure and uremia, while normal lactate levels indicate that lactic acidosis is unlikely. The patient has no history of ingesting foreign substances.

Nonketotic Hyperglycemic Hyperosmolar Ketoacidosis (NHHK) is a severe hyperosmolar state in the **absence of ketosis.** It often occurs in older adults with Type 2 diabetes mellitus. Influential factors in the development of NHHK include infection, increased glucose ingestion, and cerebrovascular accident (CVA) (which inhibits the body's ability to recognize and respond to NHHK). Because this patient has ketone bodies in her urine and serum, NHHK can be ruled out. Ketones are not found in NHHK because insulin is adequate to suppress lipolysis in these patients, **preventing hepatic ketogenesis.** Blood **glucose** levels and **serum osmolality** are significantly **higher,** above 800 mg/dL and 350 mOsm/kg, respectively, in NHHK than in DKA (Table 10-2).

TABLE 10-2 Effects of Metabolic and Respiratory Acid/Base Disturbances

Primary Disorder	pH	H⁺	HCO₃⁻	PCO₂
Metabolic acidosis	↓	↑	↓*	↓
Metabolic alkalosis	↑	↓	↑*	↑
Acute respiratory acidosis	↓	↑	↑	↑ᵃ
Chronic respiratory acidosis	↓	↑	↑↑	↑ ᵃ
Acute respiratory alkalosis	↑	↓	↓	↓ ᵃ
Chronic respiratory alkalosis	↑	↓	↓↓	↓ ᵃ

ᵃ Primary disorder.

Related Basic Science

The endocrine pancreas and hormone regulation

The **islets of Langerhans** comprise the endocrine portion of the pancreas and are responsible for regulating levels of blood glucose. Many factors influence the islets (Table 10-3). Most islets exist in the tail of the pancreas. The β **(beta)** cells, which constitute about 70% of the total islet cells, secrete **insulin.** The α **(alpha)** cells, which comprise about 20%, secrete **glucagon.** The Δ (delta) cells, approximately 10% of the endocrine pancreas, release somatostatin, which inhibits the secretion of growth hormone.

The body's response to starvation

The liver is responsible for maintaining blood glucose levels via input from hormones released by the endocrine pancreas. About 2 to 3 hours after a meal, the liver initiates **glycogenolysis.** Approximately 4 to 6 hours of **fasting** leads to **gluconeogenesis,** which becomes the major process for maintaining blood glucose levels after 30 hours (by that point liver glycogen stores are depleted). The rising level of glucagon also initiates **ketone body formation.** During the **starved** state (after 3 to 5 days of fasting), muscle decreases its use of ketone bodies and depends primarily on FAs for fuel. The liver, however, continues to convert FAs to ketone bodies (Figure 10-4), resulting in an increased concentration of ketone bodies in the blood. Protein degradation provides amino acids for gluconeogenesis; however, after a certain point, protein degradation begins to involve enzymes, compromising vital body functions. Since liver gluconeogenesis decreases during starvation, protein degradation also decreases. In the starved state, the **brain** uses mainly **ketone** bodies, in lieu of glucose, for energy.

Because of a lack of thiolase (an enzyme that converts ketone bodies to acetyl CoA), the liver cannot use ketone bodies as a source of energy.

Diabetes mellitus

Diabetes mellitus refers to a group of disorders that are characterized by hyperglycemia and affect 1 to 2% of people in the United States (Table 10-4). Patients with diabetes are unable to produce enough insulin to meet their metabolic needs. Consequently, they are susceptible to numerous complications (Table 10-5).

> **QUICK HIT**
> The body releases epinephrine in response to infection. Epinephrine inhibits insulin release and stimulates the activity of **hormone-sensitive lipase (HSL),** which breaks down fat. This activity increases serum levels of glucose, which can precipitate either DKA or NHHK.

> **QUICK HIT**
> RBCs cannot use ketone bodies as a source of energy and therefore must rely on glucose even during starvation states.

> **QUICK HIT**
> Because of a lack of thiolase (an enzyme that converts ketone bodies to acetyl CoA), the liver cannot use ketone bodies as a source of energy.

TABLE 10-3 **Regulation and Function of Major Endocrine Pancreas Hormones**

	Insulin	Glucagon
Major regulators	⊕ Glucose	⊖ Glucose ⊖ Insulin ⊕ Amino acids
Minor regulators	⊕ Amino acids ⊕ Neural input ⊖ Epinephrine	⊕ Cortisol ⊕ Stress ⊕ Epinephrine
Function	Stores fuel after meals Aids growth	Mobilizes fuel Maintains blood glucose levels during fasting
Metabolic pathways affected	Stimulates glucose storage as glycogen (in muscle and liver) Stimulates FA synthesis and storage Stimulates amino acid uptake Stimulates protein synthesis	Activates glycogenolysis (in the liver) during fasting Activates gluconeogenesis (in the liver) during fasting Activates FA release from adipose tissue

FA, fatty acid.

FIGURE
10-4

Ketone body synthesis and use (*CoA* = Coenzyme A; *HMG* = 3-hydroxy-3-methylglutaryl; *TCA* = the citric acid cycle

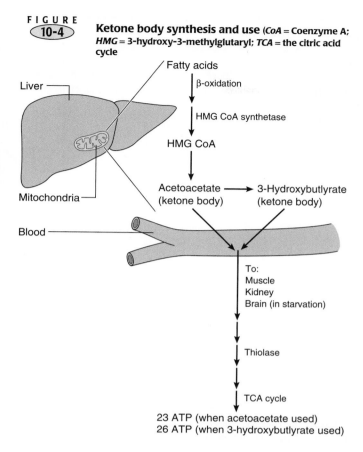

Fatty acids

β-oxidation

HMG CoA synthetase

HMG CoA

Acetoacetate ⟶ 3-Hydroxybutlyrate
(ketone body)   (ketone body)

Liver

Mitochondria

Blood

To:
Muscle
Kidney
Brain (in starvation)

Thiolase

TCA cycle

23 ATP (when acetoacetate used)
26 ATP (when 3-hydroxybutlyrate used)

TABLE 10-4 **Type 1 vs. Type 2 Diabetes Mellitus**

	Type 1	**Type 2**
% of patients	15%	85%
Cause	Possible **autoimmunity** to β cells triggered by a virus	Increased **insulin resistance** Decreased receptors Decreased conversion of proinsulin to insulin
Chromosome	6 (HLA DQ)	Unknown
Family history	Weak	Strong
Age of onset	Younger than 25 years Rapid onset	Older than 40 years Insidious onset
Body habitus	Normal to thin	Obese
Plasma insulin	Low	Normal to high
Plasma glucagon	High but suppressible	High and resistant to suppression
Pancreas morphology	Atrophy and fibrosis β cell depletion	Atrophy and amyloid deposits Variable β cell population
Acute complication	Ketoacidosis	Hyperosmolar coma
Common symptoms	**Polydipsia Polyuria Polyphagia**	Variable: from asymptomatic to polydipsia, polyuria, polyphagia
Insulin therapy	Responsive	Variable

TABLE 10-5 **Chronic Symptoms of Diabetes**

Anatomical Location	Clinical Findings
RBCs	Glycosylation (**HbA1c**)—measure of long-term diabetic control (reflects past 3 months)
Blood vessels	• **Atherosclerosis** • Coronary artery disease • Peripheral vascular disease • Gangrene
Eyes	• **Retinopathy** • Hemorrhage • Hard exudates • Cotton-wool spots • Cataracts • Glaucoma
GI tract	• Constipation • **Gastroparesis**
Kidneys	• Nephropathy • **Nodular sclerosis** • **Kimmelstiel-Wilson nodules** • Chronic renal failure • Azotemia
Penis	• Impotence from autonomic neuropathy • Retrograde ejaculation
Extremities	• Stocking/glove peripheral neuropathy • Ulcers

Insulin can be given to patients with either Type 1 or Type 2 diabetes to help control their glucose. Insulin is usually administered by **subcutaneous injection,** since the GI tract can degrade the hormone if taken orally. Many preparations of insulin exist, ranging from short acting to long acting (Regular, NPH, Semilente, Lente, and Ultralente). Patients with Type 2 diabetes can also take **oral hypoglycemic agents** to control their blood sugar (Table 10-6).

Gestational diabetes

Gestational diabetes is detected for the first time during pregnancy and usually subsides by the 6th week or later after pregnancy. Since glucose moves across the placenta by passive diffusion, fetal insulin is increased which in turn stimulates fetal growth and fat deposition. There is also an increased risk of **fetal macrosomia (large fetus).** This presents an increased risk of birth injury as an oversized fetus passes through the birth canal.

Upon delivery, there is increased risk for the infant to be hypoglycemic. In utero, when the fetal glucose levels are elevated secondary to maternal diabetes, the fetus develops **hyperinsulinemia.** Therefore, after delivery, when the fetus is no longer exposed to the elevated maternal glucose levels, the residual hyperinsulinemia can result in hypoglycemia.

QUICK HIT

Gastroparesis, most frequently a complication of Type 1 diabetes of longer than 10 years, is caused by loss of gastric phase II activity as a result of neuropathy. It can be treated with prokinetic agents like metoclopramide.

TABLE 10-6 **Oral Hypoglycemic Agents**

Category	Examples	Mechanism of Action
Sulfonylureas	Tolbutamide Glyburide Glipizide	• Stimulate insulin release from β cells • Reduce serum glucagon levels • Increase binding of insulin to target tissues
Biguanides	Metformin	• Inhibit gluconeogenesis • Reduce hepatic glucose production • Promote weight loss
α-Glucosidase inhibitors	Acarbose	• Inhibit α-glucosidase in the intestinal brush border • Decrease absorption of starch/disaccharides • Blunt rise in postprandial blood glucose
Thiazolenediones	Rosiglitazone	• Sensitize the body to insulin • Enhance insulin's actions on liver and skeletal muscle

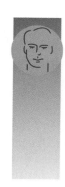

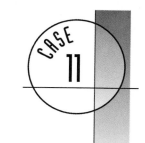

"I got tackled hard, and I think I broke my arm."

OBJECTIVES

1. Develop a differential diagnosis and an appropriate workup for acute pain in the humerus and weakness with wrist extension
2. Review the brachial plexus, its major innervations, and associated injuries
3. Learn the cutaneous innervation of the upper limbs
4. Understand the motor and sensory implications of an ulnar nerve injury
5. Review the neurological and clinical manifestations of carpal tunnel syndrome
6. Learn the mechanism of action and clinical uses for key neuromuscular blockers and local anesthetics

HISTORY AND PHYSICAL EXAMINATION

A 15-year-old boy complains of acute **pain in the distal third of the right humerus** with associated weakness of wrist extension **(wrist drop).** The patient is reluctant to move the right shoulder or elbow. He states that the injury occurred 1 hour prior to arrival, when he was tackled during a football game. He recalls getting tackled from his left side and falling hard on his right elbow. He denies any other recent history of trauma to this area. Past family, medical, and surgical histories are unremarkable. Sensory examination reveals decreased sensation on the posterior third of the arm, posterior forearm, and lateral aspect of the dorsum of the hand. Muscular examination indicates a lack of tone and strength in the wrist extensors. The forearm flexors are normal. Swelling and tenderness are noted on the posterior-lateral aspect of the distal third of the humerus.

APPROPRIATE WORKUP

Radiograph of right arm

DIFFERENTIAL DIAGNOSIS

Brachial plexus injury, humeral fracture, pathological fracture, radial/ulnar fracture, wrist fracture, or a combination of these

DIAGNOSTIC LABORATORY TESTS AND STUDIES

Right arm radiograph:
  Hand, wrist, and forearm negative for fractures
  An oblique fracture at the distal third of the humerus, involving the spiral (radial)
    groove normal bone density of the humerus with no other lesions noted

DIAGNOSIS: HUMERAL FRACTURE WITH RADIAL NERVE DAMAGE

Oblique fractures of the distal third of the humerus commonly cause injury to the radial nerve because of the involvement of the **spiral groove.** This injury occurs during high-energy trauma from contact sports or motor vehicle collisions (MVCs). The lesion presents with localized swelling and pain associated with wrist extensor weakness (**wrist drop**) and **sensory loss** over the posterior third of the arm, posterior forearm, and lateral aspect of the dorsum of the hand. Although the radial nerve innervates the triceps, this muscle is typically unaffected, because branches of the radial nerve that innervate the triceps are given off before the nerve comes in close proximity with the humerus.

EXPLANATION OF DIFFERENTIAL

Forearm fractures are common in MVCs, falls, and contact sports. **Colles fracture,** a particular type of fracture of the radius, results from falling on an outstretched hand. It is characterized by a fracture of the distal radius with dorsal angulation: **"dinner fork"** deformity. Common sites of **ulnar fractures** include the olecranon (from falling on the elbow) and the shaft (from direct lateral force during contact sports or MVCs). These lesions present with pain; loss of elbow motion, wrist motion, or both; and swelling. This patient had no pain in the forearm.

A **pathological fracture** occurs when a preexisting condition weakens bone, predisposing it to fracture. This weakened state allows a significantly less than normal force to cause a fracture. On radiographs, the bone surrounding the fracture appears abnormally radiolucent (abnormally opaque in the case of prostate metastasis). Common causes of bone lesions predisposing to fracture include **metastasized carcinomas** of the **breast, prostate,** lung, kidney, and thyroid; primary bone tumors; **osteoporosis;** osteopetrosis; Paget disease, and **hyperparathyroidism.**

In **wrist fractures,** the most commonly affected carpal bone is the **scaphoid.** Injury to the scaphoid commonly results from a fall on an outstretched hand. Signs include point tenderness in the **anatomical snuff box** and limited wrist motion because of pain. This patient had no pain in the wrist.

Related Basic Science

Brachial plexus

The brachial plexus, comprised of the ventral rami of C5-T1, innervates the upper limb. Figure 11-1 shows the general structure of the plexus and lists some major muscle groups that it innervates. Figure 11-2 outlines the sensory innervation of the upper limb.

Certain parts of the plexus and terminal nerves are especially susceptible to injury. Injury of the radial nerve represents one example, because the nerve is in close proximity to the midshaft of the humerus. Some other common injuries to the brachial plexus are listed in Table 11-1.

> **QUICK HIT**
> This lesion of the radial nerve is an example of lower motor neuron damage. The affected muscles will show flaccid paralysis and areflexia.

> **QUICK HIT**
> A patient with multiple fractures of the lower limbs who suddenly develops respiratory distress most likely has a pulmonary fat embolism from the legs.

> **QUICK HIT**
> The anatomical snuff box is bounded dorsally by the extensor pollicis longus and ventrally by the extensor pollicis brevis and abductor pollicis longus. The scaphoid and trapezium bones form the base, and the radial artery runs through the middle.

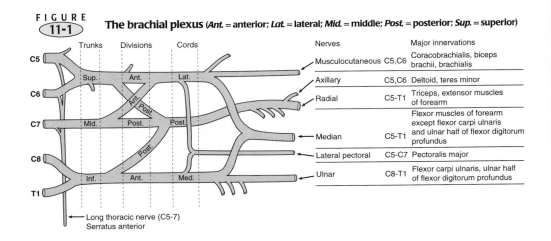

FIGURE 11-1 The brachial plexus (*Ant.* = anterior; *Lat.* = lateral; *Mid.* = middle; *Post.* = posterior; *Sup.* = superior)

Nerves		Major innervations
Musculocutaneous	C5,C6	Coracobrachialis, biceps brachii, brachialis
Axillary	C5,C6	Deltoid, teres minor
Radial	C5-T1	Triceps, extensor muscles of forearm
Median	C5-T1	Flexor muscles of forearm except flexor carpi ulnaris and ulnar half of flexor digitorum profundus
Lateral pectoral	C5-C7	Pectoralis major
Ulnar	C8-T1	Flexor carpi ulnaris, ulnar half of flexor digitorum profundus

Long thoracic nerve (C5-7)
Serratus anterior

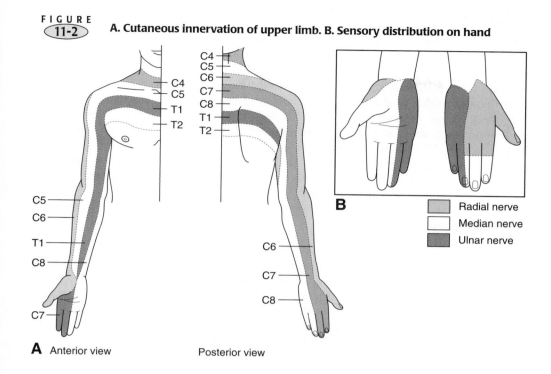

FIGURE 11-2 A. Cutaneous innervation of upper limb. B. Sensory distribution on hand

TABLE 11-1 Other Common Brachial Plexus Injuries

Nerve/Segment Involved	Cause(s)	Result	Notes
Lower trunk (C8,T1)	Birth trauma, clavicle fracture, cervical rib, scalene syndrome, hyperabduction of the arm	**Klumpke paralysis,** claw hand, paralysis of intrinsic hand muscles, paresthesias	Clavicle fracture can injure the subclavian vein.
Axillary nerve	Inferior dislocation of the shoulder, fracture of the humerus at the surgical neck	Paralysis of the deltoid and teres minor muscles, sensory loss over area of deltoid tuberosity	No ligaments or muscles support the lower part of the shoulder joint.
Upper trunk (C5,C6)	Violent downward displacement of the shoulder from birth trauma or a fall (e.g., from a horse or motorcycle)	**Erb-Duchenne paralysis,** "waiter's tip" position of the affected extremity	Arm is adducted and extended, forearm is pronated, and wrist is flexed.
Posterior cord	Pressure in the axilla	Paralysis of the extensors in the arm and forearm	Possible cause is misuse of crutches.
Long thoracic nerve	Stab wound	Paralysis of the serratus anterior muscle, **medial winging** of the scapula, inability to abduct arm above horizontal	This may result as a complication of surgery (especially of the breast).

Ulnar nerve injury

Trauma to the posterior aspect of the elbow **and fracture of the medial epicodyle** can injure the **ulnar nerve.** This lesion results in **claw hand,** which involves the fourth and fifth fingers and is characterized by hyperextension of the metacarpophalangeal joints and flexion of the interphalangeal joints. Injury to the ulnar nerve also results in hypesthesia over the area of the hand innervated by this nerve (see Figure 11-2B). Certain intrinsic hand muscles (i.e., interossei, medial two lumbricals, and adductor pollicis) that the ulnar nerve innervates are also paralyzed. Paralysis of the interossei causes the inability to abduct or to adduct the fingers. Paralysis of the adductor pollicis causes the inability to adduct the thumb. Injury to the ulnar nerve also may result from **slashing the wrists** in a suicide attempt. Such an injury causes only those deficits related to the intrinsic muscles and sensory innervation of the hand, not claw hand.

Carpal tunnel syndrome

Compression of the **median nerve** within the carpal tunnel causes this syndrome, which presents as **pain** associated with **tingling and numbness** throughout the sensory distribution of the median nerve in the hand, with sparing of the radial aspects (Figure 11-3). The radial side is unaffected, because the superficial branch of the median nerve that supplies this area enters the hand outside the carpal tunnel. The first and second lumbricals, the flexor pollicis brevis, the abductor pollicis brevis, and the opponens pollicis are also weak. If severe, **atrophy of the thenar muscles** can occur. Carpal tunnel syndrome is associated with **repetitive wrist motion,** rheumatoid arthritis, diabetes mellitus, **hypothyroidism,** acromegaly, amyloidosis, and pregnancy.

Neuromuscular blockers/Muscle relaxants

The body attempts to splint a fractured bone by inducing spasm in the surrounding muscles. Muscle relaxants are sometimes used to facilitate the setting of the broken bone. The most common use of muscle relaxants is during surgery. These agents are classified into two general classes: depolarizing and nondepolarizing. The drugs in both classes bind reversibly to the **nicotinic cholinergic receptor** of the neuromuscular (N-M) junction.

Curare, the classic nondepolarizing N-M blocker, is a competitive antagonist of acetylcholine (Ach) at the nicotinic receptor. This **competitive inhibition** can be overcome by increasing the concentration of Ach through the administration of pyridostigmine, an inhibitor of Ach-esterase.

All the curare-like agents are given by injection. They are not absorbed from the intestine and do not cross the blood-brain barrier or placenta. Onset of symptoms begins with paralysis of small, fast twitch muscles, such as the extraocular muscles. These agents next

FIGURE 11-3 **Transverse section of wrist showing carpal tunnel and its contents. Flexor digitorum profundus; flexor digitorum superficialis**

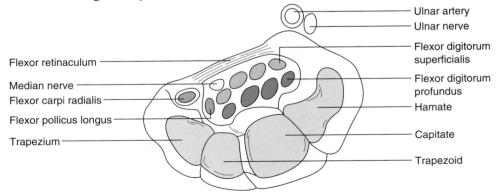

Flexor retinaculum

Median nerve

Flexor carpi radialis

Flexor pollicus longus

Trapezium

Ulnar artery

Ulnar nerve

Flexor digitorum superficialis

Flexor digitorum profundus

Hamate

Capitate

Trapezoid

(Redrawn from Moore KL. Essential Clinical Anatomy. Philadelphia: Lippincott Williams & Wilkins, 1995, p 327.)

affect the muscles of the limbs and trunk. Paralysis of the diaphragm is last. Function recovers in reverse. The curare-like agents do not impair consciousness.

Some commonly used curare-like drugs include tubo**cur**arine, miva**cur**ium, meto**cur**ine, pan**cur**onium, ve**cur**onium, and atra**cur**ium. Each has unique properties that make it suited for certain situations.

Other centrally acting muscle relaxants act by different mechanisms. **Cyclobenzaprine,** which is structurally like the tricyclic antidepressants, is good for acute local muscle spasm. It causes sedation and antimuscarinic side effects. **Diazepam,** a benzodiazepine, "acts at the GABAa receptor" to increase the amplitude of the chloride current. **Baclofen** acts at the GABAb receptor and causes less sedation than diazepam. Both of the GABA-mimetics are best used for the diffuse muscle spasms associated with cerebral palsy, spinal cord injury, and amyotrophic lateral sclerosis.

Succinylcholine is classified as a depolarizing N-M blocker. It causes first a Phase I block, when the drug binds to the nicotinic N-M receptor and activates it. The result is transient muscle fasciculations. Unlike Ach, which quickly dissociates from the receptor and is broken down by Ach-esterase, succinylcholine remains at high concentrations at the N-M junction and continues to activate the nicotinic receptor. Eventually **Phase II block** ensues, in which the membrane has repolarized but the receptor is still blocked. Phase II block causes flaccid paralysis.

Succinylcholine has a rapid onset and short duration of action. The diaphragm is often spared from complete paralysis. Certain adverse effects must be considered when using this agent. Succinylcholine can cause massive potassium release from damaged muscle, leading to **hyperkalemia** and dysrhythmia. When used with the anesthetic halothane, succinylcholine can cause **malignant hyperthermia.**

Local anesthetics

These drugs can be identified by the suffix "-caine." Some commonly used local anesthetics include **lidocaine,** procaine, tetracaine, and bupivacaine. By **blocking sodium channels,** these agents inhibit nerve conductance. Pain fibers, because they are small and unmyelinated, are affected first. Systemic absorption of the anesthetic from the site is undesirable, because it decreases the local anesthetic effect and causes systemic side effects. These side effects begin as slurred speech and tremors and progress to **seizures** and **convulsions.** A period of cardiorespiratory depression and hypothermia follows.

Halothane, aminoglycoside antibiotics (e.g., gentamicin), and calcium channel blockers (e.g., verapamil) enhance the effect of curare.

Vecuronium has few cardiovascular side effects, while pancuronium causes tachycardia. Tubocurarine and metocurine can cause histamine release and hypotension. Atracurium degrades in the blood, and, unlike the other drugs listed, the dose does not need to be lowered in patients with renal failure.

Malignant hyperthermia occurs only in certain susceptible individuals and is characterized by widespread muscle spasms and increased body temperature. Treatment includes a cooling blanket, oxygen, and **dantrolene.** Dantrolene is a noncentrally acting muscle relaxant that inhibits calcium release from the sarcoplasmic reticulum.

Epinephrine is often injected with local anesthetics to constrict the nearby vessels and limit the systemic distribution of the drug.

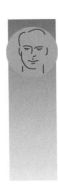

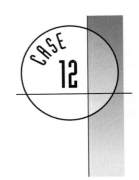

"I'm having bad stomach cramps and diarrhea with blood and mucus."

OBJECTIVES

1. Develop a differential diagnosis and an appropriate workup for abdominal pain with bloody and mucoid diarrhea
2. Review common causes and clinical presentation of bacterial enteritis
3. Review causes and treatment of constipation
4. Describe common intestinal parasites and their clinical features
5. Understand the mechanism of action, therapeutic effect, and side effects of metronidazole

HISTORY AND PHYSICAL EXAMINATION

A 30-year-old man complains of 5 days of abdominal **cramps,** weight loss, and **diarrhea containing mostly blood and mucus.** The patient took a trip to Mexico 3 weeks before the onset of symptoms. He says that he and his wife stopped in a small rural town outside Tijuana. The town did not have running water, but had a well; the only toilet in town was an outhouse. Other than this episode, the patient denies any remarkable history of GI symptoms. He is taking no antibiotics or steroids and has not changed his diet. Physical examination reveals slight **hypotension** (105/68 mm Hg), **tachycardia** (93 beats per minute), a dry oral mucosa **(dehydration)**, no fever, and hyperactive bowel sounds. Digital rectal examination yields no evidence of hemorrhoids but is heme positive.

> **QUICK HIT**
> Severe diarrhea can result in the loss of brush border enzymes, causing a temporary enzyme deficiency. Therefore, patients suffering or recovering from diarrhea cannot tolerate dairy products because they are temporarily lactase deficient.

APPROPRIATE WORKUP

Stool analysis for toxins, cysts, and trophozoites

DIFFERENTIAL DIAGNOSIS

Parasitic enteritis (*Entamoeba histolytica*, Cryptosporidium, *Giardia lamblia*), viral enteritis, inflammatory bowel disease, bacterial enteritis (*Escherichia coli*, Salmonella, Shigella, *Yersinia enterocolitica, Campylobacter jejuni*).

> **QUICK HIT**
> Patients taking clindamycin or other broad-spectrum antibiotics (e.g., cephalosporins) can develop pseudomembranous colitis from overgrowth of *C. difficile,* a Gram-positive, spore-forming, anaerobic rod. Also called *C. diff* colitis, it presents as diarrhea, fever, and toxicity. Treatment is metronidazole or oral vancomycin.

DIAGNOSTIC LABORATORY TESTS AND STUDIES

Stool analysis:
Positive results for *E. histolytica* cysts and trophozoites

FIGURE 12-1 Life cycle of *Entamoeba histolytica* cyst

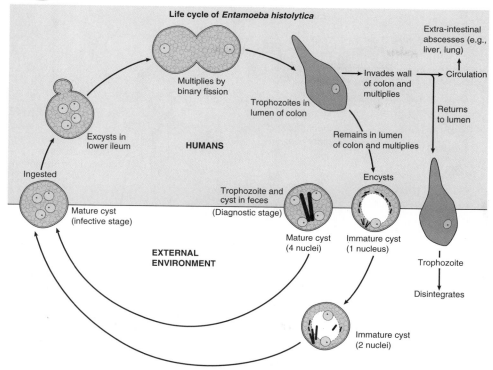

Life cycle of *Entamoeba histolytica*

Multiplies by binary fission

Trophozoites in lumen of colon

Invades wall of colon and multiplies

Extra-intestinal abscesses (e.g., liver, lung)

Circulation

Returns to lumen

Remains in lumen of colon and multiplies

Excysts in lower ileum

HUMANS

Encysts

Ingested

Mature cyst (infective stage)

Trophozoite and cyst in feces (Diagnostic stage)

Mature cyst (4 nuclei)

Immature cyst (1 nucleus)

Trophozoite

Disintegrates

EXTERNAL ENVIRONMENT

Immature cyst (2 nuclei)

(Adapted from Koneman EW et al. Color Atlas and Textbook of Diagnostic Microbiology. Philadelphia: Lippincott Williams & Wilkins, 1997, p 1083.)

DIAGNOSIS: PARASITIC ENTERITIS (AMEBIASIS)

Up to 90% of cases of **amebiasis** are **asymptomatic.** Symptomatic cases present with **dysentery** and can progress to invasive disease with **flask-shaped ulcers** in the intestinal mucosa and **disseminated abscesses in the liver** and elsewhere. The disease is usually self-limited but tends to be more severe in children and patients taking glucocorticoids. Diagnosis is made based on symptoms and identification of *E. histolytica* **trophozoites or cysts** in the stool. *E. histolytica* is a protozoan spread by fecal–oral transmission and by consumption of contaminated food or water. The cyst form is nonmotile and has four nuclei (Figure 12-1).

EXPLANATION OF DIFFERENTIAL

Cryptosporidium is a parasite that causes diarrhea in **immunocompromised patients** (especially those with AIDS). Transmission is by the fecal–oral route, and outbreaks have been linked to poorly purified tap water. The diarrhea is **watery and profuse.** The disease is mild to moderately severe but self-limited in healthy hosts. In immunocompromised patients, the chronic diarrhea and water loss can be debilitating. Diagnosis is based on symptoms and identification of **oocysts in the stool.** This patient's diarrhea was not profuse or watery, and no cryptosporidium oocysts were seen in the stool.

   Giordia lamblia is a parasite that is spread by the fecal–oral route and by contaminated water. Patients typically complain of **greasy, malodorous stools, cramps, and flatulence.** Outbreaks of Giardiasis are associated with **camping** and **daycare centers.** Chronic infestation can lead to malabsorption symptoms, especially megaloblastic anemia resulting from folate deficiency. Diagnosis is made by identification of the organism in a stool sample (Figure 12-2). This patient had no *G. lamblia* in his stool sample. Giardiasis is treated with **metronidazole.**

QUICK HIT
C. difficile produces two toxins. One is an enterotoxin that causes GI upset. The other is an exotoxin that leads to mucosal cell death and pseudomembrane formation.

QUICK HIT
Vibrio parahaemolyticus secretes a toxin that is similar to choleragen and causes diarrhea, nausea, and vomiting. *V. parahaemolyticus* is transmitted in undercooked shellfish.

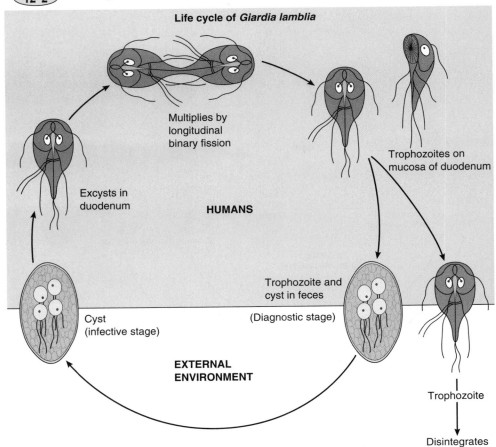

FIGURE 12-2 Life cycle of *Giardia lamblia*

(Adapted from Koneman EW et al. Color Atlas and Textbook of Diagnostic Microbiology. Philadelphia: Lippincott Williams & Wilkins, 1997, p 1090.)

Viral enteritis is typically characterized by the acute onset of copious watery diarrhea. Accompanying symptoms often include nausea, vomiting, and fever. The two most common viruses implicated are **Norwalk virus** and **rotavirus.** Norwalk virus typically causes mild diarrhea in adults. Rotavirus, on the other hand, can cause severe diarrhea in infants.

Inflammatory bowel disease, which specifically includes Crohn disease and ulcerative colitis, presents as relapsing episodes of diarrhea containing blood, mucus, and pus. Patients have no pathogenic microbes in their stool, do not respond to antimicrobial therapy, and often have characteristic extraintestinal manifestations (including sacroiliitis and uveitis).

Table 12-1 lists the details of **bacterial enteritis.**

QUICK HIT

Diarrhea with eosinophilia is typical of both parasitic infestation and inflammatory bowel disease.

TABLE 12-1 Bacterial Enteritis

Bacteria	Primary Mechanism of Disease (Toxin/ Invasion/Both)	Clinical Features	Notes
Vibrio cholera	Toxin	• Disease is spread by fecally contaminated water. • Primary symptom is copious watery diarrhea (**"rice water stools"**). • Death from dehydration can occur quickly.	Choleragen toxin activates adenylate cyclase and raises cAMP levels, which causes secretion of Cl⁻ and an osmotic diarrhea.

(Continued)

TABLE 12-1 **Bacterial Enteritis** (*continued*)

Bacteria	Primary Mechanism of Disease (Toxin/Invasion/Both)	Clinical Features	Notes
Staphylococcus aureus		• Toxin is preformed. • **Onset** of food poisoning is **rapid.** • Vomiting, cramping, and diarrhea begin **2–6 hr** after ingestion and **resolve within 24 hr.**	Disease occurs with **contaminated foods** that are not properly refrigerated.
Clostridium difficile		• **Pseudomembranous colitis** results when use of **broad-spectrum antibiotics** (esp. **clindamycin**) suppresses the normal gut flora. • Treatment is oral **vancomycin or metronidazole.**	Two toxins are produced: an **enterotoxin** that causes diarrhea and a cytotoxin that causes pseudomembrane formation.
Enterotoxigenic *Escherichia coli*		Bacteria cause **traveler's diarrhea,** which is copious diarrhea **without mucous or blood,** lasting 2–3 days.	• **Heat labile toxin increases cAMP,** with increased Cl⁻ secretion and osmotic diarrhea. • **Heat stable toxin increases cGMP** and inhibits electrolyte transport from the gut lumen leading to diarrhea.
Enterohemorrhagic *E. coli*		• Primary symptom is copious **bloody diarrhea.** • Usual cause is contaminated **ground beef.**	Toxin acts by the same mechanism as the Shiga toxin.
Salmonella	Invasion	• Enterocolitis follows ingestion of contaminated **poultry or eggs.** • Neutrophils are found in the stool.	Infection is primarily in the small intestine.
Shigella	Both	Mucosal invasion and toxin production cause **dysentery,** with diarrhea containing blood, mucus, and pus.	Shiga toxin is a six subunit that inactivates the 28s ribosomal subunit and stops protein synthesis.
Campylobacter jejuni		• Symptoms include enterocolitis with **severe abdominal pain and bloody diarrhea.** • Transmission is from person to person and from animal reservoirs.	• Toxin increases cAMP and osmotic diarrhea. • *C. jejuni* infection can precipitate the initial attack of **spondylitis in HLA-B27 positive patients.**

cAMP, cyclic adenosine monophosphate; cGMP, cyclic guanosine monophosphate.

TABLE 12-2	Causes of Constipation		
Causes	**Neurologic Derangement**	**Drugs**	**Miscellaneous**
Specific examples	• Diabetes mellitus • Multiple sclerosis • Hirschsprung disease • Chagas disease • Spinal cord injury	Antimuscarinics: • Atropine • Ipratropium • Scopolamine Drugs with antimuscarinic side effects: • Opioids • TCAs	• Scleroderma • Hypothyroidism • Cushing syndrome • Hypercalcemia • Postoperative ileus • Mechanical obstruction (e.g., tumor, hernia, adhesions, volvulus, intussusception)

TCA, tricyclic antidepressant.

Related Basic Science

Constipation

Constipation is defined as decreased stool frequency and increased difficulty with defecation. It is the functional opposite of diarrhea. The causes of constipation are many and varied. Table 12-2 categorizes some common causes. Constipation can be treated by increasing fiber and fluid intake and with laxatives, magnesium-containing antacids, or muscarinic agonists such as bethanechol.

> **QUICK HIT**
> Alternating episodes of diarrhea and constipation should suggest partial colonic obstruction caused by a tumor or irritable bowel syndrome.

Intestinal parasites

Three of the most common intestinal parasites (*E. histolytica*, *G. lamblia*, Cryptosporidium) are discussed in the case presentation and differential. Other parasites infect the GI tract; however, they do not cause significant diarrhea. Table 12-3 summarizes the characteristics of these parasites.

> **QUICK HIT**
> *Ascaris lumbricoides, Ancylostoma duodenale,* and *Necator americanus* all have larval stages that penetrate the skin and travel in the lymphatic system and blood to the lungs. The larvae enter the alveoli and are coughed up and swallowed. All three of these parasites can therefore cause pneumonitis with cough.

Metronidazole

Metronidazole is the primary drug used to treat infections with *E. histolytica*, *G. lamblia*, and *Trichomonas vaginalis*. This drug also is used to treat infections caused by certain anaerobic bacteria, including *Clostridium difficile* and *Bacteroides fragilis*. Metronidazole forms cytotoxic compounds that bind to DNA and proteins. It is given orally and metabolized by hepatic mixed function oxidases. Therefore, drugs that activate these liver enzymes, such as phenobarbital and rifampin, shorten the half-life of metronidazole. Conversely, cimetidine and other drugs that inhibit these hepatic enzymes extend the drug's half-life.

The side effects of metronidazole include **GI upset,** oral yeast infections, and **neurologic signs,** including **dizziness, vertigo, and paresthesias.** When neurologic signs occur, the drug is usually discontinued. The drug can cause a **disulfiram-like reaction** when taken with alcohol.

TABLE 12-3	Intestinal Parasites	
Parasite	**Clinical Presentation**	**Notes**
Enterobius vermicularis (pinworm)	Common symptom is **perianal itching;** disease is fairly benign.	Transmission is hand to mouth; infection is most common **in children.**
Trichuris trichiura (whipworm)	Infection can be asymptomatic or progress to **anemia,** abdominal pain, diarrhea, or rectal prolapse.	Transmission is fecal–oral; infection affects mainly young children in the southeastern United States.

(Continued)

TABLE 12-3 Intestinal Parasites (*continued*)

Parasite	Clinical Presentation	Notes
Ascaris lumbricoides	Larvae in the lungs cause fever and **cough;** adult worms in the intestines can cause fever and **obstruction.**	Infection is very common worldwide.
Ancylostoma duodenale, Necator americanus (hookworms)	Infections usually are asymptomatic; **skin rash** can develop where larvae penetrate; **pneumonitis** and **anemia** may develop secondary to chronic blood loss.	Chronic infection with blood loss from intestinal mucosal bite sites can lead to poor growth in children.
Strongyloides stercoralis	Infection usually is asymptomatic but can cause **skin lesions** at the point of entry, **pneumonitis,** and **diarrhea/malabsorption.**	Patient can undergo **autoinfection;** larvae produced penetrate the gut wall before they are passed.
Taenia saginata (beef tapeworm)	Infection is usually asymptomatic; diarrhea and weight loss can occur.	Larvae are contracted by eating **undercooked beef.**
Taenia solium (pork tapeworm)	Infection usually is asymptomatic; diarrhea and weight loss can occur; **cysticercosis** presents as lesions in eyes and brain.	Intestinal infection follows ingestion of larvae in **undercooked pork;** cysticercosis follows ingestion of the eggs in contaminated food or water.
Diphyllobothrium latum (fish tapeworm)	Infection usually is asymptomatic; diarrhea, malabsorption, or **B_{12} deficiency** can occur.	Larvae are ingested in **undercooked fish.**

"I get out of breath even with the slightest activity and I can't fit into my shoes anymore."

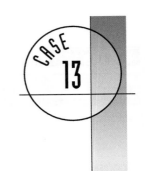

OBJECTIVES

1. Develop a differential diagnosis and an appropriate workup for dyspnea on exertion and pitting edema
2. Understand the defining characteristics for each diagnosis in the differential
3. Review the types and causes of shock
4. Learn the normal pressures of the heart chambers
5. Compare and contrast the pathophysiologies of neonatal versus adult respiratory distress syndrome

HISTORY AND PHYSICAL EXAMINATION

A 40-year-old female complains of dyspnea on exertion and has recently noticed extended **shortness of breath** even with trivial activity. She is unusually tired and has experienced temporary periods of blackout when moving from a sitting or lying position to standing. She also complains of **increasing swelling in her lower extremities** making it difficult to wear her normal shoe size. Finally, she complains of tenderness in her right upper abdomen. She is currently on no medicines and does not smoke or drink.

Her vital signs are as follows: pulse, 100; respiratory rate, 18: temperature, 99°F; BP 125/78. Examination reveals **jugular venous distension,** a right ventricular heave, and **loud P2.** A **holosystolic murmur** is heard at the lower, left sternal border that becomes louder on inspiration. Her breath sounds are normal without wheezes or crackles. There is right upper quadrant tenderness and the liver edge is palpable. Her feet and ankles are swollen and there is 2+ pitting edema to the mid-calf.

APPROPRIATE WORKUP

Chest X-ray, ECG, Doppler echocardiography with contrast, complete blood count, liver function tests, plasma D-dimer, cardiac catheterization, arterial blood gas, pulmonary function tests, ventilation perfusion scan, spiral CT, and angiogram

DIFFERENTIAL DIAGNOSIS

Idiopathic pulmonary arterial hypertension (PAH), left ventricular failure, congenital heart disease, pulmonary embolism, obstructive sleep apnea, interstitial lung disease

DIAGNOSTIC LABORATORY TESTS AND STUDIES

Chest radiograph:
Enlarged right ventricle and main pulmonary artery (Figure 13-1)

EKG:
Right axis deviation and right ventricular hypertrophy

Doppler echocardiography with contrast:
Left ventricular size and function normal; right atrial and ventricular hypertrophy with pericardial effusion; underfilling of left ventricle; elevated systolic pulmonary artery pressure; no shunting of contrast

Complete blood count = normal
Liver function tests = normal
Plasma D-dimer = normal

Cardiac catheterization:
Pulmonary arterial pressure = 65/25 mm Hg (H)
Mean pulmonary capillary wedge pressure = 10 mm Hg (N)
Mean right atrial pressure = 13 mm Hg (H)
Mean right ventricular end-diastolic pressure = 12 mm Hg (H)
Mean left atrial pressure = 8 mm Hg (N)
Cardiac output = 4 L/min (L)
Pulmonary vascular resistance = 7.2 mm Hg/L/min (H)

Arterial blood gas:
pO_2 = 70 mm Hg (L)
pCO_2 = 31 mm Hg (L)
Alveolar-arterial (A-a) gradient = 36 mm Hg (H)

Pulmonary function tests:

	Percent of Predicted	Normal Ranges
FVC	95%	
FEV_1	105%	80–120%
TLC	95%	
DLCO	60%	

Ventilation Perfusion Scan = normal
Spiral CT and angiogram = normal

DIAGNOSIS: IDIOPATHIC PULMONARY ARTERIAL HYPERTENSION (PAH)

Pulmonary hypertension may occur as a **primary disorder** of the pulmonary arteries or it may be **secondary to cardiac or pulmonary diseases.** Primary (unexplained or idiopathic) pulmonary hypertension is of unknown etiology found most frequently in women between 20 to 40 years old. Given this patient's findings, primary PAH, although rare, is the most likely diagnosis.

FIGURE 13-1 Chest radiograph. A chest radiograph from a patient with primary pulmonary hypertension, illustrating enlarged proximal pulmonary arteries and right ventricle (arrows)

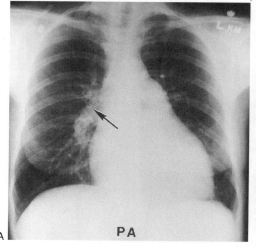
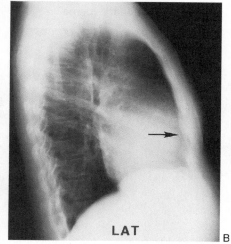

A — PA
B — LAT

(From Crapo JD, Glassroth J, Karlinsky JB, King TE, Jr. Baum's Textbook of Pulmonary Diseases, 7th Ed. Philadelphia: Lippincott Williams & Wilkins, 2004.)

Sustained pulmonary hypertension causes muscular hypertrophy and hyperplasia of pulmonary arteries which becomes fixed over time and increases pressures to even higher levels. The pathologic changes that accompany this remodeling include intimal hyperplasia, partial or complete obliteration of the lumen of small arteries or arterioles, thickening of the wall of larger elastic pulmonary arteries, and right ventricular hypertrophy. As in this patient, once symptoms develop, they are most often due to right ventricular failure rather than pulmonary hypertension. Symptoms of **RV failure** include **RUQ pain** (distension of the liver capsule), **edema of the lower extremities, dyspnea on exertion, and easy fatigue** (restricted cardiac output).

A number of factors may contribute to secondary pulmonary hypertension acutely or chronically. They are as follows, in order of decreasing likelihood:

LV disease/dysfunction (i.e., an undiscovered congenital problem such as ASD, valvular problems such as AS, MS, MR, cardiomyopathy)
Pulmonary disorders (i.e., chronic lung disease/hypoxemia/sleep disordered breathing)
Embolic disease
Idiopathic PAH
Miscellaneous

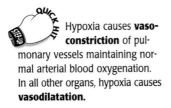

Hypoxia causes **vasoconstriction** of pulmonary vessels maintaining normal arterial blood oxygenation. In all other organs, hypoxia causes **vasodilatation.**

EXPLANATION OF DIFFERENTIAL

The most common cause of pulmonary arterial hypertension is pulmonary venous hypertension caused by **dysfunction of the left heart** leading to **elevated left atrial pressures** and progressive venous pressure elevation back into the pulmonary capillaries, arterioles, and arteries. Eventually, **right ventricular dysfunction** can occur with peripheral edema, ascites, and a pulsatile liver. A palpable right ventricular heave may also be present.

Chronically elevated pressures cause thickening of artery and arteriole walls. The most important clinical result of increased pulmonary venous pressure is **pulmonary edema** (Figure 13-2), *not* pulmonary hypertension. Clinical presentation includes increased dyspnea on exertion, orthopnea, and paroxysmal nocturnal dyspnea. Often a **history of smoking** can be elicited. Physical exam would reveal **basal crepitations, tachycardia, and a third heart sound.** The chest radiograph would have revealed **left ventricle enlargement** with or without interstitial edema. The pulmonary artery would not be

FIGURE 13-2 **Pulmonary edema**

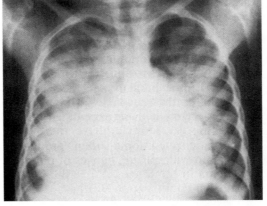

(From Swischuk LE. Emergency Radiology of the Acutely Ill or Injured Child, 2nd Ed. Philadelphia: Lippincott Williams & Wilkins, 1986.)

enlarged. ECG would have indicated left axis deviation and left ventricular hypertrophy. **Echocardiography** is also very helpful in confirming left ventricular disease.

Congenital intracardiac left-to-right shunts, such as with a patent ductus arteriosus (PDA) or atrial/ventricular septal defects (ASD/VSD), increase pulmonary arterial flow. Right-sided cardiac pressure may become so elevated that it exceeds left-sided pressure and the shunt reverses, becoming a right-to-left shunt. This conversion of the shunt direction is referred to as **Eisenmenger syndrome.**

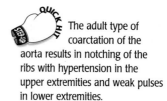 Mitral valve stenosis can also cause left heart dysfunction progressing to right ventricular dysfunction in late stages.

Some cases of congenital heart disease become apparent in infancy. Small interventricular defects may not present until adulthood, such as an atrial or ventricular septal defect. **Systolic murmurs** are usually heard in atrial septal defects and ventricular septal defects. **Atrial septal defects** are associated with **wide, fixed splitting of the second heart sound. Cyanosis** and **digital clubbing** are common late-stage manifestations. A chest radiograph would show enlargement of the right ventricle and a large pulmonary artery. ECG would reveal right bundle branch block in atrial septal defects and left-sided heart enlargement in large ventricular septal defects. An **echocardiography with Doppler flow** is diagnostic. Treatment is often **surgical repair.**

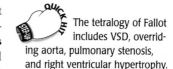 A PDA is associated with a continuous, "machine-like" murmur on auscultation.

Pulmonary emboli can also raise pulmonary artery pressure. **Sickle cell disease** patients can have elevated pulmonary arterial pressures by occluding smaller branches of the pulmonary arterial tree over a long time period. The total cross-sectional area of the pulmonary arterial tree may be reduced by processes that scar or destroy capillaries within alveolar walls. This process is common to **emphysema** and **interstitial fibrosis.** In both disorders, it is unusual for the **pulmonary arterial pressures to be very high at rest,** but significant elevations develop with exercise since recruitment and distension of the bronchopulmonary tree are limited. On physical exam, there may be **elevated jugular venous pressure,** an apparent right ventricular heave, palpable pulse in the second intercostal space, and a **right ventricular S3 gallop.** Since pulmonary emboli can result in **right heart failure,** systemic symptoms such as hepatomegaly, ascites, and peripheral edema may also be seen. A **positive plasma D-dimer** test has high sensitivity for an acute pulmonary embolus. A chest X-ray with a pulmonary embolism is presented in Figure 13-3.

The adult type of coarctation of the aorta results in notching of the ribs with hypertension in the upper extremities and weak pulses in lower extremities.

The tetralogy of Fallot includes VSD, overriding aorta, pulmonary stenosis, and right ventricular hypertrophy.

FIGURE 13-3   **Pulmonary embolism**

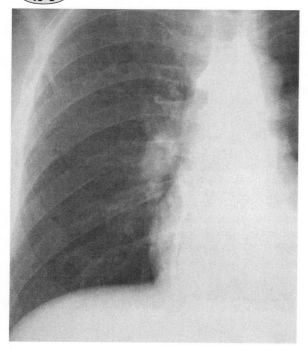

(From Khan GP, Lynch JP. **Pulmonary Disease Diagnosis and Therapy: A Practical Approach.** Philadelphia: Lippincott Williams & Wilkins, 1997, p 15.)

Sickle cell disease can also result in complications such as aplastic crises with parvovirus B19 infection, autosplenectomy with increased risk of infection from encapsulated organisms, *Salmonella* osteomyelitis, and painful crises when sickled cells occlude vasculature.

The deepest sleep stage is REM with loss of motor tone, dreaming, erections, and increased brain oxygen use. It has the same EEG pattern of beta waves in an awake and alert person.

Obstructive sleep apnea is airway obstruction that occurs **during sleep**, causing excessive **daytime sleepiness** with **impairment of concentration, mood, or work performance.** Unlike central sleep apnea, obstructive sleep apnea involves respiratory effort against a **closed airway.** There is cyclic oxygen desaturation and carbon dioxide retention during sleep caused by repeated episodes of hypopnea and apnea. There is often excessive adrenergic stimulation complicated by hypertension. Obstructive sleep apnea is associated with **obesity, loud snoring,** and even sudden **death.** Treatment includes **weight loss, continuous positive airway pressure (CPAP), and palatal surgery.**

Interstitial lung disease is characterized by **inflammation** and **derangement of the alveolar walls** and damage to the lung parenchyma by varying degrees of **inflammation and fibrosis.** The disease can be chronic and insidious with dyspnea being the most common presenting symptom. Chronic cough, wheezing, and hemoptysis may also be reported. On physical exam, an **S3 gallop** and right ventricular lift is often noted.

Asbestosis caused by inhaling asbestos fibers can result in **diffuse pulmonary interstitial fibrosis.** There is an increased risk of developing **bronchogenic carcinoma** and **mesothelioma,** a malignant tumor of serosal surfaces. **Ferruginous bodies** can be seen in the lung which are asbestos fibers coated with hemosiderin (Figure 13-4). Other interstitial lung diseases include adult/neonatal respiratory distress syndrome, sarcoidosis, pneumoconiosis (i.e., coal miner's silicosis, asbestosis), idiopathic pulmonary fibrosis, Goodpasture syndrome, Wegener granulomatosis, and eosinophilic granuloma. These are restrictive lung diseases with a normal or an increased FEV_1/FVC ratio.

FIGURE 13-4

(See also Color Plate 13-4.) Ferruginous bodies. Iron stains the beaded iron coat of an asbestos body bright blue around a clear asbestos fiber core, highlighting the asbestos body against a pale pink background

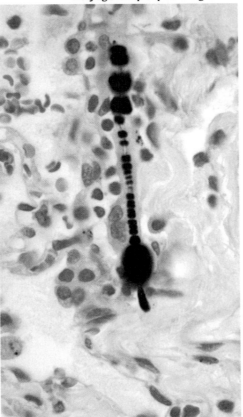

(From Cagle PT. Color Atlas and Text of Pulmonary Pathology. Philadelphia: Lippincott Williams & Wilkins, 2005.)

TABLE 13-1 Shock

Type of Shock	Mechanism	Clinical Causes
Cardiogenic	Pump failure	Cardiac arrhythmias; heart failure; intracardiac obstruction; myocardial infarction
Hypovolemic	Volume loss	Blood, electrolyte, fluid, or plasma loss; burns; severe vomiting; or diarrhea
Obstructive	Extracardiac obstruction of blood flow	Aortic dissection; cardiac tamponade; pulmonary embolism
Septic	Increased venous capacitance	Gram-negative endotoxemia; direct toxic injury; DIC
Neurogenic	Massive peripheral vasodilation	Severe cerebral, brain stem, or spinal cord injury
Anaphylactic	Increased venous capacitance stimulated by histamine release	Type I hypersensitivity reaction to exogenous stimulus (e.g., food allergy, bee sting)

DIC = diffuse intravascular coagulation.

Related Basic Sciences

Shock

Shock is defined as a metabolic state in which **oxygen supply is not adequate** to meet oxygen demand. Classic signs and symptoms of shock include tachycardia, hypotension, mental status changes, weak pulses, cool extremities, and oliguria. Table 13-1 summarizes the types of shock, their mechanisms, and frequent causes.

Normal pressures in the heart

It is important to be familiar with the normal pressures in the atria and ventricles of the heart to be able to detect pathologies. **Pulmonary capillary wedge** pressure is a good estimate of the **left atrial pressure.** All pressures are measured with a Swan-Ganz catheter. Pressures in Figure 13-5 are in mm Hg.

FIGURE 13-5 Normal pressures in the heart

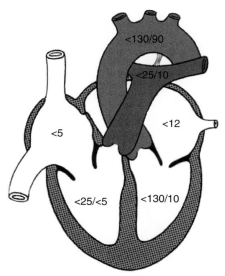

<130/90

<25/10

<5

<12

<25/<5

<130/10

(Adapted from Sadler T. Langman's Medical Embryology, 9th Ed. Image Bank. Baltimore: Lippincott Williams & Wilkins, 2003.)

QUICK HIT Cor pulmonale refers to right-sided heart disease secondary to pulmonary hypertension caused by disease of the lungs or pulmonary vasculature. This term does not include right ventricular disease secondary to left-sided heart disease or congenital heart disease.

QUICK HIT Kartagener syndrome is due to a dynein arm defect which results in immotile cilia. The constellation of findings includes: situs inversus, recurrent sinusitis, bronchiectasis, and infertility.

QUICK HIT Goodpasture syndrome involves the kidney (renal lesions→ hematuria) and lungs (pulmonary hemorrhages → hemoptysis). Antiglomerular basement membrane antibodies result in a linear staining on immunofluorescence.

QUICK HIT Wegener granulomatosis is associated with focal necrotizing vasculitis of the small- to medium-sized vessels, acute necrotizing granulomas of the upper and lower respiratory tract, and necrotizing glomerulonephritis. **C-ANCA** is a strong marker of the disease along with hematuria and a chest radiograph with large, nodular densities.

TABLE 13-2 Adult Respiratory Distress Syndrome (ARDS) and Neonatal Respiratory Distress Syndrome (NRDS)

	ARDS (Diffuse Alveolar Damage)	NRDS (Hyaline Membrane Disease)
Age Group	*Adults*	*Premature infants*
Causes	**Shock, infection, trauma,** oxygen toxicity (free radical damage), or aspiration	**Lack of surfactant** production
Pathophysiology	Impaired gas exchange caused by pulmonary hemorrhage, pulmonary edema, or atelectasis	Increased work to expand lungs; infant can clear lungs of fluids, but cannot fill lungs with air; atelectasis
Features	Respiratory insufficiency; cyanosis; hypoxemia; heavy, wet lungs; diffuse pulmonary infiltrates on radiograph; hyaline membranes in alveoli; pneumothorax may result—may be rapid and fatal	Respiratory insufficiency; cyanosis; hypoxemia; heavy, wet lungs; diffuse pulmonary infiltrates on radiograph; hyaline membranes in alveoli

Reprinted with permission from Mehta S, Milder EA, Mirarchi AJ. Step-Up: A High-Yield, Systems-Based Review for the USMLE Step 1 Examination. Philadelphia: Lippincott Williams & Wilkins, 2000, p 75.

Adult versus neonatal respiratory distress syndrome

Both types can lead to respiratory failure and death. The distinct causes, pathophysiologies, and features are compared in Table 13-2.

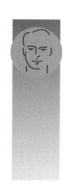

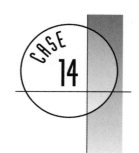

"My toe has hurt so badly over the past 2 days that I can't sleep at night. Nothing helps at all!"

OBJECTIVES

1. Develop a differential diagnosis and an appropriate workup for severe pain in the metatarsophalangeal (MTP) joint
2. Compare and contrast purine and pyrimidine metabolism and associated pathologies
3. Learn the key reactants, rate-limiting steps, and products of the urea cycle
4. Understand the biochemical deficiency, clinical presentation, and treatment of severe combined immunodeficiency (SCID)
5. Review the mechanisms of action, and side effects for common drugs used to treat gout

HISTORY AND PHYSICAL EXAMINATION

A 53-year-old African American man presents with severe pain in his **great toe** that began 2 days ago after an **extravagant meal** with his publisher. The pain has kept him from falling asleep the past two nights. He denies pain elsewhere, but reports similar bouts of pain when he had uric acid **kidney stones** several years ago. He denies any trauma to his toe. The patient's diet includes various **meats,** few vegetables, and large amounts of **wine.** Upon physical examination, he has a low-grade fever. His left great toe is erythematous, swollen, tender to touch, and painful with passive and active movement.

APPROPRIATE WORKUP

Blood chemistries, urinalysis, and joint aspirate

DIFFERENTIAL DIAGNOSIS

Lesch-Nyhan syndrome, osteoarthritis, primary gout, pseudogout, sarcoidosis, septic arthritis, trauma

DIAGNOSTIC LABORATORY TESTS AND STUDIES

Blood chemistry:
  WBCs = 12,000/μL (H)
  Uric acid = 10 mg/dL (H)
  ESR = 32 mm/hr (H)
Urinalysis:
  Uric acid crystals = Positive (H)
Joint aspirate:
  Cloudy
  Xanthochromic

Needle-like, strongly negatively birefringent monosodium urate crystals
Gram stain negative for organisms
Decreased glucose
Elevated WBCs

DIAGNOSIS: PRIMARY GOUT

Primary gout results from **hyperuricemia,** which can be caused by overproduction (10%) or underexcretion (90%) of uric acid. Overproduction can be further subdivided into primary (i.e., associated with purine pathway enzymatic defects) or secondary (i.e., associated with increased cell turnover due to alcohol use, malignancy, hemolysis, or chemotherapy). The basis for hyperuricemia in underexcreters is often decreased renal excretion of uric acid secondary to renal disease or pharmacologic agents (e.g., salicylates, diuretics).

Hyperuricemia results in accumulation of uric acid in joints. This accumulation incites a **phagocytic response** and subsequent inflammation. The inflammatory response produces metabolites of **oxygen** that damage tissue and cause the release of lysosomal enzymes. The subsequent **decrease in local pH** results in further deposition of urate crystals. Acute attacks of gout can be brought on by **salicylates, diuretics**, and, as in this case, **alcohol consumption** and **high-protein** meals. **Men** are more commonly afflicted with gout, while women are spared until after menopause.

Primary gout has four phases: asymptomatic hyperuricemia, **acute gouty arthritis,** intercritical gout, and **chronic gout.** The acute attack is the primary manifestation of gout and is marked by an extremely painful, acute onset of arthritis, often involving the first metatarsophalangeal joint (i.e., **podagra**). The chronic stage is marked by urate crystal deposition (i.e., **tophi**) in the synovium of the olecranon, bursa, and pinna of the ear. The **gold standard** for diagnosis of gout is analysis of **synovial fluid aspirate.** Elevated uric acid in the blood is neither sensitive nor specific for gout.

EXPLANATION OF DIFFERENTIAL

Lesch-Nyhan syndrome is an **X-linked disorder** associated with a deficiency of hypoxanthine-guanine phosphoribosyltransferase **(HGPRT).** HGPRT is involved in the **"salvage" pathway** (Figure 14-1) for purines, where unused purine compounds are converted to triphosphates and used by the body for energy. Deficiency in HGPRT results in increased levels of hypoxanthine and guanine, which are then converted to uric acid. An individual with Lesch-Nyhan syndrome may present with **hyperuricemia,** severe mental retardation, and self-mutilation.

Osteoarthritis (OA), also referred to as **degenerative joint disease,** is the **most common** form of joint disease. Patients complain of use-related pain (as opposed to night or rest pain) affecting multiple, **asymmetric** joints; **brief early morning stiffness;** functional limitation; and joint deformity. Weight-bearing joints (e.g., knees, hips, spine) are most often affected. The hands are also commonly involved. The joint aspirate is straw colored with minimal WBCs and **no crystals.**

Pseudogout also presents with acute swelling, pain, and erythema of a joint. However, the joint aspirate shows **weakly positively birefringent, rod-shaped crystals.** These crystals are a result of calcium pyrophosphate deposition disease **(CPPD),** which can be secondary to hyperparathyroidism, hypothyroidism, and hemochromatosis. Radiographs of the larger joints affected show **linear calcification.** The goal in treatment of pseudogout is pain relief with nonsteroidal anti-inflammatory drugs (NSAIDs) and joint injections.

Sarcoidosis is a systemic, noncaseating, granulomatous disease of unknown etiology that involves the proximal interphalangeal joint and knee joints. Systemic manifestations

> **QUICK HIT**
>
> The purines are guanine (G) and adenine (A). The pyrimidines are cytosine (C), thymine (T), and uracil (U). A binds to T and G binds to C in DNA. U replaces T in RNA.

FIGURE 14-1 **Purine "salvage" pathway** (*AMP* = adenosine monophosphate; *APRT* = adenine phosphoribosyltransferase; *GMP* = guanosine monophosphate; *HGPRT* = hypoxanthine-guanine phosphoribosyltransferase; *IMP* = inosine monophosphate; *PPi* = pyrophosphate; *PRPP* = phosphoribosyl pyrophosphate.)

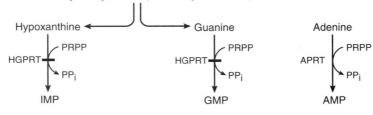

of sarcoidosis include respiratory complications, lymphadenopathy, ocular lesions, splenomegaly, and erythema nodosum. Affected tissues have overwhelming infiltration of T lymphocytes and phagocytes.

Septic arthritis is primarily caused by **gonorrhea** in sexually active young adults and *Staphylococcus aureus* in other groups. Alcoholics, diabetics, intravenous drug users, and immunosuppressed individuals are at an increased risk. Septic arthritis presents with pain and erythema of a joint. Opaque synovial fluid demonstrates considerable leukocytosis and infectious organisms.

Trauma can result in bacterial seeding of a joint and precipitate septic arthritis. Injury to interarticular structures can cause pain, and the resultant bleeding can cause swelling. Large joints (e.g., knees) are often susceptible to trauma. However, this patient's history is inconsistent with having received trauma to a joint.

Related Basic Science

Purine and pyrimidine metabolism

The metabolism of purine and pyrimidine synthesis plays a role in uric acid formation and gout. Purine and pyrimidine biosynthesis usually takes place in the liver and, to some extent, in the brain. The nucleotides produced in the liver are converted to nucleosides and bases that travel via RBCs to tissues, where they are reconverted to nucleotides. The committed step in **purine biosynthesis** is the synthesis of 5′-phosphoribosylamine from phosphoribosyl pyrophosphate (PRPP) and glutamine. 5′-Phosphoribosylamine is converted to inosine monophosphate (IMP), which is the parent compound of guanosine monophosphate (GMP) and adenosine monophosphate (AMP). The committed step in **pyrimidine biosynthesis** is the synthesis of carbamoyl phosphate in the cytosol, catalyzed by carbamoyl phosphate synthetase II (CPSII).

The catabolism of purine nucleotides leads to the production of uric acid (Figure 14-2). During pyrimidine degradation, the carbons from the compound are

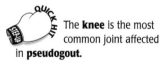

Rheumatoid arthritis (RA) can also lead to joint destruction. Often, RA causes a **symmetric** polyarthritis of peripheral joints. In contrast to OA, RA patients have an extended period of joint stiffness in the morning and have extra-articular manifestation of the disease. Rheumatoid factor is present in 85% of patients with RA.

"Bony" swelling of the distal interphalangeal joints in OA is referred to as **Heberden** nodes. Swollen proximal interphalangeal joints are called **Bouchard** nodes.

The **knee** is the most common joint affected in **pseudogout.**

Sarcoidosis most commonly afflicts **young, African American women.**

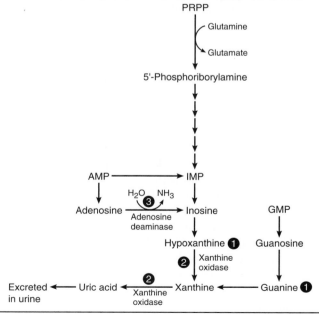

FIGURE
14-2

Purine catabolism (*AMP* = adenosine monophosphate; *GMP* = guanosine monophosphate; *IMP* = inosine monophosphate; *PRPP* = phosphoribosyl pyrophosphate.)

❶ The levels of hypoxanthine and guanine are increased in Lesch-Nyhan syndrome, resulting in increased uric acid production (see Figure 14-1).

❷ Xanthine oxidase is inhibited by allopurinol (treatment for gout). Hypoxanthine and xanthine are more soluble than uric acid (and can be excreted in urine).

❸ Adenosine deaminase deficiency causes severe combined immunodeficiency (SCID).

FIGURE 14-3

The urea cycle (*AMP* = adenosine monophosphate; *ATP* = adenosine triphosphate; *P$_i$* = phosphate; *PP$_i$* = pyrophosphate.)

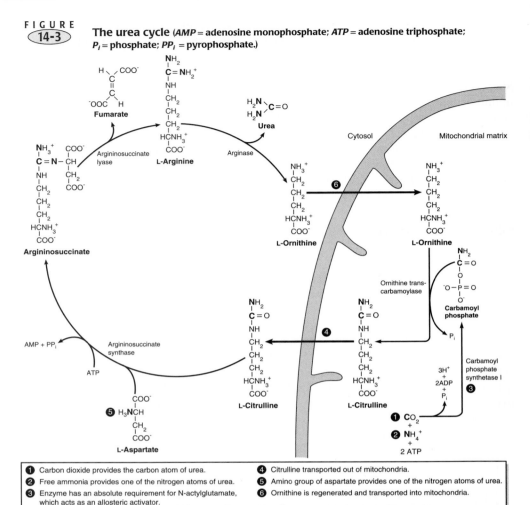

① Carbon dioxide provides the carbon atom of urea.
② Free ammonia provides one of the nitrogen atoms of urea.
③ Enzyme has an absolute requirement for N-actylglutamate, which acts as an allosteric activator.
④ Citrulline transported out of mitochondria.
⑤ Amino group of aspartate provides one of the nitrogen atoms of urea.
⑥ Ornithine is regenerated and transported into mitochondria.

(Reprinted with permission from Harvey RA, Champe PC. Biochemistry: Lippincott's Illustrated Reviews, 2nd Ed. Philadelphia: J.B. Lippincott, 1994, p 237.)

released as carbon dioxide and the nitrogens are excreted as urea through the urea cycle (Figure 14-3).

The urea cycle

Urea is the major disposal form of amino groups and nitrogen generated by the body. Urea is produced by the liver and excreted by the kidneys. The first two steps in the synthesis of urea occur in the mitochondria, whereas the remaining reactions occur in the cytosol. A portion of the urea synthesized in the liver diffuses into the GI tract (as opposed to being filtered and excreted by the kidneys), where it is cleaved to carbon dioxide and ammonia by bacterial urease. Ammonia can then be reabsorbed. Renal failure can lead to increased urea in the GI tract and, subsequently, increased ammonia in the blood. Ammonia is toxic for the body. Administration of **neomycin,** an aminoglycoside, reduces the number of intestinal bacteria, thus decreasing ammonia production.

Adenosine deaminase (ADA) deficiency

ADA deficiency is an autosomal recessive disease that results in a buildup of adenosine, AMP, and deoxyadenosine triphosphate (dATP). Elevated levels of dATP inhibit DNA synthesis by inhibiting ribonucleotide reductase. ADA deficiency leads to severe combined immunodeficiency **(SCID)** (i.e., dysfunction of T and B cells). Death often occurs before 2 years of age; however, **gene therapy** is now a possible treatment for SCID.

Therapeutic strategies for gout

The therapeutic strategies for gout (Table 14-1) are aimed at lowering the uric acid level, thus preventing urate crystal deposition. This can be accomplished by interfering with uric acid synthesis, increasing uric acid secretion, or inhibiting leukocyte entry into the affected joint. NSAIDs can be given for pain relief and inflammation during acute gouty attacks. Other medications are used prophylactically.

QUICK HIT Aspirin and uric acid use the same secretion method in the proximal tubule. Therefore, aspirin should not be given to treat acute gouty pain because it will prevent uric acid secretion. Instead, other NSAIDs should be administered.

QUICK HIT Allopurinol is often given to patients undergoing chemotherapy as a significant amount of DNA is degraded, increasing purine catabolism, and hence uric acid production.

TABLE 14-1 **Treatment Strategies for Gout**

Therapeutic Agent	Effect	Mechanism	Side Effects
Colchicine	Relieves pain in acute attacks, reduces frequency of acute attacks, **decreases movement of granulocytes** into affected area	Binds to and depolymerizes **tubulin, disrupts cellular mobility** of granulocytes, inhibits synthesis and release of leukotrienes	Nausea, vomiting, diarrhea, **agranulocytosis,** aplastic anemia, alopecia, contraindicated in pregnancy
Probenecid	**Uricosuric** agent, effective in chronic gout, relieves pain and frequency of attacks	Blocks proximal tubular reabsorption of uric acid	Blocks tubular secretion of penicillin
Sulfinpyrazone	**Uricosuric** agent, effective in chronic gout, relieves pain and frequency of attacks	Blocks proximal tubular reabsorption of uric acid	Gastric distress
Allopurinol	Decreases uric acid production, effective in chronic gout	Purine analog, competitively **inhibits xanthine oxidase**	Hypersensitivity reactions, GI symptoms

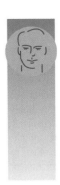

"I have a funny-looking, pinkish bump on my nose that keeps growing. It has recently started bleeding every once in a while for no particular reason."

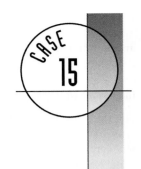

OBJECTIVES

1. Develop a differential diagnosis and an appropriate workup for an ulcerating pearl-like papule
2. Compare and contrast the two types of growth patterns (benign radial versus aggressive vertical) of melanocytes
3. Review skin histology and types of pain fibers
4. Understand the skin's role in thermal regulation and the role of the posterior hypothalamus
5. Learn the causes of fever and the role of the anterior hypothalamus

HISTORY AND PHYSICAL EXAMINATION

A 43-year-old **White** man complains of a 2-cm, ulcerated nodule on the tip of his nose. He claims that he first noticed the lesion about 1 year ago, when it presented as a 3-mm, shiny, **pearl-like papule.** He does not remember an incident of trauma or infection in that area. The patient states that over the past 3 months the lesion has occasionally bled, but healed quickly. He has been using over-the-counter cortisone cream for the past few months with no result. The patient has smoked one pack of cigarettes a day for the past 15 years, and admits to having one can of beer every other day. He has been employed as a construction worker for the past 20 years. Physical examination reveals a firm, nontender nodule. No other skin lesions are found on his body.

APPROPRIATE WORKUP

Skin biopsy

DIFFERENTIAL DIAGNOSIS

Actinic keratosis, basal cell carcinoma, malignant melanoma, squamous cell carcinoma

DIAGNOSTIC LABORATORY TESTS AND STUDIES

Skin biopsy:
Histologic examination of the biopsy reveals a nodular lesion composed of hyperchromatic cells growing into the dermis.
The cells at the periphery of the lesion are arranged radially, with their long axes in parallel arrangement.

FIGURE
15-1 (See also Color Plate 15-1A–B.) A. The gross appearance of basal cell carcinoma. B. The microscopic appearance of basal cell carcinoma

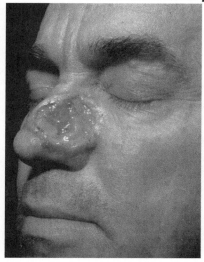
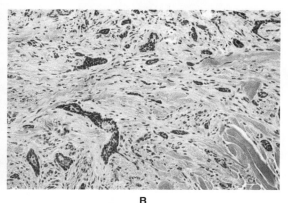

A   B

(Reprinted with permission from Rubin E, Farber JL. Pathology, 3rd Ed. Philadelphia: Lippincott-Raven Publishers, 1999, p 1292.)

DIAGNOSIS: BASAL CELL CARCINOMA (FIGURE 15-1)

Basal cell carcinoma is the **most common** of all the skin tumors. It typically affects fair-skinned people older than 40 years of age with a history of excessive **sunlight** exposure. Men are affected more often than women. Lesions usually arise on the face, neck, and upper trunk, and do not involve mucosal surfaces. Basal cell carcinoma is a slow-growing tumor that presents as a **pearl-like papule,** which may ulcerate at later stages (see Figure 15-1A). Histologically, the lesion appears as a dark cluster with palisading peripheral cells arising from the basal layer of the epidermis (see Figure 15-1B). Basal cell carcinoma **rarely metastasizes** because the metastasized cells do not have access to the required growth factors produced from the tumor's stroma. However, it is very destructive locally and must be removed.

EXPLANATION OF DIFFERENTIAL

Actinic keratosis (Figure 15-2) is a **premalignant** lesion (i.e., a precursor to squamous cell carcinoma) primarily caused by excessive **sunlight** exposure. It presents as rough, scaly, poorly demarcated plaques on the face, neck, upper trunk, or extremities (see Figure 15-2A). It is commonly described as having a **wart-like appearance** due to the excessive buildup of keratin. Histologically, the lesion is characterized by cytologic atypia in lower layers of the epidermis with nuclei present in a diffusely thickened stratum corneum (see Figure 15-2B). Alternatively, diffuse thinning of the epidermal surface can occur.

    Malignant melanoma (Figure 15-3) arises anywhere melanocytes are found (i.e., skin, mucous membranes, CNS). It can develop at any age, and typically affects fair-skinned people. Predisposing factors include excessive sunlight exposure, family history, preexisting nevi (i.e., dysplastic nevi), and carcinogen exposure. The **S-100** tumor marker is also associated with malignant melanoma. Typically, melanoma presents as a flat, dark brown or black lesion with alternating hypopigmentation (see Figure 15-3A). The most important clinical characteristic is a new or preexisting **pigmented lesion that changes color or enlarges.** There are two main growth patterns of melanoma (Table 15-1). The gross and histologic appearance of this patient's lesion indicates the diagnosis of basal cell carcinoma and rules out malignant melanoma.

    Squamous cell carcinoma (Figure 15-4) is very common. Like basal cell carcinoma, it **rarely metastasizes** and typically affects fair-skinned men with a history of excessive

QUICK HIT

Seborrheic keratosis is a benign neoplasm typically found in the elderly. It is characterized by raised papules and plaques that appear to be **"pasted on."**

FIGURE
15-2
(See also Color Plates 15-2A and 15-2B.) A. The gross appearance of actinic keratosis. B. The microscopic appearance of actinic keratosis

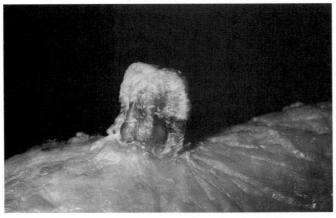

A

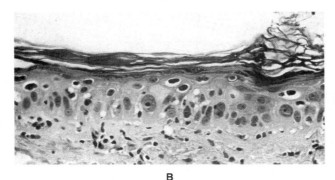

B

A: (Reprinted with permission from Fitzpatrick TB, Johnson RA, Wolff K, Suurmond D. Color Atlas and Synopsis of Clinical Dermatology, 4th Ed. New York: McGraw-Hill, 2001, p 251.) B: (Reprinted with permission from Rubin E, Farber JL. Pathology, 3rd Ed. Philadelphia: Lippincott-Raven Publishers, 1999, p 1293.)

FIGURE
15-3
(See also Color Plates 15-3A and 15-3B.) A. The gross appearance of malignant melanoma. B. The microscopic appearance of malignant melanoma

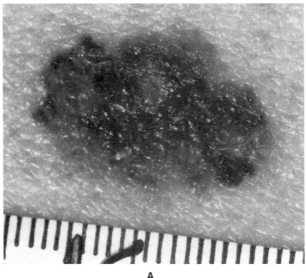

A

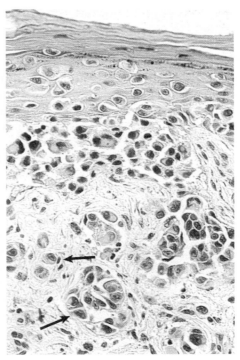

B

(Reprinted with permission from Rubin E, Farber JL. Pathology, 3rd Ed. Philadelphia: Lippincott-Raven Publishers, 1999, pp 1281–1282.)

TABLE 15-1	Growth Patterns of Melanocytes	
Growth Pattern	**Description**	**Tendency to Metastasize**
Benign radial growth	Growth occurs in any direction, but predominantly in lateral directions	Does not readily metastasize
Aggressive vertical growth	Growth occurs into the deeper layers of the skin and beyond	Readily metastasizes

exposure to **sunlight.** However, squamous cell carcinoma differs from basal cell carcinoma in several ways: it usually affects men older than 55 years of age; it can involve both the skin and mucous membranes; and it is associated with excessive exposure to chemical carcinogens (e.g., arsenic), radiation, and X-rays. It typically presents on sun-exposed areas (e.g., face, back of hands) as a slow-growing, **ulcerating, scaling nodule** (see Figure 15-4A). Microscopically, the lesion demonstrates invasion of the dermis by islands of neoplastic cells with **whorls of keratin** (i.e., **"pearls"**) (see Figure 15-4B). Biopsy is the definitive way to differentiate between squamous cell carcinoma and basal cell carcinoma.

Related Basic Science

Skin

The skin can be divided into two layers: epidermis and dermis. The epidermis is composed of a **stratified, keratinized squamous epithelium** derived from ectoderm. The dermis is composed of dense, irregular, collagenous connective tissue derived from mesoderm (Figure 15-5). Melanocytes, which are interspersed in the epidermis, are derived from neural crest cells. Langerhans cells, found in the stratum spinosum, have major histocompatibility complex (MHC) II receptors and act as antigen-presenting cells (APCs) to $CD4^+$ T cells. Functions of the skin include temperature regulation, waterproofing, vitamin D synthesis, and protection.

Pain receptors are **free nerve endings** found throughout the body, especially in the skin. Pain receptors are activated by mechanical, thermal, or chemical stimuli. The receptors have very slow adaptation or no adaptation to painful stimuli. **Type A-delta** (group III) fibers are fast pain fibers that carry acute pain information. **Type C** (group IV) fibers are slow pain fibers that carry chronic pain information. Because type C fibers are unmyelinated, they are more quickly blocked by local anesthetics (e.g., lidocaine). Pain information (i.e., nociception) is carried by the lateral spinothalamic tract.

QUICK HIT Xeroderma pigmentosum is an autosomal recessive disorder characterized by the failure of **DNA repair** mechanisms, resulting in a strong disposition to develop skin cancer.

QUICK HIT Keloids are raised, firm lesions on the skin caused by excessive scarring after minor trauma or surgery. Keloids are more common in African Americans.

FIGURE 15-4 (See also Color Plates 15-4A and 15-4B.) A. The gross appearance of squamous cell carcinoma. B. The microscopic appearance of squamous cell carcinoma

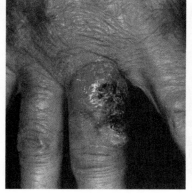

A

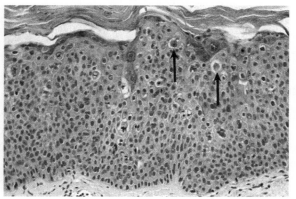

B

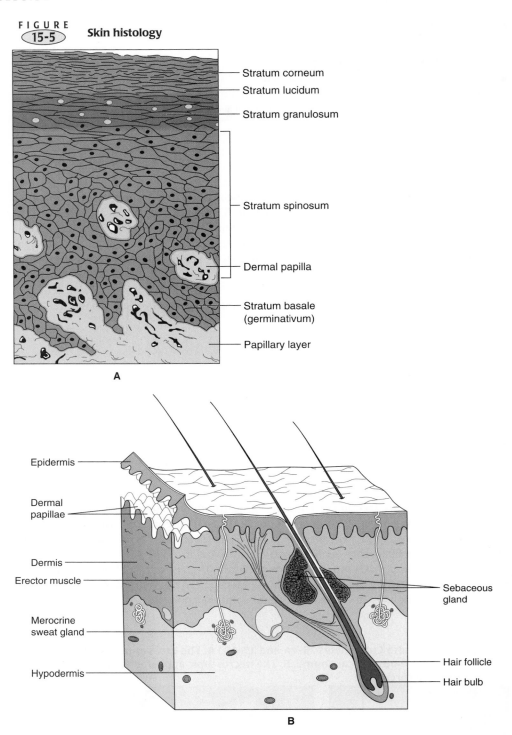

FIGURE
15-5   **Skin histology**

A

B

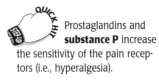

Prostaglandins and **substance P** increase the sensitivity of the pain receptors (i.e., hyperalgesia).

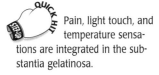

Pain, light touch, and temperature sensations are integrated in the substantia gelatinosa.

Thermal regulation

The skin is an integral part of thermal regulation, especially in heat dissipation. Increases in ambient temperature and core temperature (as with exercise) are sensed by the skin and posterior hypothalamus, respectively. The **posterior hypothalamus** coordinates the heat dissipating response. A decrease in sympathetic tone to the blood vessels of the skin allows blood to flow through **arteriovenous (AV) shunts** close to the surface of the skin, allowing heat to escape. Sympathetic muscarinic input to the sweat glands activates sweating and evaporative heat loss.

Heat-producing mechanisms are activated in response to a drop in temperature. The **anterior hypothalamus,** which is constantly comparing the body temperature to the body's desired set temperature, coordinates this response. The posterior hypothalamus is directed to activate the shivering response, which is the most potent heat-generating mechanism. Other responses include an increase in basal metabolic rate mediated by thyroid hormone. Sympathetic activation constricts the AV shunts in the skin and activates brown fat.

Fever results from activation of the heat-producing mechanisms after a rise in the hypothalamic set temperature. This occurs during infection as endogenous pyrogens (i.e., interleukins [IL] 1 and 6) are released from cells of the immune system. **IL-1** and **IL-6** increase production of prostaglandins in the anterior hypothalamus, which is the signal to raise the set temperature. By blocking cyclooxygenase, **aspirin** inhibits prostaglandin production and can reduce a fever. **Steroids** can have the same effect by blocking phospholipase A_2 and the release of arachidonic acid.

Understanding these temperature control mechanisms helps explain characteristics of different disease states. For example, hyperthyroid patients are heat intolerant while hypothyroid patients are cold intolerant. Patients in heart failure are heat intolerant because sympathetic tone is increased as the body attempts to maintain cardiac output. Sympathetic activation of brown fat, cutaneous vasoconstriction, and sweating all occur, which explains why heart failure patients can have cold, clammy skin.

Atropine blocks activation of sweat glands and can cause an increase in body temperature called an "atropine fever."

The severe muscle contractions of malignant hyperthermia cause a rapid rise in body temperature. This syndrome occurs in certain susceptible people after administration of halothane and succinylcholine. It is treated with dantrolene, a muscle relaxant.

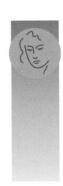

"I found a lump in my breast while I was in the shower last week."

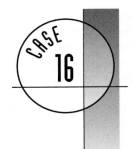

OBJECTIVES

1. Develop a differential diagnosis and an appropriate workup for a breast lesion
2. Compare and contrast key features of tumors of the breast
3. Understand the leading types of cancers and cancer-related deaths by gender
4. Review the role of oncogenes in causing breast cancer
5. Learn the anatomy and development of the breast
6. Review the stages of psychologic development according to Freud, Erikson, and Piaget
7. Understand the physiology associated with milk production and release

HISTORY AND PHYSICAL EXAMINATION

A distraught **58**-year-old woman presents to the office complaining of a hard, bumpy **mass** in her **left breast** that she first noticed during a self-examination in the shower last week. She denies having any breast or nipple discharge, but has noticed some **puckering** of the nipple since early last month. She is 3 years postmenopause and **does not take hormone replacement therapy.** Menses began at either 11 or 12 years of age. Her mother died of **breast cancer** at 48 years of age. The patient has **never been pregnant** and has no history of fibrocystic changes or cancers. On physical examination, the patient has puckering of her left nipple and dimpling of the skin on the same breast. A hard, nodular, **nontender** mass is palpable in the upper left quadrant of her left breast.

APPROPRIATE WORKUP

Mammogram, breast biopsy, estrogen receptor test

DIFFERENTIAL DIAGNOSIS

Breast cancer, fat necrosis, fibroadenoma, fibrocystic disease of the breast, mastitis

DIAGNOSTIC LABORATORY TESTS AND STUDIES

Mammogram:
　　Spiculated density with irregular infiltration of surrounding tissue
　　Calcifications
Biopsy (Figure 16-1):
　　Large cells in nests, cords, and sheets
Estrogen receptor (ER) positive
　　Anaplastic cells with a high mitotic index

F I G U R E
16-1
Breast cancer: invasive ductal carcinoma

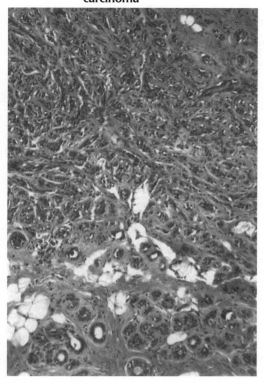

(Reprinted with permission from Mehta S, Milder EA, Mirarchi AJ. Step-Up: A High-Yield, Systems-Based Review for the USMLE Step 1 Examination. Philadelphia: Lippincott Williams & Wilkins, 2000, p 351.)

DIAGNOSIS: BREAST CANCER (INVASIVE DUCTAL CARCINOMA)

Breast cancer is the **most common cancer** in women (1 in 9) and the second leading cause of cancer death in women (Table 16-1). **Invasive ductal carcinoma** of the breast is the **most common** type of breast cancer in women, accounting for nearly 70 to 80% of cases. Risk factors for breast cancer include **family history, age over 45, early menarche, late menopause,** fibrocystic disease with atypical hyperplasia, **obesity,** diet high in animal fat, genetics (i.e., genes BRCA1 and BRCA2), **first pregnancy after 30, nulliparity,** and amplification of the oncogene HER-2/*neu*. Sites of metastasis of breast cancer, in order of decreasing frequency, are the lungs, bones, liver, adrenal glands, and brain. Sites of nodal spread, in order of decreasing frequency, are the axillary, internal mammary, and supraclavicular nodes.

TABLE 16-1 Cancer Statistics Based on Gender

Gender	Leading Types of Cancer	Leading Causes of Cancer-Related Death
Women	Breast cancer Lung cancer Colon cancer	Lung cancer Breast cancer Colon cancer
Men	Prostate cancer Lung cancer Colon cancer	Lung cancer Prostate cancer Colon cancer

Cancers are listed in decreasing order of frequency.

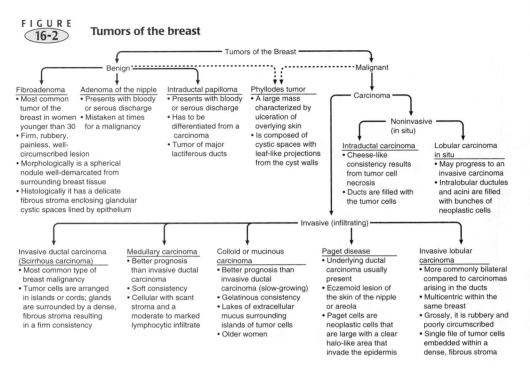

FIGURE 16-2 **Tumors of the breast**

The tumor associated with invasive ductal carcinoma tends to be a very **hard, circumscribed** mass averaging 1 to 2 cm in size. It often forms in the **upper outer quadrant** of the breast. If the tumor infiltrates the chest wall, **skin dimpling** and nipple retraction can occur. Malignant cells, which appear as nests, cords, tubules, and glands, are highly atypical and can invade connective tissue, nerves, and vasculature (see Figure 16-1).

Regular **mammography** has been shown to reduce mortality, but has a 15% false-negative rate. Because of the false-negative rate of mammography and because there are a number of histologic types of breast cancer (Figure 16-2), all masses must be **biopsied.**

In addition to histologic appearance, breast cancers can be classified by their estrogen-receptor **(ER) status.** ER-positive tumors are more common in postmenopausal patients and have a better prognosis because they are more responsive to therapy. ER-negative tumors are more prevalent in premenopausal women. Treatment for ER-positive cancers can include **tamoxifen,** a competitive inhibitor of the ER. A combination regimen of cyclophosphamide, methotrexate, and 5-fluorouracil is advised for patients with ER-negative tumors.

EXPLANATION OF DIFFERENTIAL

Fat necrosis should be considered when a patient has a recent history of **trauma,** surgery, or radiation to the breast and presents with a painful lump. Although fat necrosis can lead to skin retraction, an indurated lesion, fibrosis, and calcification, the **presence of pain** is the defining feature.

Fibroadenoma is the **most common benign breast tumor,** and it is more common in women younger than 30 years of age. Clinically, patients present with a round, painless, clearly demarcated nodule that is freely moveable. The mass contains fibrous and glandular tissue. This benign breast tumor is hormonally influenced and can grow in size at the end of the menstrual cycle or during pregnancy. On a mammogram, **"popcorn"** calcifications are evident.

Fibrocystic disease of the breast is the **most common disorder** of the breast and the most common cause of palpable breast masses in patients 25 to 50 years of age. Patients often present with **lumpy** breasts that have **bilateral, mid-menstrual cycle tenderness.** There is no increased cancer risk in women with fibrocystic changes; however, the risk of cancer is increased if the hyperplastic epithelium demonstrates atypia. Histologically, fibrosis or cysts may be present. The cysts may be filled with blue fluid (i.e., **blue dome** cyst).

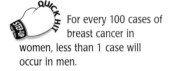

For every 100 cases of breast cancer in women, less than 1 case will occur in men.

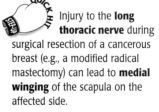

Acanthosis nigricans is a thickened, hyperpigmented zone of skin in flexural regions (e.g., axillae). It is often an outward marker for underlying malignant conditions (e.g., adenocarcinoma of the breast or stomach).

Injury to the **long thoracic nerve** during surgical resection of a cancerous breast (e.g., a modified radical mastectomy) can lead to **medial winging** of the scapula on the affected side.

Mastitis is infection and inflammation of the breast. The most common offending organism is ***Staphylococcus aureus,*** which gains entry to the breast via cracks or fissures in the nipple. Patients present with purulent discharge from the nipple, which is most often a complication of **lactation** after pregnancy. Patients can also have local inflammation, soreness, and redness. Administration of **antibiotics** may contain the infection, but abscess formation may lead to fibrous scarring and nipple retraction.

Related Basic Science

Oncogenes and breast cancer

Oncogenes are in a family of genes that normally code for proteins involved in cell growth or regulation (e.g., growth factors, protein kinases). However, if oncogenes become mutated or activated by contact with retroviruses, they may result in malignant processes. Oncogenes often work together to produce cancer. Their effect may be amplified by inherited mutations or jumping genes. One common oncogene associated with breast cancer is HER-2/*neu*. This oncogene is frequently amplified and correlates with a less favorable diagnosis. The BRCA1 gene on the long arm of chromosome 17 has been linked to many cases of early breast cancer found in particular families. Other oncogenes involved in disease processes include *BCR-ABL* [t(9;22)] in chronic myelogenous leukemia (CML), c-*myc* [t(8;14)] in Burkitt lymphoma, and N-*myc* in neuroblastoma.

Only one copy of a mutant oncogene needs to be present to result in cancerous growth. The **"two-hit" hypothesis** applies to mutations of **tumor suppressor genes** (e.g., p53, Rb). All individuals have two copies of tumor suppressor genes. Both copies need to be defective or mutated for the body to lose the ability to suppress cell growth, resulting in cancer. Mutations involving the **Rb** gene result in retinoblastoma and can increase the risk of developing osteosarcoma. Loss of the **p53** tumor suppressor gene is found in 70% of colon cancers, 50% of breast cancers, and 50% of lung cancers. Mutation of the WT-1 tumor suppressor gene leads to Wilms tumor.

The breast

The **mammary glands** are modified **apocrine sweat glands** that develop under the influence of sex hormones (Figure 16-3). During embryologic development in both men and women, multiple glands develop along paired epidermal thickenings called the mammary ridges (i.e., **milk lines**). As fetal development proceeds, only one group of cells develops into a breast on each side.

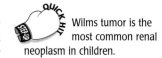 Wilms tumor is the most common renal neoplasm in children.

In women, breast development and lobule formation begin with puberty under hormonal (i.e., estrogen) control. **Thelarche** (i.e., externally recognizable breast development) starts at approximately 11 years of age. From puberty onward, thelarche can be divided into five separate **Tanner stages.** Menarche usually begins 2 years after the first phase of thelarche.

Psychologic stages of development (Figure 16-4)

The physical changes that occur during puberty coincide with psychologic and behavioral changes. **Freud** labeled this period as the genital phase of development. **Erikson** determined that the identity of the individual is established during puberty. **Piaget** felt that adolescence is the period during which abstract and concrete thinking formally develop together.

Milk production and release

The synthesis and release of milk during and after pregnancy is under the influence of a number of hormones acting in concert (Figure 16-5). During pregnancy, progesterone, prolactin, and chorionic somatomammotropin stimulate breast growth and the capacity for milk synthesis.

Progesterone and estrogen levels are maintained by human chorionic gonadotropin **(hCG)**, a hormone produced by the placenta that is similar to luteinizing hormone (LH). However, unlike LH secretion, placental secretion of hCG is not inhibited by high levels

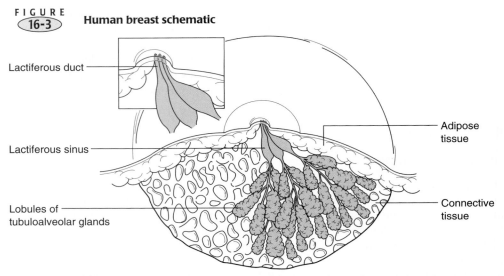

FIGURE
16-3   **Human breast schematic**

Lactiferous duct

Adipose tissue

Lactiferous sinus

Connective tissue

Lobules of tubuloalveolar glands

(Reprinted with permission from Ross MH, Romrell LJ, Kaya GI. Histology: A Text and Atlas, 3rd ed. Baltimore: Williams & Wilkins, 1995, p 710.)

> **QUICK HIT**
> Along with intrauterine pregnancy, elevated levels of hCG can be seen in patients with hydatidiform moles, choriocarcinoma, gestational tumors, **ectopic pregnancy,** and pseudocyesis.

of progesterone or estrogen. hCG maintains the **corpus luteum,** which produces progesterone, until 8 to 10 weeks' gestation, at which time the **placenta** becomes the major producer of progesterone. The high levels of progesterone and estrogen during pregnancy **inhibit milk release.** The inhibitory effect of these two hormones is lost after delivery of the placenta, allowing for milk release.

FIGURE
16-4   **Stages of development**

	Infancy (0–1y)	Toddler (1–3y)	School age (3–11y)	Adolescence (11–20y)	Early adulthood (20–40y)	Middle adulthood (40–60y)	Late adulthood (60–80y)
Freud	Oral	Anal	Phallic-oedipal (3–6y); latency (6–11y)	Genital			
Erikson	Trust vs mistrust	Autonomy vs shame and doubt	Initiative vs guilt (3–6y); industry vs inferiority	Identity vs role confusion	Intimacy vs isolation	Generativity vs stagnation	Ego integrity vs despair
Piaget	Sensorimotor (0–2y)	Preoperational (2–7y)	Concrete operations (7–11y)	Formal operations			
Characteristics	Reflexes: • Palmer grasp (0–2m) • Rooting (0–3m) • Babinski (0–12m) Milestones: • Turn over (5m) • Sit (6m) • Walk (12m)	Terrible two's ("no"); band-aid (2–4y); parallel play (2–4y); balance on one foot (2y); climb stairs (3y)	Cooperative play (4–7y); conservation of mass (7–11y); button clothes (4y); throw a ball (4y);	First menstruation (11y); first ejaculation (13y); peer pressure	New family; children; role in society solidified; period of reassessment	Height of career; mid-life crises; menopause (45–55y)	Depression (ECT); women outlive men by 6–8 years; Kübler-Ross (stages of grief and dying) • Denial • Anger • Bargaining • Depression • Acceptance

y = years of age; m = months old

(Reprinted with permission from Mehta S, Milder EA, Mirarchi AJ. Step-Up: A High-Yield, Systems-Based Review for the USMLE Step 1. Philadelphia: Lippincott Williams & Wilkins, 2000, p 176.)

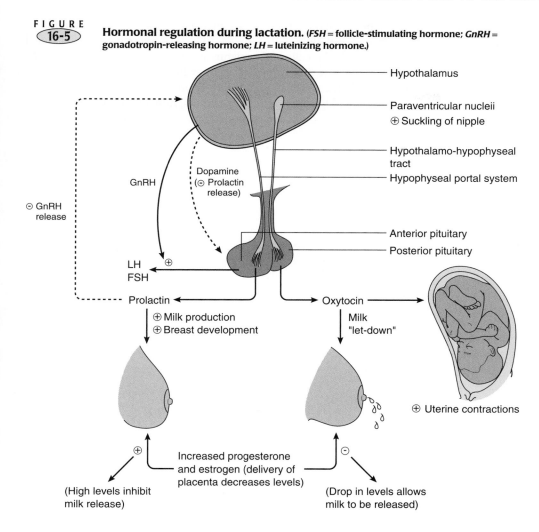

FIGURE 16-5 Hormonal regulation during lactation. (*FSH* = follicle-stimulating hormone; *GnRH* = gonadotropin-releasing hormone; *LH* = luteinizing hormone.)

Prolactin is the primary hormone responsible for **lactogenesis** and, along with estrogen, **breast development** (see Figure 16-5). Its secretion from the **anterior pituitary** is regulated by the inhibitory influence of **dopamine** from the hypothalamus. Prolactin is also responsible for **inhibiting ovulation** by inhibiting the release of gonadotropin-releasing hormone (GnRH) from the hypothalamus, thus preventing the release of LH. Destruction of the anterior pituitary can lead to failure to lactate as a result of loss of prolactin. On the other hand, excess prolactin from a prolactinoma, inhibition of dopamine due to antipsychotics, or hypothalamic destruction can lead to amenorrhea, decreased libido, and galactorrhea.

Oxytocin, produced by the **paraventricular nuclei** of the hypothalamus and released by the posterior pituitary, serves two functions: **ejection of milk** from the breast and **contraction of the smooth muscle of the uterus** (see Figure 16-5). **Suckling** of the breast activates afferent fibers in the nipple, which carry the signal to the hypothalamus and trigger the release of oxytocin. In the absence of suckling, the mere thought, sight, or sound of the infant can stimulate oxytocin release. **Milk let-down** is a result of oxytocin contracting the myoepithelial cells of the breast. A similar contraction is seen in the uterus, where oxytocin is thought to play a role in parturition. During pregnancy, oxytocin receptors on the uterus are upregulated; therefore, the hormone can be used to induce labor and reduce postpartum bleeding.

QUICK HIT Lactose, one of the proteins composing breast milk, is synthesized by the action of α-**lactalbumin** (protein B). Prolactin stimulates protein B synthesis in mammary glands.

QUICK HIT Women who exclusively breast-feed may experience lactation amenorrhea and temporary infertility due to high levels of serum prolactin (maintained by the act of breast-feeding), which suppresses GnRH and LH release.

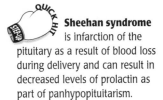

Sheehan syndrome is infarction of the pituitary as a result of blood loss during delivery and can result in decreased levels of prolactin as part of panhypopituitarism.

Approaching the end of pregnancy, there is an increase in the immunoglobulin A (**IgA**)-secreting lymphocyte population of the breast. The IgA secreted into the local bloodstream is absorbed by epithelial cells of the mammary glands and deposited into the milk. IgA is responsible for **passive immunity** in the newborn through breast-feeding. Furthermore, **colostrum** (i.e., the earliest mammary gland secretion after birth) has increased immunoglobulins. In addition to immunoglobulins, human milk is composed of long-chain fatty acids (i.e., palmitic, oleic, and linoleic acids) and lipases.

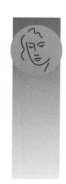

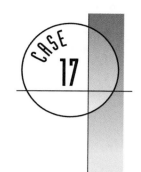

"It is really hard to breathe!"

OBJECTIVES

1. Develop a differential diagnosis and an appropriate workup for increased dyspnea
2. Review the three lung zones and the relative changes in ventilation (V) and perfusion and the overall V/Q ratios
3. Compare and contrast common causes for respiratory and metabolic alkalosis and acidosis
4. Review primary and secondary causes of hypercoagulable states
5. Review the anatomy and associated pathologies of the lower extremity
6. Learn common tumors of the bone and cartilage

HISTORY AND PHYSICAL EXAMINATION

A 42-year-old African American woman complains of sudden onset of **shortness of breath**, inspiratory chest pain, cough, and hemoptysis. The patient underwent an uneventful right anterior cruciate ligament (ACL) repair on her left knee 4 days before, but has not been discharged because of a low-grade **fever** that occurred on **postoperative** day 2. She has been **immobile** due to pain. The patient does not have a history of smoking and denies any illegal drug use. She has no known allergies and has an unremarkable medical and surgical history. Physical examination reveals a low-grade **fever, tachypnea** with decreased breath sounds on the right, **tachycardia** with a prominent S2, and an edematous right lower extremity.

APPROPRIATE WORKUP

Blood chemistries, arterial blood gases (ABG), chest X-ray, EKG, Doppler ultrasound, and V/Q scan

DIFFERENTIAL DIAGNOSIS

Adult respiratory distress syndrome, myocardial infarction (MI), pneumonia, pneumothorax, pulmonary embolism (PE)

DIAGNOSTIC LABORATORY TESTS AND STUDIES

Blood chemistry:
 WBCs = 9,000/μL (N)
 Hgb = 13.4 g/dL (N)
 Platelets = 150,000/L (N)
 CK = 60 U/L (N)
 Troponin I = <0.4 mg/mL (N)
ABG:
 pH = 7.50 (H)
 $PaCO_2$ = 30 mm Hg (L)

PaO_2 = 60 mm Hg (L)
A-a gradient = 52 (H)
Chest radiograph:
 Atelectasis in the right lung
EKG:
 Sinus tachycardia
 S1Q3T3 (large S wave in lead I, Q wave in lead III, and an inverted T wave in lead III)

Doppler ultrasound:	V/Q scan:
Right thigh shows **thrombosis** of femoral vein	Mismatch right upper lobe
Left lower extremity normal	**V/Q ratio markedly elevated**

DIAGNOSIS: PE SECONDARY TO DVT FOLLOWING AN OPERATION

There are three major risk factors that predispose a patient to **PE** (Figure 17-1) and deep venous thrombosis (DVT) as outlined by the **Virchow triad**: stasis, vessel wall damage, and blood hypercoagulability. Clinically, these risk factors can result from the postoperative state, atrial fibrillation, obesity, pregnancy, oral contraceptive use, cancer, protein C and S deficiency, immobilization, thrombocytosis, and advanced age.

Sudden-onset dyspnea is the most frequent presenting symptom of PE, while **tachypnea** is the most common sign. Patients can present with pleuritic chest pain manifested by inspiratory pain, cough, and hemoptysis. Associated syncope, hypotension, and cyanosis may indicate a massive PE, which can result in sudden death.

The ABG classically shows **hypoxia** (decreased PO_2), **hyperventilation** (decreased PCO_2), and a respiratory alkalosis (elevated pH). A normal A-a gradient rules out PE as a diagnosis. The chest radiograph is often normal. A **V/Q** scan is helpful, but **pulmonary angiography** is the **gold standard.** Because the V/Q scan in this patient shows a high probability for PE and the Doppler ultrasound is positive for DVT, pulmonary angiography is not necessary to confirm the diagnosis; treatment with **heparin** is initiated. Spiral CT and D-dimers are evolving diagnostic modalities, while low-molecular-weight heparin and warfarin (coumadin) are common therapeutic modalities for PE.

FIGURE
17-1   **Pulmonary embolism**

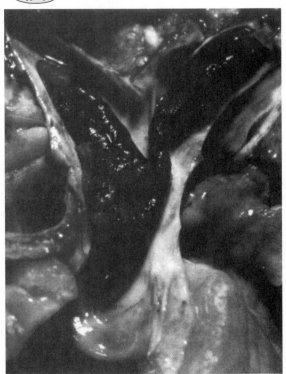

(Reprinted with permission from Mehta S, Milder EA, Mirarchi AJ. Step-Up: A High-Yield, Systems-Based Review for the USMLE Step 1. Philadelphia: Lippincott Williams & Wilkins, 2000, p 362.)

EXPLANATION OF DIFFERENTIAL

Adult respiratory distress syndrome can be a result of **trauma, aspiration,** and **sepsis,** which can injure the alveolocapillary membrane, leading to the deposition of neutrophils, blood products, and protein-rich fluid in the alveolar space. The typical presentation of this syndrome includes severe **hypoxemia unresponsive to oxygen** administration and a normal pulmonary artery wedge pressure. The chest radiograph demonstrates complete **"white out"** of the lung fields in advanced stages.

Patients having an **MI** classically complain of crushing **substernal chest pain,** nausea, vomiting, diaphoresis, and shortness of breath. Physical examination findings may vary, but often include murmurs, hypotension, and tachycardia. The **EKG** is often diagnostic with ST segment and T-wave changes. Cardiac enzymes (e.g., **troponin I,** CK-MB) are elevated after an MI.

Pneumonia can also present with cough, dyspnea, fever, and an abnormal chest radiograph. Furthermore, hospitalized patients are at high risk for developing pneumonia from nosocomial agents, such as *Staphylococcus aureus* and **gram-negative rods** (e.g., *Klebsiella, Pseudomonas*). Patients with pneumonia often show consolidation on a chest radiograph and have a less abrupt onset of symptoms, an elevated WBC count, and a positive sputum culture.

Pneumothorax (i.e., **accumulation of air** in the pleural space) can lead to collapse of the lung. Pneumothorax often results from trauma, but can be **spontaneous** if bullae (usually in the upper lobe and often from emphysema) rupture. It can also occur secondary to pulmonary diseases, such as tuberculosis, malignancy, emphysema, and pulmonary infarction. Patients complain of sudden-onset dyspnea and chest pain. The physical examination is diagnostic with **decreased breath sounds** and **hyperresonance** over the affected side. The chest radiograph may demonstrate a thin line parallel to the chest wall demarcating the shrinking lung from the wall. The ABG shows a decreased PO_2 and an increased PCO_2.

Related Science

Lung zones (Figure 17-2)

The V/Q ratio compares alveolar ventilation to the rate of pulmonary blood flow. Decreased ventilation (e.g., a foreign body in the airway) creates a **shunt,** which allows blood to go directly from the venous circulation to the arterial circulation without being oxygenated and makes the **V/Q** ratio abnormally **low.** On the other hand, decreased perfusion (e.g., PE) creates **dead space** where no gas exchange can occur, even though the alveolus is being adequately ventilated, resulting in an **elevated V/Q** ratio. V/Q mismatches can result in an abnormal ABG, which can detect major disturbances in respiratory function, such as respiratory alkalosis or acidosis (Table 17-1). See Appendix B for normal ABG values.

The **A-a gradient,** which is the difference between the oxygen content in the alveolus (A) and the alveolar arteriole (a), can assess more subtle abnormalities of gas exchange. The normal range of the A-a gradient is between 0 and 30. An increased gradient signifies that capillary oxygen is low. The A-a gradient is calculated by subtracting the arteriolar oxygen content from the alveolar oxygen content (i.e., **$PAO_2 - PaO_2$**). PaO_2 is capillary oxygen pressure, which is measured with an ABG. The PAO_2 is the alveolar oxygen pressure, which is a calculated value: **$PAO_2 = (760 \text{ mm Hg} - 47 \text{ mm Hg}) \cdot FIO_2 - (PaCO_2/0.8)$,** where

> **QUICK HIT** A symptom is based on the patient's history, while a sign is a physical finding upon examination.

> **QUICK HIT** Patients presenting with chest pain and shortness of breath need to be evaluated for the following life-threatening conditions: MI, PE, pneumothorax, esophageal rupture, and aortic aneurysm.

> **QUICK HIT** A **tension pneumothorax** is a life-threatening condition in which pressure builds in the pleural space owing to air being allowed to enter, but not leave. Clinically, the **trachea is deviated** away from the affected side, there are **decreased breath sounds** and hyperresonance on the affected side, and there is **jugular venous distention.** Immediate treatment is with a **large-bore needle** in the **second intercostal space** on the affected side to decompress the chest, followed by placement of a chest tube.

---

760 mm Hg = total atmospheric pressure at sea level

47 mm Hg = partial pressure of completely humidified air as found in the alveoli

FIO_2 = percent of air that is oxygen (normally 21% at sea level)

$PaCO_2$ = partial pressure of carbon dioxide in the capillaries (normally 40 mm Hg)

0.8 = ratio of volume of carbon dioxide produced to the volume of oxygen consumed

FIGURE
(17-2) **Pulmonary circulation**

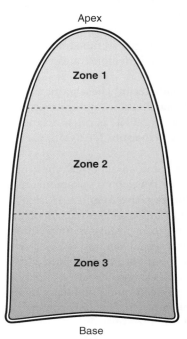

Apex

Zone 1

Zone 2

Zone 3

Base

Zone 1
- Lowest blood flow
- Alveolar pressure > Arterial pressure > Venous pressure
- Capillaries collapse due to high alveolar pressure
- Ventilation (V) is decreased less than blood flow [also called perfusion (Q)]

so: $\frac{V}{Q} = \frac{\downarrow}{\downarrow\downarrow} = \uparrow$ (Ventilation in excess of profusion)

Zone 2
- Blood flow is higher than Zone 1, but lower than Zone 3
- Arterial pressure > Alveolar pressure > Venous pressure
- Capillaries remain open because arterial pressure is greater than alveolar pressure
- Ventilation (V) is approximately equivalent to perfusion (Q)

so: $\frac{V}{Q} \approx 1$

Zone 3
- Highest blood flow
- Arterial pressure > Venous pressure > Alveolar pressure
- Capillaries remain open because arterial pressure is higher than both alveolar and venous pressure
- Ventilation (V) is increased less than perfusion (Q)

so: $\frac{V}{Q} = \frac{\uparrow}{\uparrow\uparrow} = \downarrow$ (Profusion in excess of ventilation)

(Reprinted with permission from Mehta S, Milder EA, Mirarchi AJ. Step-Up: A High-Yield, Systems-Based Review for the USMLE Step 1. Philadelphia: Lippincott Williams & Wilkins, 2000, p 69.)

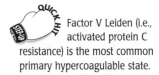

Hypoxemia results in vasodilation systemically, but causes vasoconstriction in the lungs in an effort to maintain the V/Q ratio.

Factor V Leiden (i.e., activated protein C resistance) is the most common primary hypercoagulable state.

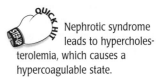

Nephrotic syndrome leads to hypercholesterolemia, which causes a hypercoagulable state.

Trousseau syndrome is characterized by increased susceptibility to thrombophlebitis due to malignancy, often of the pancreas.

Hypercoagulable states

Hypercoagulability is part of the Virchow triad for clotting. Hypercoagulable states can include intrinsic blood disorders, hereditary disorders of enhanced thrombosis, and acquired disorders of enhanced thrombosis. Table 17-2 lists some of the more common causes of primary and secondary hypercoagulable states.

Structures of the lower extremities

The deep veins of the lower extremities (i.e., **femoral, popliteal,** and **iliac** veins) are the most common sites of thromboembolic formation. Thrombus of the superficial veins of the lower extremities is common, but usually clinically insignificant. **Fat** from a **long bone fracture** or after liposuction can also cause a thromboembolic event, as can septic emboli from endocarditis.

TABLE 17-1 Common Causes of Alkalosis and Acidosis

Respiratory		Metabolic	
Acidosis	**Alkalosis**	**Acidosis**	**Alkalosis**
COPD	Emotion and pain	Diabetes	Vomiting
Respiratory center depression	Pneumonia	Renal failure	Nasogastric suction
Trauma	CHF	Lactic acidosis	Hypokalemia
Polio	PE	Diarrhea	Diuretics

CHF, congestive heart failure; COPD, chronic obstructive pulmonary disease; PE, pulmonary embolism.

TABLE 17-2 Hypercoagulable States

Primary (Inherited)	Secondary (Acquired)
Antithrombin III deficiency	Antiphospholipid antibodies (lupus anticoagulant)
Protein C deficiency	Malignancy
Protein S deficiency	Pregnancy
Activated protein C resistance (factor V Leiden)	Oral contraceptive use
	Sepsis
	Nephrotic syndrome
	Postoperative state
	Immobility

Constriction or clotting of the arterial vessels of the lower extremities (Figure 17-3) can lead to **intermittent claudication.** Intermittent claudication typically occurs as a result of atherosclerosis of the major arteries supplying specific muscles (Table 17-3). It presents as attacks of pain, primarily in the calf muscles, brought on by walking. Rest relieves pain from intermittent claudication.

FIGURE 17-3 Lower limb vasculature. A. Anterior view. B. Posterior view.

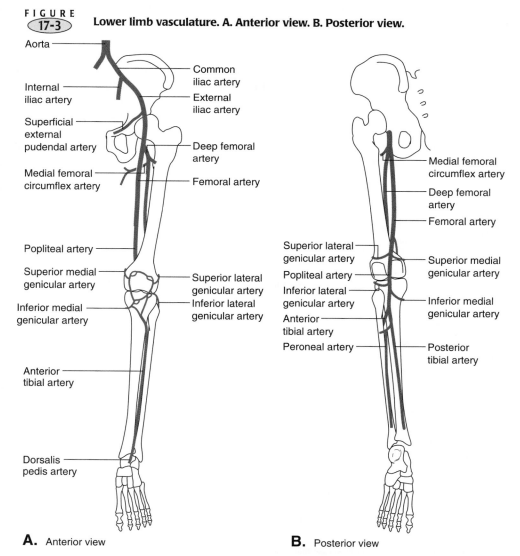

A. Anterior view **B.** Posterior view

(Adapted with permission from Moore K. Clinically Oriented Anatomy. Baltimore: Williams & Wilkins, 1995, p 406.)

TABLE 17-3	Lower Limb Musculature, Function, Innervation, and Blood Supply			
Joint	**Major Movements**	**Primary Muscles**	**Innervation**	**Blood Supply**
Hip	Flexion Extension Abduction Adduction	Iliopsoas m. Gluteus maximus m. Gluteus medius m. Adductor longus m.	Femoral n. Inferior gluteal n. Superior gluteal n. Obturator n.	Femoral a. Inferior gluteal a. Superior gluteal a. Deep femoral a.
Knee	Flexion Extension	Hamstring mm. Quadriceps m.	Sciatic n. Femoral n.	Deep femoral a. Femoral a.
Ankle	Dorsiflexion Plantarflexion	Tibialis anterior m. Gastrocnemius m. Soleus m.	Deep fibular n. Tibial n.	Anterior tibial a. Posterior tibial a.

QUICK HIT Footdrop is an inability to dorsiflex. The lesion is due to paralysis of the anterior tibial muscle from injury to the common or deep peroneal nerve.

Lower extremity complications

Plantar fasciitis can also cause lower extremity pain, usually of the foot or heel, and is characterized by inflammation of the plantar fascia. It is most frequently found in older, overweight individuals who complain of heel pain on standing or walking. A radiography may reveal **plantar bone spur formation.**

ACL tears occur when the knee is hyperextended or when excessive force is placed on the knee from the lateral side. Commonly, the medial meniscus and the medial collateral ligament are torn with the ACL (**terrible triad**) if there is excessive medial rotation of the femur associated with the lateral force (Figure 17-4). Injury to these structures occurs most often in contact sports (e.g., football). A **positive anterior drawer sign** is seen on physical examination.

Aside from ligamentous damage, the lower extremities are often the site of primary bone and cartilage tumors (Figure 17-5).

QUICK HIT Tears of the medial meniscus occur with tears of the medial collateral ligament because this ligament is firmly attached to the medial meniscus.

QUICK HIT The lateral collateral ligament is rarely injured because it is much stronger than the medial collateral ligament.

FIGURE 17-4 **Tear of the anterior cruciate ligament**

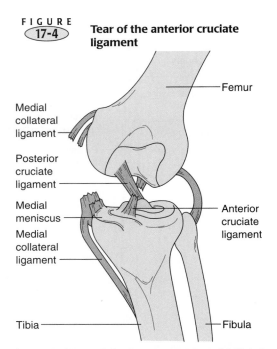

Medial collateral ligament

Posterior cruciate ligament

Medial meniscus

Medial collateral ligament

Tibia

Femur

Anterior cruciate ligament

Fibula

(Adapted with permission from Moore K. Essential Clinical Anatomy. Baltimore: Williams & Wilkins, 1995, p 272.)

FIGURE 17-5   Tumors of bone and cartilage

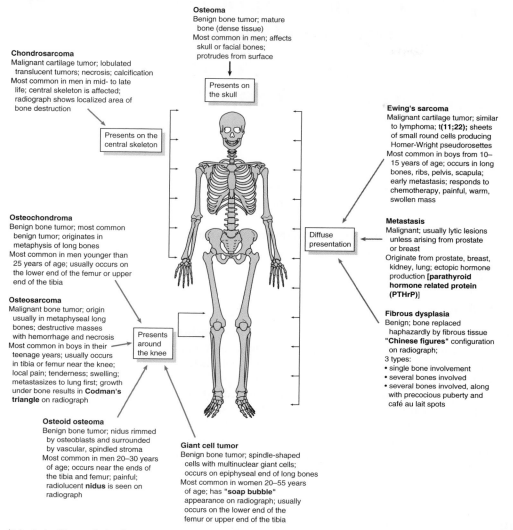

Osteoma
Benign bone tumor; mature bone (dense tissue)
Most common in men; affects skull or facial bones; protrudes from surface

Presents on the skull

Chondrosarcoma
Malignant cartilage tumor; lobulated translucent tumors; necrosis; calcification
Most common in men in mid- to late life; central skeleton is affected; radiograph shows localized area of bone destruction

Presents on the central skeleton

Ewing's sarcoma
Malignant cartilage tumor; similar to lymphoma; t(11;22); sheets of small round cells producing Homer-Wright pseudorosettes
Most common in boys from 10–15 years of age; occurs in long bones, ribs, pelvis, scapula; early metastasis; responds to chemotherapy, painful, warm, swollen mass

Osteochondroma
Benign bone tumor; most common benign tumor; originates in metaphysis of long bones
Most common in men younger than 25 years of age; usually occurs on the lower end of the femur or upper end of the tibia

Metastasis
Malignant; usually lytic lesions unless arising from prostate or breast
Originate from prostate, breast, kidney, lung; ectopic hormone production [**parathyroid hormone related protein (PTHrP)**]

Diffuse presentation

Osteosarcoma
Malignant bone tumor; origin usually in metaphyseal long bones; destructive masses with hemorrhage and necrosis
Most common in boys in their teenage years; usually occurs in tibia or femur near the knee; local pain; tenderness; swelling; metastasizes to lung first; growth under bone results in **Codman's triangle** on radiograph

Presents around the knee

Fibrous dysplasia
Benign; bone replaced haphazardly by fibrous tissue
"Chinese figures" configuration on radiograph;
3 types:
• single bone involvement
• several bones involved
• several bones involved, along with precocious puberty and café au lait spots

Osteoid osteoma
Benign bone tumor; nidus rimmed by osteoblasts and surrounded by vascular, spindled stroma
Most common in men 20–30 years of age; occurs near the ends of the tibia and femur; painful; radiolucent **nidus** is seen on radiograph

Giant cell tumor
Benign bone tumor; spindle-shaped cells with multinuclear giant cells; occurs on epiphyseal end of long bones
Most common in women 20–55 years of age; has **"soap bubble"** appearance on radiograph; usually occurs on the lower end of the femur or upper end of the tibia

(Adapted with permission from Moore K. Essential Clinical Anatomy. Baltimore: Williams & Wilkins, 1995, p 10.)

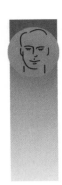

"For months I've been having diarrhea and hot flashes. Lately, I've been having trouble catching my breath."

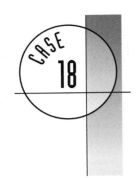

OBJECTIVES

1. Develop a differential diagnosis and an appropriate workup for dyspnea, diarrhea, and hot flashes
2. Review the function of serotonin, associated pathologies, and treatment for normalizing serotonin levels
3. Understand the location and physiology of smooth muscle

HISTORY AND PHYSICAL EXAMINATION

A 60-year-old man presents with a 6-month history of **watery diarrhea** and **hot flashes** (episodic flushing of the skin). He reports that the diarrhea has been getting worse and is sometimes accompanied by nausea and vomiting. He can think of no dietary changes that might be causing these episodes. On questioning, the patient recalls instances of **black, tarry stools (melena).** He recalls no history of heartburn, polyuria, or bloody stools. He is taking no antibiotics; his only medication is a multivitamin. All vital signs are within normal limits. Chest examination reveals diffuse wheezes heard over both lungs. A pulmonic ejection murmur is heard over the right sternal border at the second intercostal space. The liver is palpable two finger widths below the costal margin (slight **hepatomegaly**). There is no splenomegaly or abdominal tenderness, but hyperactive bowel sounds are heard.

APPROPRIATE WORKUP

Blood chemistries, stool analysis, urinalysis, and abdominal CT

DIFFERENTIAL DIAGNOSIS

Carcinoid tumor, Crohn disease, infectious diarrhea, irritable bowel syndrome, VIPoma, hyperthyroidism

> **QUICK HIT**
> GI bleeding in or above the duodenum generally causes melena (tarry black stools), while bleeding below the duodenum typically causes hematochezia (red blood in the stool).

DIAGNOSTIC LABORATORY TESTS AND STUDIES

Blood chemistry:
WBCs = 7000/μL (N)
Hgb = 14.0 g/dL (N)
Hct = 42% (N)
platelet count = 150,000/mm^3 (N)
K$^+$ = 4.0 mEq/L (N)
pH = 7.41 (N)

Stool analysis:
Positive results for heme
No evidence of parasites

Urinalysis:
Positive results for 5-hydroxyin-doleacetic acid (5-HIAA)

Abdominal CT:
Nodular masses in duodenum
Nodular liver metastases
No other abnormalities

DIAGNOSIS: CARCINOID TUMOR

Tumors rarely affect the small bowel, but 50% of all cases are **carcinoid tumors.** Carcinoid tumors arise from **neuroendocrine** cells and can occur in the small bowel, large bowel, pancreas, liver, bile ducts, or lungs. These tumors most often arise in the appendix, from which they never metastasize. From other regions of the bowel, however, a carcinoid tumor may **metastasize to the liver.** These tumors produce serotonin (5-HT), which is broken down in the liver to 5-HIAA. 5-HIAA appears in the urine. Until the tumor metastasizes to the liver, 5-HT does not reach the general circulation or cause systemic symptoms. With metastasis to the liver, **5-HT** in the systemic circulation causes the **carcinoid syndrome** (cyanosis/flushing, diarrhea, nausea, vomiting, cramps, bronchoconstriction, systemic fibrosis involving the valves of the right side of the heart, and hepatomegaly). Only a small fraction of carcinoid cases presents with this syndrome. The common presentation of a carcinoid tumor includes symptoms related to bleeding (anemia) and **obstruction** (vomiting). Carcinoid tumors sometimes produce gastrin or insulin. For this reason, octreotide (a somatostatin analog) is sometimes part of the initial treatment.

EXPLANATION OF DIFFERENTIAL

Crohn disease, like ulcerative colitis, is an inflammatory bowel disease and is more common in people of Jewish descent. Diarrhea and abdominal pain can be the presenting symptoms. Other accompanying systemic signs include arthritis, ankylosing spondylitis, iritis, and erythema nodosum. The systemic signs in this patient do not include those specified above, and 5-HIAA is not found in the urine of patients with inflammatory bowel disease.

Giardia lamblia and *Entamoeba histolytica* could cause chronic diarrhea, but these would be identified in the stool. Except in the case of certain parasites, infectious diarrhea rarely lasts as long as 6 months.

Irritable bowel syndrome is the most common GI disease diagnosed in general practice. It can present with cramps, constipation, **alternating bouts of constipation and diarrhea,** or chronic diarrhea. The disease is more common in women than in men and usually develops before 30 years of age. Only rarely does this disease have associated systemic symptoms, which can include back pain, weakness, and fainting.

VIPoma, a rare tumor of the pancreatic islets, secretes vasoactive intestinal peptide (VIP). The **WDHA** syndrome (watery diarrhea, hypokalemia, achlorhydria) and sometimes renal failure are associated with this tumor. This patient's potassium level was normal, and the abdominal CT showed no pancreatic abnormalities.

Hyperthyroidism could also have a similar presentation of diarrhea, hot flashes, tachycardia, and palpitations. However, on blood analysis, an elevation in T_3 and T_4 (total and free) and decrease in TSH would be observed. Case 63 provides more details on this diagnosis.

Related Basic Science

Serotonin and disease

Serotonin is a neurotransmitter whose function is not completely understood. Outside the CNS, serotonin contributes to vasoconstriction following damage to blood vessels. Derangements of serotonin function have been implicated in many disease states; therefore, some drugs specifically target serotonin receptors. Serotonin is produced from tryptophan in a reaction requiring tetrahydrobiopterin (BH_4) (Figure 18-1).

A strong association has been found between low levels of serotonin and **depression.** Reduced serotonin may allow levels of catecholamine to drop, leading to depression. The selective serotonin reuptake inhibitors **(SSRIs)** combat this effect by blocking the reuptake of serotonin, therefore increasing the effective concentration. SSRIs, including fluoxetine,

> **QUICK HIT**
> The gut pathogen that most typically causes watery diarrhea is *Vibrio cholera* (rice-water stools.)

> **QUICK HIT**
> Nerves and smooth muscle cells in the gut produce VIP, which causes relaxation of GI smooth muscle, production of pancreatic HCO_3^-, and inhibition of gastric H^+ secretion.

> **QUICK HIT**
> In the CNS, serotonin is produced only in the raphe nuclei of the brainstem and the pineal gland.

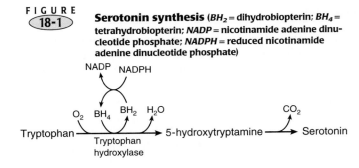

FIGURE
18-1
Serotonin synthesis (*BH$_2$* = dihydrobiopterin; *BH$_4$* = tetrahydrobiopterin; *NADP* = nicotinamide adenine dinucleotide phosphate; *NADPH* = reduced nicotinamide adenine dinucleotide phosphate)

SSRIs have also been used to treat obsessive-compulsive disorder, anorexia, bulimia, and panic disorder.

sertraline, and paroxetine, have been successful in treating depression. The common side effects of these drugs include sexual dysfunction, nausea, and tremors.

The tricyclic antidepressants (TCAs) block not only serotonin reuptake but also norepinephrine reuptake, muscarinic receptors, α_1 receptors, and histamine receptors. These other actions cause a constellation of side effects, which have made the SSRIs a more attractive alternative for depression therapy.

Serotonin also plays a role in migraine headaches. **Migraines** are most common in **women** and patients with a family history of migraines. Characteristics of a migraine attack include **unilateral, pounding pain, often accompanied by nausea and photophobia;** an aura may or may not precede a migraine. In all types of migraine, intracranial and extracranial **vasodilation** seems to be involved in causing the attack.

Perhaps the most effective drug used for migraines is **sumatriptan,** a serotonin agonist at the 5-HT$_{1D}$ receptor. If taken early, this drug can abort an attack. Other drugs used in migraine therapy include the ergot alkaloids (**ergotamine** and **methysergide**), nonsteroidal anti-inflammatory drugs (NSAIDs), and β-blockers (**propranolol**). The ergot derivatives are serotonin antagonists and cause general vasoconstriction. Caffeine enhances their effectiveness by increasing their absorption; caffeine itself is a cerebral vasoconstrictor. Ergotamine and NSAIDs are used in acute attacks, while propranolol and methysergide are used as prophylaxis. The ergot drugs should not be used during pregnancy or in patients with vascular disease.

Smooth muscle

The intestinal wall contains several layers of smooth muscle (inner circular and outer longitudinal). Smooth muscle is also found in the ureter, bladder, eye, uterus, airways, and walls of blood vessels. Smooth muscle, unlike skeletal and cardiac muscle, can sustain high levels of contraction without consuming much energy. Histologically, smooth muscle **lacks the sarcomere** organization of cardiac and skeletal muscle. The sarcomeres are the structural units of these other muscle types and produce a striated appearance under the light microscope. Just like cardiac and skeletal muscle, smooth muscle has myosin, actin, and tropomyosin; however, **troponin is absent.**

Calcium is involved in excitation–contraction coupling in all muscle types, but the mechanisms differ. In smooth muscle, stimulation causes calcium to enter the cytoplasm from outside the cell through voltage-gated channels and also to be released from the sarcoplasmic reticulum through inositol triphosphate (IP$_3$)-gated channels. Calcium binds **calmodulin,** and this complex activates **myosin light-chain kinase** (MLCK). Activated MLCK phosphorylates light chain 20 (LC$_{20}$), which then allows myosin to bind actin and contraction to occur. With contraction, ATP is consumed rapidly, and the muscle shortens. Myosin light-chain phosphatase then dephosphorylates LC$_{20}$, resulting in **latch-bridge** formation. In this state, contraction is maintained with a minimal use of ATP. As stimulation ceases, calcium levels fall, the latch-bridge dissociates, and the muscle relaxes (Figure 18-2).

FIGURE 18-2

Smooth muscle contraction (*IP$_3$* = inositol triphosphate; *LC$_{20}$* = light chain 20; *MLCK* = myosin light-chain kinase; *SR* = sarcoplasmic reticulum)

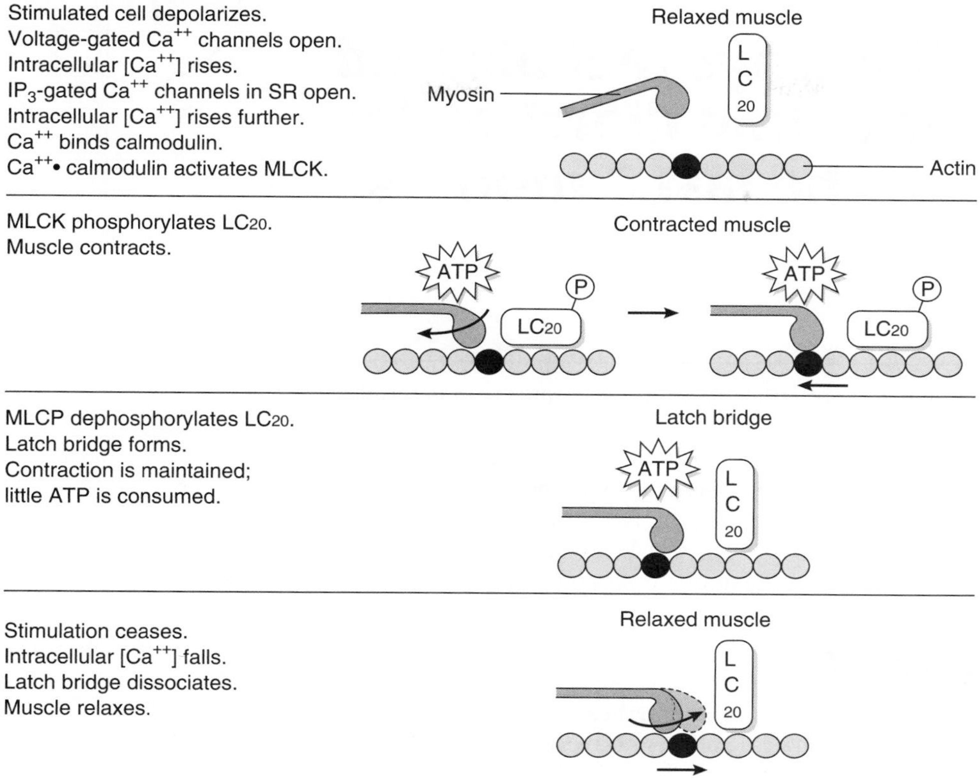

Stimulated cell depolarizes.
Voltage-gated Ca^{++} channels open.
Intracellular [Ca^{++}] rises.
IP$_3$-gated Ca^{++} channels in SR open.
Intracellular [Ca^{++}] rises further.
Ca^{++} binds calmodulin.
Ca^{++}• calmodulin activates MLCK.

Relaxed muscle

Myosin

L C 20

Actin

MLCK phosphorylates LC20.
Muscle contracts.

Contracted muscle

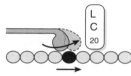

ATP   LC20   (P)   →   ATP   LC20   (P)

MLCP dephosphorylates LC20.
Latch bridge forms.
Contraction is maintained;
little ATP is consumed.

Latch bridge

ATP   L C 20

Stimulation ceases.
Intracellular [Ca^{++}] falls.
Latch bridge dissociates.
Muscle relaxes.

Relaxed muscle

L C 20

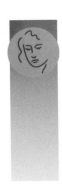

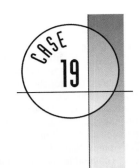

"I always feel bloated and have had diarrhea for the last 3 months."

OBJECTIVES

1. Develop a differential diagnosis and an appropriate workup for chronic diarrhea and flatulence
2. Compare and contrast key features of Crohn disease and ulcerative colitis
3. Understand the causes, diagnosis, and treatment of megaloblastic anemia
4. Learn the lipoproteins and their functions
5. Review familial dyslipidemia
6. Compare and contrast the physiology and treatment of emesis and diarrhea

HISTORY AND PHYSICAL EXAMINATION

A 41-year-old female presents with a 4-month history of **diarrhea**, abdominal pain, and **flatus**. She also reports feelings of extreme weakness and **easy fatigue**. She describes her stools as watery, **grayish in color, frothy, and foul smelling.** She has not noticed any blood or mucus in her stools. She also reports an **unintentional 10-pound loss** over the past 2 months. The patient also complains of extremely cold hands and feet. Abdominal exam reveals a protuberant and tympanic abdomen. An examination of her skin reveals **hyperkeratosis and ecchymoses.**

Her physician suggested she maintain a strict diet with **no wheat, barley, or rice** for the next week.

APPROPRIATE WORKUP

CBC, blood chemistries, D-xylose test, small intestinal biopsy before and after diet control

DIFFERENTIAL DIAGNOSIS

Celiac disease, Whipple disease, tropical sprue, Crohn disease, ulcerative colitis, giardiasis

DIAGNOSTIC LABORATORY TESTS AND STUDIES

CBC: microcytic, hypochromic anemia
Blood chemistry:
Platelets = 240,000/ μL (N)
Prothrombin time (PT) = 20 seconds (H)
Partial thromboplastin time (PTT) =
    30 seconds (N)
Bleeding time = 6 minutes (N)
D-xylose test = abnormal

Small intestinal biopsy (pre):
Villous atrophy of intestinal mucosa,
    elongated crypts, and lymphocytic
    infiltration of the lamina propria
    (Figure 19-1)
Small intestinal biopsy (post):
    Abundant villi throughout the intestinal
    mucosa

FIGURE 19-1 (See also Color Plate 19-1.) Small intestinal biopsy (pre).

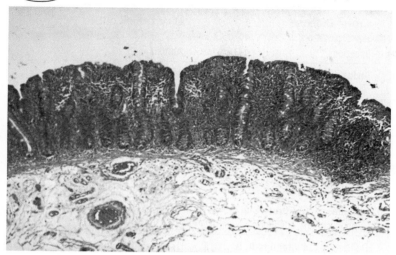

(From Rubin MD, Farber JL. Pathology, 3rd Ed. Philadelphia: Lippincott Williams & Wilkins, 1999.)

DIAGNOSIS: CELIAC DISEASE

Celiac disease (also known as celiac sprue or nontropical sprue) is a **hypersensitivity reaction** of the intestinal mucosa to **gliadin,** a glycoprotein component of gluten, which is present in wheat, barley, and rice. Patients with this disease are required to maintain a **strict diet,** avoiding these foods. Resolution of mucosal damage to the small intestine can occur as soon as a few weeks after maintaining this diet.

Celiac disease is increased in incidence in association with **HLA-DR3** and **HLA-DQw2.** This finding and the presence of antibodies directed against gliadin suggest a **genetic** and **immune-mediated** mechanism. Pathologic findings include **blunting of villi, lymphocytic infiltration** in the lamina propria, and an **abnormal D-xylose test.** This leads to malabsorption of fats and results in **steatorrhea.**

Dermatitis herpetiformis is also associated with celiac sprue. Like the vesicles in herpes simplex, the lesions are arranged in groups and manifest as pruritic erythematous papules on the extensor surfaces of the extremities, trunk, buttocks, scalp, and neck.

Finally, this patient's CBC panel reveals **microcytic, hypochromic anemia** due to a **lack of intestinal iron absorption.** This patient's cool extremities may be related to her anemia. The protuberant and tympanic abdomen is due to distention of intestinal loops with fluids and gas. Osteopenia **(calcium malabsorption)** can cause bone pain for several reasons, including defective calcium transport by the small intestine, vitamin D deficiency, and binding of luminal calcium and magnesium to unabsorbed dietary fatty acids.

The prothrombin time (PT) is prolonged because of **malabsorption of vitamin K.** This patient's ecchymoses is most likely also due to her vitamin K malabsorption while the hyperkeratosis is due to vitamin A malabsorption. Stool examination with the classic Sudan stain reveals **bulky, greasy stools** suggesting **malabsorption of fat.** The oral D-xylose tolerance test can reveal carbohydrate malabsorption. D-Xylose is absorbed preferentially in the proximal small intestine and excreted unmetabolized in the urine. In untreated celiac sprue, urinary D-xylose excretion and peak blood xylose levels are depressed.

EXPLANATION OF DIFFERENTIAL

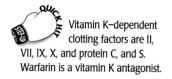

Vitamin K–dependent clotting factors are II, VII, IX, X, and protein C, and S. Warfarin is a vitamin K antagonist.

Whipple disease presents with similar signs and symptoms. However, the intestinal biopsy would reveal lipid vacuolation with infiltration of PAS-positive macrophages and small

Vitamin A is a constituent of retinal (a visual pigment). Deficiency can result in xerophthalmia, keratomalacia, and dry skin.

Classical peripheral neurologic findings suggesting hypocalcemia are the Chvostek or Trousseau signs. The Chvostek sign is elicited by tapping over the facial nerve ~2 cm anterior to the tragus of the ear. Depending on the calcium level, a graded twitching response will occur. The Trousseau sign is observed after inflating the blood pressure cuff above the systolic pressure, causing local ulnar and median nerve ischemia, resulting in carpal spasm.

Crypt abscesses are aggregates of neutrophils in intestinal crypts, or crypts of Lieberkühn.

Metronidazole can also be used to treat *Entamoeba, Trichomonas, Gardnerella vaginalis, Helicobacter pylori* (part of triple therapy).

TABLE 19-1 **Comparison of Crohn Disease and Ulcerative Colitis**

	Crohn Disease	**Ulcerative Colitis**
Etiology	Infectious	Autoimmune
Clinical presentation	Abdominal pain with mild, **nonbloody diarrhea**	Abdominal pain with **bloody and mucoid diarrhea**
Areas involved	**Skip lesions** usually of the small intestine, terminal ileum, and colon	**Continuous lesions** from the colon to the rectum
Gross appearance	**Transmural inflammation** with cobblestone mucosa, creeping fat, and "string sign" on x-ray (wall thickening)	Inflammation and ulceration **limited to the mucosal and submucosal layers;** loss of haustrations ("lead pipe" on barium enema)
Microscopic	**Lymphocytic infiltrate** with noncaseating granulomas	**Crypt abscesses** and pseudopolyps
Complications	Deficiencies **in vitamins A, B_{12}, D, E, and K;** fistulas; migratory polyarthritis	**Toxic megacolon;** colorectal carcinoma; primary sclerosing cholangitis; ankylosing spondylitis
Treatment	Sulfasalazine, antidiarrheal drugs, and glucocorticoids	

bacilli of ***Tropheryma whippelii. Tropical sprue*** presents with the same symptoms *and* intestinal biopsy findings as celiac disease. However, tropical sprue does not resolve with a gluten-free diet. **Crohn disease and ulcerative colitis** are compared in Table 19-1.

Giardiasis is considered to be the most common protozoal pediatric infection in the U.S. Stool culture would reveal **flagellated, binucleate, pear-shaped trophozoites.** The patient would present with **chronic, nonbloody/nonmucoid diarrhea** that is foul smelling. The treatment of choice is **metronidazole.**

Related Basic Sciences

Megaloblastic anemia

Macrocytic, megaloblastic anemia is due to a **deficiency in vitamin B_{12}.** A **Schilling test** can be used to detect B_{12} deficiency. In addition to hematologic effects, vitamin B_{12} deficiency can result in **neurologic symptoms** since B_{12} is a cofactor for **homocysteine methylation** and **methylmalonyl-CoA conversion to succinyl-CoA.** This can be corrected with **folic acid** supplementation. In this smear of peripheral blood with megaloblastic anemia, the erythrocytes are large, often oval, and are associated with poikilocytosis and teardrop shapes. The **neutrophils are hypersegmented** (Figure 19-2).

Lipoproteins

Refer to Table 19-2 for lipoprotein functions and dyslipidemia.

Emesis versus diarrhea

See Table 19-3 for physiology and treatment of vomiting versus diarrhea

Vitamin B_{12} deficiency can be caused by pernicious anemia (lack of intrinsic factor), absent or inflamed terminal ileum (Crohn disease), sprue, enteritis, and *Diphyllobothrium latum.*

FIGURE
19-2

(See also Color Plate 19-2.) Megaloblastic anemia. In this smear of peripheral blood, the erythrocytes are large, often with an oval shape, and are associated with poikilocytosis and teardrop shapes. The neutrophils are hypersegmented.

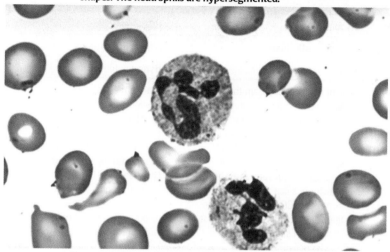

(From Rubin MD, Farber JL. Pathology, 3rd Ed. Philadelphia: Lippincott Williams & Wilkins, 1999.)

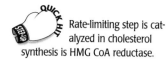 Rate-limiting step is catalyzed in cholesterol synthesis is HMG CoA reductase.

LDL and HDL carry cholesterol in the opposite directions. LDL transfers hepatic cholesterol to the periphery while HDL transfers cholesterol from the periphery to the liver. Elevated LDL levels are a risk factor for atherosclerosis and coronary artery disease (CAD) while high HDL levels are protective against atherosclerosis.

There is a normal anion gap with diarrhea since lost HCO_3^- ions are replaced by chloride ions.

TABLE 19-2 Lipoproteins Functions and associated Dyslipidemia

Lipoprotein	Function	Dyslipidemia
Chylomicron	Transfers **dietary triacylglycerol** to peripheral tissues; synthesizes in intestinal epithelial cells	Type I: hyperchylomicronemia; due to deficiency in lipoprotein lipase or apolipoprotein C-II (an activator of lipoprotein lipase)
HDL	Transfers cholesterol **from the periphery to the liver;** transfers apoprotein C-II and E for chylomicron and VLDL metabolism	—
VLDL	Transfers **hepatic triglycerides to periphery;** digested by **lipoprotein lipase** (VLDL → IDL); synthesized in the liver	Type IIb: combined hyperlipidemia (LDL, VLDL) Type III: dysbetalipoproteinemia (IDL, VLDL) Type IV: hypertriglyceridemia (VLDL) Type V: mixed hypertriglyceridemia (VLDL, chylomicrons)
LDL	Transfers **hepatic cholesterol to periphery**	Type IIa: hypercholesterolemia (LDL); excess causes atherosclerosis and xanthomas Type IIb: combined hyperlipidemia (LDL, VLDL)
IDL	Formed from degradation of VLDL; transfers cholesterol and triglycerides to liver where VLDL → LDL	Type III: dysbetalipoproteinemia (IDL, VLDL)

TABLE 19-3 Physiology and Treatment of Vomiting versus Diarrhea

	Vomiting	Diarrhea
Loss	H^+ ions	HCO_3^- ions
Primary acid-base disorder	Metabolic **alkalosis**	Metabolic **acidosis**
Compensation	**Hypo**ventilation	**Hyper**ventilation
Associated physiology	Loss of chloride ions from the stomach along with H^+ ions results in volume contraction and hypochloremia $\rightarrow \downarrow$ renal perfusion pressure $\rightarrow$ renin-angiotensin-aldosterone (RAA) system activated $\rightarrow$ Volume contraction **worsens metabolic alkalosis** since angiotensin II increases HCO_3^- reabsorption in the kidney and aldosterone causes increased distal H^+ secretion	Diarrhea $\rightarrow$ volume contraction $\rightarrow \downarrow$ arterial pressure $\rightarrow$ activate baroreceptor reflex $\rightarrow \uparrow$ sympathetic firing $\rightarrow \uparrow$ **pulse rate and cutaneous vasoconstriction** Diarrhea $\rightarrow$ volume contraction $\rightarrow \uparrow$RAA system $\rightarrow$ increased distal potassium secretion $\rightarrow$ **hypokalemia**
Treatment	**NaCl** to correct volume contraction and **potassium** to replace K^+ lost in urine	**Replace lost fluids** and **electrolytes**, especially Na^+, K^+, and HCO_3^-

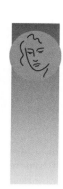

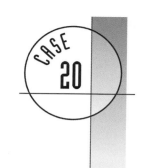

"I get tired easily. I am losing weight, and am often nauseated."

OBJECTIVES

1. Develop a differential diagnosis and an appropriate workup for fatigue, weight loss, and skin pigmentation
2. Review the structure and function of the adrenal gland
3. Understand the effects of adrenal hypofunction with direct damage to the gland and over- and underproduction of hormones

HISTORY AND PHYSICAL EXAMINATION

A 39-year-old woman complains of **nausea** and **becoming easily fatigued** for the past 3 months. During this same period, **she has lost 10 pounds.** Upon questioning, she states that she also has been **vomiting** excessively, and generally **"doesn't have much of an appetite."** She denies smoking or a family history of cancer. The patient has not been sexually active for the past 2 years; for 15 years before, she was married and in a monogamous relationship. Her blood pressure is 100/70 mm Hg reclined and 80/60 mm Hg standing (orthostatic hypotension). She is 5'5" and weighs 105 pounds. **Increased pigmentation** is noted on her knuckles, knees, and elbows, as well as on her palmar creases. Her areolae are bluish-black. Axillary and pubic hair is sparse. There is no lymphadenopathy.

APPROPRIATE WORKUP

Blood chemistries, HIV test, PPD test, chest X-ray, and abdominal CT

DIFFERENTIAL DIAGNOSIS

Addison disease, AIDS, occult cancer, hemochromatosis, pituitary hypofunction

DIAGNOSTIC LABORATORY TESTS AND STUDIES

Blood chemistry:
Hgb = 16 g/dL (H)
Hct = 53% (H)
Na^- = 110 mEq/L (L)
K^+ = 6.1 mEq/L (H)
HCO_3^- = 19 mEq/L (L)
BUN = 24 mg/dL (H)
Fasting glucose = 45 mg/dL (L)
Serum ferritin = 200 ng/mL (N)
Plasma cortisol (morning) = 3 mg/dL (L)
plasma corticotropin (ACTH)
    (morning) = 200 pg/mL (H)

HIV test:
Negative result
Purified protein derivative (PPD) test:
Negative results
Chest radiograph:
Normal lungs
Small heart
CT:
Noncalcified and small adrenal glands

DIAGNOSIS: ADDISON DISEASE

Primary adrenocortical insufficiency, or **Addison disease,** results from dysfunction or destruction of the adrenal cortices. The cause is unknown, but an **autoimmune** process may be responsible for approximately 70% of cases. **Tuberculosis (TB)** and other granulomatous infections, tumors, and amyloidosis can also cause adrenal destruction.

Clinical manifestations result from **deficiencies of cortisol, aldosterone,** and **dehydroepiandrosterone (DHEA),** which are the products of the adrenal cortex. Skin **hyperpigmentation** is usually seen in skin creases and on exposed areas, mucous membranes, bony prominences, and scars. The hyperpigmentation results from increased melanocyte-stimulating hormone (MSH), a by-product of adrenocorticotropic hormone (ACTH) synthesis by the pituitary gland. When the adrenal cortex is impaired, cortisol synthesis is decreased. Because cortisol controls ACTH production by negative feedback, ACTH levels increase.

The lack of cortisol production also contributes to orthostatic hypotension. Cortisol has a mild pressor effect on the heart and vasculature. Hypoglycemia also develops, because cortisol aids in gluconeogenesis. Cortisol deficiency can also produce GI symptoms (e.g., nausea, vomiting, and anorexia) and subsequent weight loss. A life-threatening shock state of vascular collapse may result because increased cortisol is necessary in times of stress.

Aldosterone, the final step in the renin–angiotensin–aldosterone (RAA) system, maintains blood pressure by stimulating sodium resorption in the distal tubule. Aldosterone deficiency causes sodium loss, hyponatremia, hypovolemia, decreased cardiac output, decreased renal blood flow, and azotemia. Such changes cause weakness, hypotension, and weight loss. Because aldosterone also stimulates potassium secretion, aldosterone deficiency can also cause hyperkalemia, which can lead to cardiac dysrhythmia.

Definitive diagnosis of Addison disease is achieved with cortisol and ACTH testing: **cortisol levels are low and ACTH levels are high.** Hyponatremia, hyperkalemia, hypoglycemia, and increased eosinophil count are present but not specific to Addison disease. A small heart may be seen on chest radiograph. Treatment of Addison disease is with glucocorticoid and mineralocorticoid replacement therapy.

QUICK HIT

High doses of exogenous steroids suppress the release of CRH and ACTH, and rapid withdrawal of these drugs can precipitate hypoglycemia and shock. It takes time for the adrenals to begin synthesizing cortisol again, so the dose of steroids must be slowly tapered down.

EXPLANATION OF DIFFERENTIAL

Approximately 17% of patients with **AIDS** have cortisol resistance and adrenal insufficiency and can present with associated symptoms. The negative HIV test results rule out AIDS in this case.

Cancer may produce symptoms of fatigue, unexplained weight loss, and anorexia. **Bronchogenic carcinoma,** which is more common in **smokers** than nonsmokers, can also present with increased pigmentation. The normal lungs on chest radiograph in combination with the physical examination point away from cancer.

Hemochromatosis, a disease of **increased iron storage,** is usually familial and idiopathic. It can also occur secondary to conditions that require regular transfusions, such as β-thalassemia major. Typical presenting manifestations include **cirrhosis, diabetes mellitus,** and **increased skin pigmentation (termed bronze diabetes).** Ferritin levels generally also are increased. If diagnosed early, hemochromatosis can be treated by regular phlebotomy to remove excess iron.

Pituitary hypofunction, or **secondary adrenocortical insufficiency,** can present with many of the same symptoms and signs as Addison disease because the adrenal cortex is under the control of the pituitary gland. ACTH levels, however, would be decreased, and skin pigmentation would not be increased. Aldosterone would not be decreased with pituitary hypofunction because the RAA system works independently of the pituitary gland.

Related Basic Science

Adrenal gland

The two adrenal glands sit atop the kidneys. The cortex is derived from mesoderm of the posterior body wall, while the medulla is derived from neural crest cells. Because they are involved in steroid hormone synthesis, the cells of the cortex have abundant smooth endoplasmic reticulum (ER). The **chromaffin cells** of the medulla produce **epinephrine (EPI) and norepinephrine (NEPI)** and are under the control of the sympathetic nervous system.

The adrenal cortex is organized into cords of cells and divided into three zones. The outermost zone is called the **zona glomerulosa.** The cells of the zona glomerulosa produce **aldosterone** and are under the control of the RAA system. In the middle is the zona fasciculata, while the innermost zone is called the **zona reticularis.** These inner two zones of the cortex are under pituitary control through ACTH. ACTH release is itself under the control of **corticotropin-releasing hormone (CRH)** from the hypothalamus. The fasciculata cells, which make cortisol, are the most numerous in the adrenal cortex. The reticularis cells make DHEA, a weak androgen, and small amounts of other sex steroids. Figure 20-1 summarizes the organization and functions of the adrenal cortex.

The adrenal medulla is part of the **sympathetic nervous system,** which tends to act on the body in a coordinated fashion. The parasympathetic system, on the other hand, can activate discrete organ systems (such as stimulating intestinal motility without affecting heart rate). The **sympathetic preganglionic cell** is **cholinergic,** derived from **neuroectoderm,** and found in the intermediolateral cell column of the spinal cord at thoracic and upper lumbar levels. This neuron synapses via a **nicotinic receptor** on a postganglionic neuron in the sympathetic chain. The **postganglionic cell** is derived from **neural crest,** and is usually **adrenergic (releases NEPI).**

The **chromaffin cells** of the adrenal medulla are modified **postganglionic cells.** As such, they are derived from **neural crest cells** and innervated by sympathetic preganglionic nerves that pass through the sympathetic chain and synapse directly on the chromaffin cells. These cells of the adrenal medulla act just like sympathetic postganglionic cells, except they produce **mostly EPI** and release it into the systemic circulation.

FIGURE 20-1   **The adrenal cortex**

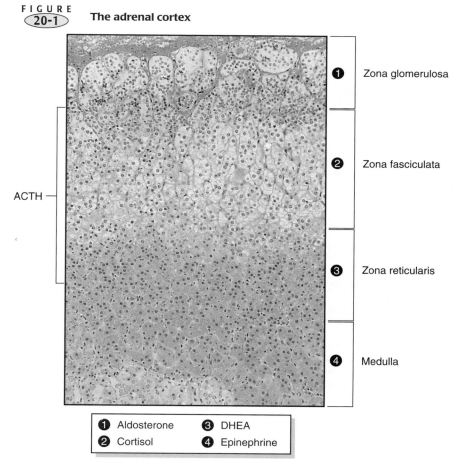

ACTH

- ❶ Zona glomerulosa
- ❷ Zona fasciculata
- ❸ Zona reticularis
- ❹ Medulla

❶ Aldosterone		❸ DHEA	
❷ Cortisol		❹ Epinephrine	

(From Berman I. Color Atlas of Basic Histology, 2nd Ed. New York: McGraw-Hill, 1998, p 261.)

QUICK HIT
Other exceptions to the normal structure of the sympathetic nervous system are the dopaminergic innervation of the renal vasculature and the muscarinic innervation of sweat glands.

Adrenal hypofunction

Adrenal hypofunction can progress slowly or acutely and can result from damage to the adrenal gland itself or to the pituitary. Also, a deficiency in the production of one hormone can cause overproduction of another, as in the case of the adrenogenital syndromes (Figure 20-2).

Addison disease affects the adrenal gland directly. **Waterhouse-Friderichsen syndrome,** which is acute adrenal insufficiency and circulatory collapse from hemorrhagic necrosis of the adrenals, is another example of direct damage. This syndrome is usually associated with meningococcemia secondary to meningococcal meningitis. Damage to the pituitary can indirectly compromise adrenal function. Destruction of the pituitary is called pituitary cachexia or Simmonds disease. For example, a nonsecretory **pituitary adenoma** can grow and crush other parts of the gland. ACTH levels fall and adrenal production of cortisol decreases. Ischemic damage to the pituitary caused by bleeding and shock during childbirth may cause postpartum pituitary necrosis, or **Sheehan syndrome.** In this disease, gonadotropin-releasing hormone (GnRH) and thyrotropin typically decrease first, followed by a fall in ACTH levels.

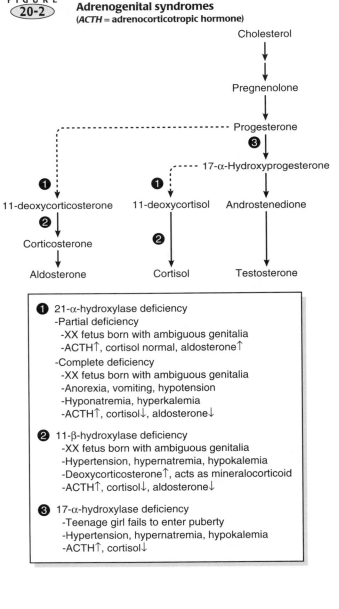

FIGURE 20-2

Adrenogenital syndromes
(*ACTH* = adrenocorticotropic hormone)

❶ 21-α-hydroxylase deficiency
 -Partial deficiency
  -XX fetus born with ambiguous genitalia
  -ACTH↑, cortisol normal, aldosterone↑
 -Complete deficiency
  -XX fetus born with ambiguous genitalia
  -Anorexia, vomiting, hypotension
  -Hyponatremia, hyperkalemia
  -ACTH↑, cortisol↓, aldosterone↓

❷ 11-β-hydroxylase deficiency
 -XX fetus born with ambiguous genitalia
 -Hypertension, hypernatremia, hypokalemia
 -Deoxycorticosterone↑, acts as mineralocorticoid
 -ACTH↑, cortisol↓, aldosterone↓

❸ 17-α-hydroxylase deficiency
 -Teenage girl fails to enter puberty
 -Hypertension, hypernatremia, hypokalemia
 -ACTH↑, cortisol↓

Deficiencies in the enzymes involved in cortisol synthesis can lead to **congenital adrenal hyperplasia** syndromes. Cortisol is responsible for feedback inhibition of the release of both CRH and ACTH. With deficient cortisol synthesis, ACTH levels rise, causing hyperplasia of the adrenal cortex. The precursors of cortisol can accumulate and spill into adrenal androgen synthesis pathways, leading to virilization of the female fetus. The different forms of congenital adrenal hyperplasia are also called the adrenogenital syndromes.

A complete or partial deficiency of 21-α-hydroxylase causes the most common adrenogenital syndrome (about 95% of cases). In half of these cases, 21-α-hydroxylase is only partially deficient (simple virilizing form), and the hyperplastic adrenal cortex can maintain normal cortisol levels. The adrenal androgens are overproduced, however, leading most notably to virilization of the female genitalia (enlarged clitoris with fusion of the labia). Complete deficiency of 21-α-hydroxylase (salt-wasting form) hampers production of both cortisol and aldosterone. Girls with this deficiency are born with ambiguous genitalia, hyponatremia, and hypotension. Figure 20-2 summarizes the adrenal hormone synthetic pathways and the result of deficiencies in these pathways.

QUICK HIT

Patients with partial 21-α-hydroxylase deficiency have elevated aldosterone levels but have normal sodium and volume status. This is because aldosterone is elevated to balance the effects of increased progesterone and 17-hydroxyprogesterone, both of which act as mineralocorticoid antagonists.

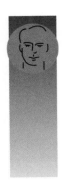

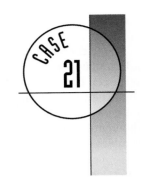

"My skin is changing color!"

OBJECTIVES

1. Develop a differential diagnosis and an appropriate workup for change in skin color
2. Understand iron absorption, transfer, and storage
3. Learn drugs and diseases that decrease iron absorption
4. Review iron-associated pathologies and the trends in iron studies
5. Compare and contrast the fed versus fasting states biochemically
6. Be able to identify basic anatomic structures on an abdominal CT

HISTORY AND PHYSICAL EXAMINATION

A 40-year-old Caucasian male presents with generalized joint pain and fatigue for the past 5 months. He has also noticed that his **skin is tanned** despite the fact he has little sun exposure. He is concerned that he and his wife have been **unable to conceive** for the past year and a half. His mother died during childbirth and his father passed away due to cardiac and liver complications at the age of 60. Sometimes he experiences his "heart beating funny" and, to improve his health, has recently joined a local gym. He does not smoke but drinks socially on the weekends. He has never had a blood transfusion.

Palpation of joints reveals tenderness and swelling over all major joints. Abdominal exam is significant for **hepatosplenomegaly and ascites**. There is also **atrophy of both testicles**. An eye exam was unremarkable.

APPROPRIATE WORKUP

Blood chemistries, liver biopsy, abdominal CT, and EKG

DIFFERENTIAL DIAGNOSIS

Hemochromatosis, Wilson disease, hemolytic anemia, β-thalassemia

DIAGNOSTIC LABORATORY TESTS AND STUDIES

Blood chemistry:
    Glucose = 310 mg/dL (H)
    Iron = 750 g/dL (H)
    Ferritin = 365 ng/mL (H)
    Iron binding capacity = 190 µg/dL (L)
    Testosterone = 280 ng/dL (L)
    Reticulocyte count = 1.0% (N)

Liver biopsy:
    Elevated hepatic iron content
        (150 µmol/g of dry weight)
CT, abdomen:
    Increased liver density
EKG:
    Figure 21-1: EKG

FIGURE 21-1 EKG. Atrial fibrillation

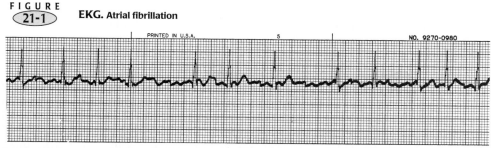

(From Smeltzer SC, Bare BG. Textbook of Medical-Surgical Nursing, 9th Ed. Philadelphia: Lippincott Williams & Wilkins, 2000.)

DIAGNOSIS: HEMOCHROMATOSIS

Hemochromatosis is the **abnormal accumulation of iron** in parenchymal organs, leading to organ toxicity. Iron accumulation can reach up to 50 g. However, since only a few extra milligrams are absorbed per day, it may take many years before the symptoms of hemochromatosis are evident. Hemochromatosis is the most common inherited liver disease in Caucasians and the most common **autosomal recessive** genetic disorder. This genetic defect results in **increased intestinal absorption of iron** in excess of iron loss. It can also be acquired in the presence of hemolytic anemia. Patients exposed to **repeated perfusions**, such as with **sickle cell disease** and **β-thalassemia**, are at increased risk of accumulating excessive iron. In addition, certain types of anemias (i.e., sideroblastic anemia) can stimulate excessive intestinal absorption of iron.

This patient also presents with ascites. Deposition of excessive iron within the liver causes **cirrhosis** leading to **hypoalbuminemia** and **portal hypertension**, both of which contribute to ascites. He complained of palpitations as well, which may be due to iron deposition in the heart which can lead to **restrictive cardiomyopathy** and **pulmonary edema** due to impaired cardiac output. The EKG in Figure 21-1 is classic for **atrial fibrillation** with no discrete P waves in between irregularly spaced QRS complexes. The blood glucose levels are elevated because increased iron is deposited in the pancreas, destroying islet cells and causing type 2 diabetes mellitus. Finally, this patient presents with testicular atrophy and a history of impotence. This also is due to increased iron stores deposited in the hypothalamus causing decreased secretion of GnRH and hence decreased pituitary LH and FSH secretion. This patient's initial change in skin pigmentation is due to deposition of iron in the form of hemosiderin in the skin which produces a "bronze" skin discoloration. Arthropathy is due to iron accumulation in joint tissues. Hemochromatosis can be treated with the **iron chelator deferoxamine. Repeated phlebotomy** can also reduce total body iron stores.

EXPLANATION OF DIFFERENTIAL

Wilson disease is also an **autosomal recessive** disease but manifests earlier in life (between the ages of 6 and 29 years). Insufficient synthesis of **ceruloplasmin** and impaired biliary copper excretion results in **copper deposition** specifically in the **liver, cornea, and lenticular nuclei.** As a result, **degeneration of the putamen and globus pallidus** (part of the lenticular nuclei) creates a Parkinson-like syndrome with dysarthria, spasticity, and tremors. A liver biopsy would reveal **elevated copper,** piecemeal necrosis, and lymphocytosis which can progress to **cirrhosis.** In this patient, the eye exam was unremarkable. Patients with Wilson disease can present with deposits of copper in the corneal limbus, called **Kayser-Fleischer rings.** In the patient's blood chemistries, free serum copper would be elevated while total serum copper levels would be low. Ceruloplasmin, which is deficient in Wilson disease, normally binds plasma copper. In its absence, total plasma copper is low while free plasma copper is elevated which is associated

QUICK HIT Patients with hemochromatosis are predisposed to developing portal hypertension and hence esophageal varices. This can also develop in alcoholics.

QUICK HIT Hemochromatosis is more likely to present in women postmenopausally. Prior to menopause, women's menstruation and subsequent iron loss keeps iron levels controlled.

QUICK HIT There is an increased incidence of hepatocellular carcinoma with hemochromatosis, hepatitis B and C, Wilson disease, alcoholic cirrhosis, carcinogens, and α_1-antitrypsin deficiency.

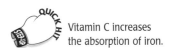

Patients with hemochromatosis can develop primary hypothyroidism due to iron deposition in the thyroid gland. Secondary hypothyroidism can develop if iron deposits accumulate in the pituitary reducing TSH secretion.

Because the liver is the major site of detoxification of drugs and poisons, it is are rich in smooth endoplasmic reticulum with detoxification as its primary purpose.

Wilson disease leads to **copper** accumulation in the liver (increased ceruloplasmin) whereas **hemochromatosis** causes **iron** to accumulate in the liver (increased hemosiderin).

Vitamin C increases the absorption of iron.

Antacid overdose can present with the following side effects:

Aluminum hydroxide: constipation
Magnesium hydroxide: diarrhea
Calcium carbonate: hypercalcemia

Cimetidine, a H_2-receptor blocker, is a potent p-450 inhibitor, and can cause gynecomastia, galactorrhea, decreased sperm count and decreased renal excretion of creatinine.

with the pathology of Wilson's disease. Treatment includes copper chelation with lifelong use of **D-penicillamine. Oral zinc,** which competes with copper for intestinal absorption, can also be used with copper chelation therapy.

Hemolytic anemia would have presented with a different blood chemistry profile. The patient's **reticulocyte count would have been elevated** as his bone marrow attempts to replace lost RBCs in conditions such as glucose-6-phosphate dehydrogenase (G6PD) deficiency, congenital spherocytosis, and Rh-hemolytic disease of the newborn. Hemolysis can be intravascular or extravascular. **Intravascular hemolysis** occurs when RBCs are lysed within blood vessels which spill hemoglobin into the bloodstream (hemoglobinemia) and urine (hemoglobinuria). Splenic macrophages or liver Kuppfer cells that destroy RBCs result in **extravascular hemolysis.**

β-Thalassemia is due to impaired synthesis of the beta subunit of hemoglobin. Homozygous β-thalassemia is clinically more severe with earlier presentation whereas heterozygous β-thalassemia is less severe and would have presented later in life. Anemia is usually microcytic with accelerated destruction of deformed RBCs (polymerization and precipitation of excessive alpha globin subunits). The blood chemistry would have been **normal for iron, TIBC, and ferritin.** On eye exam, **scleral icterus** may be noted as unconjugated hyperbilirubinemia secondary to RBC hemolysis deposits in the sclera.

Related Basic Sciences

Iron Absorption, Transfer, and Storage

Iron is absorbed in the proximal duodenum. Gastric acid lowers the pH in the proximal duodenum, enhancing the solubility and uptake of ferric iron (Fe^{3+}) and converting it to ferrous iron (Fe^{2+}), which is more readily absorbed by enterocytes. When gastric acid production is impaired (i.e., with proton pump inhibitors), iron absorption is reduced substantially. Iron is transported in the blood bound to serum protein **transferrin,** endocytosed into cells, and stored intracellularly complexed to the protein ferritin. If **ferritin** is saturated, it is degraded to hemosiderin. **Total iron-binding capacity (TIBC)** indicates the maximum amount of iron needed to saturate plasma or serum transferring. Therefore, TIBC is usually elevated when total body iron stores are low. See Table 21-1 for drugs and diseases that decrease iron absorption.

Trends of Iron Studies in Iron-Associated Pathologies

Trends of iron studies in iron associated pathologies are listed in Table 21-2.

Fed vs. Fasting State

Please refer to Figure 21-2.

TABLE 21-1 Drugs and Diseases That Decrease Iron Absorption	
Drugs	Antacids
	Histamine H_2-receptor blockers
	Proton pump inhibitors
	Tetracyclines
	Levodopa/methyldopa
	Penicillamine
	Quinolones
Diseases	Celiac disease
	Crohn disease
	Pernicious anemia
	Gastric surgery

TABLE 21-2 **Iron Studies in Iron-Associated Pathologies**

Disease	Iron	Ferritin	TIBC
Hemochromatosis[a]	↑	↑	↓
Iron deficiency	↓	↓	↑
Anemia of chronic disease	↓/N	↑	↓
Thalassemia major	N	N	N
Sideroblastic anemia	↑	↑	↓

[a]Measuring transferrin saturation in hemochromatosis patients is the initial test of choice.
↑, increased, ↓, decreased, N, normal.

CT of the abdomen

It important to be familiar with the basic anatomic structures on a CT of the abdomen. Questions may require identification of a structure on a CT and relate to associated pathologies.

FIGURE 21-2 **Fed versus fasting state**

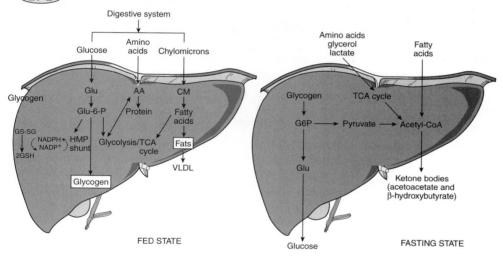

FIGURE
21-3   **Abdominal CT**

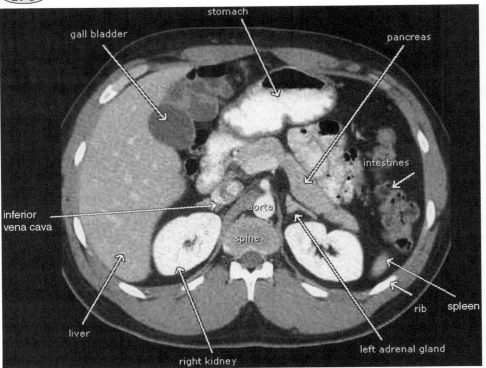

(From Dean D, Herbener TE. Cross-sectional Human Anatomy. Baltimore: Lippincott Williams & Wilkins, 2000.)

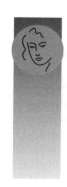

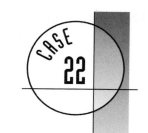
"When I urinate, it hurts and burns."

OBJECTIVES

1. Develop a differential diagnosis and an appropriate workup for dysuria
2. Compare and contrast the clinical presentation and lab findings of acute and chronic renal failure
3. Understand the clinical features, pathogenesis, and progression of acute tubular necrosis and interstitial nephritis
4. Learn key features of common urinary tract infectious agents

HISTORY AND PHYSICAL EXAMINATION

An 18-year-old woman comes to the ED complaining of severe diffuse abdominal pain for the past few hours. For the past several days, she states that she has had a **painful, burning sensation** when she **urinates.** In addition, the **urge to urinate comes on suddenly,** and when she is finished urinating, she feels like she **did not completely empty her bladder.** She denies any changes in bowel movements, but she has noted a **red tinge** to her urine. She **denies flank pain.** She has had multiple **sexual partners** over the past few months and states that her partners do not always wear condoms. She denies the use of tobacco products or illegal drugs, but states that she drinks five or six wine coolers on the weekends. She is taking no medications and has no allergies. She has a history of treated chlamydial and gonorrheal infections. Currently, she has a **low-grade fever** and is normotensive with tachycardia and tachypnea. The patient experiences some mild, lower pelvic discomfort with palpation, but has no costovertebral angle tenderness.

APPROPRIATE WORKUP

Blood chemistries, abdominal ultrasound, urinalysis, and culture

DIFFERENTIAL DIAGNOSIS

Appendicitis, ectopic pregnancy, incarcerated hernia, pelvic inflammatory disease (PID), pyelonephritis, UTI

DIAGNOSTIC LABORATORY TESTS AND STUDIES

Blood chemistry:
WBC = 9,000/mm^3 (N), β-HCG negative
Urinalysis:
Pyuria (12 neutrophils/hpf)
Bacteriuria (150,000 bacteria/mL)
No WBC casts
Culture:
Gram-positive cocci in clusters (catalase positive, coagulase negative)

Ultrasound (US):
No signs of obstruction in abdomen
No ectopic pregnancy in fallopian tubes
Normal appearance of uterus and ovaries

DIAGNOSIS: URINARY TRACT INFECTION WITH *STAPHYLOCOCCUS SAPROPHYTICUS*

UTIs are most commonly caused by *Escherichia coli;* however, in young sexually active women, *S. saprophyticus* is a common cause. UTIs are **more common in women** because the female urethra is shorter and in closer proximity to the anus than in men (Figure 22-1). Risk factors for developing a UTI include obstruction leading to urinary stasis, vesicoureteral reflux, catheterization, pregnancy, and diabetes mellitus. The typical presentation of a UTI is **burning and pain during urination, urgency, sensation of incomplete bladder emptying, blood** in the urine, and **abdominal pain** or cramping. Urinalysis often reveals **pyuria** (>5 neutrophils per high power field on microscope) and **bacteriuria** (>100,000 bacteria/mL).

FIGURE 22-1 Important anatomical structures of the perineum

A. **Male perineum**

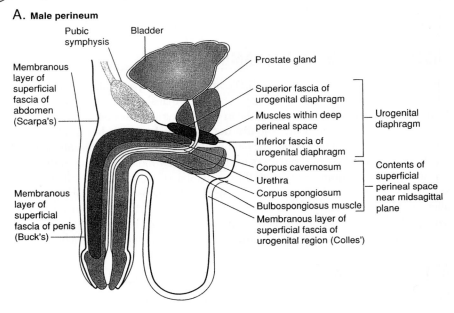

B. **Female perineum**

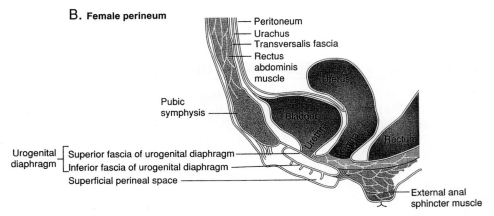

(From Mehta S, Milder EA, Mirarchi AJ. Step-Up: A High-Yield, Systems-Based Review for the USMLE Step 1. Philadelphia, Lippincott Williams & Wilkins, 2000, p 156.)

EXPLANATION OF DIFFERENTIAL

Appendicitis results from an **obstruction of the lumen of the appendix,** most commonly from a **fecalith.** Once the obstruction is established, bacteria proliferate and invade the mucosa. The patient presents with **anorexia, nausea,** and **abdominal pain.** The abdominal pain typically starts out diffuse or at the umbilicus, but can localize to the right lower quadrant as the inflammation progresses (**McBurney point**). An **abdominal US** can be used to identify an obstruction or rule out gynecologic causes for the pain.

Ectopic pregnancies result from implantation of an embryo in **extrauterine locations,** most often the **fallopian tubes.** As the fetus grows, it may cause pain, discomfort, local rupture, hemorrhage, shock, or death. Patients often have a history suggestive of pregnancy, but may also complain of lower abdominal pain or vaginal bleeding. β-**Human chorionic gonadotropin (hCG)** would be **positive** in patients with an ectopic pregnancy, and an **US** examination would localize the pregnancy to an extrauterine location.

Incarcerated hernias result from occlusion of blood flow to bowel protruding through a weak area in the abdominal wall, such as the groin. Incarcerated hernias can cause diffuse, **"crampy"** abdominal pain, abdominal distention, a **silent abdomen** (no bowel sounds), and an **elevated WBC count.** Groin hernias are 25 times **more likely in men** than women and can be further classified as inguinal or femoral. Indirect inguinal hernias are more common and more often become incarcerated than direct hernias. The terms **"direct"** and **"indirect"** refer to the **location** (**medial** or **lateral,** respectively) of the hernia with respect to the **inferior epigastric** vessels. Femoral hernias are more common in women.

PID, an infection of the reproductive organs and their supportive tissues, is commonly caused by *Neisseria gonorrhoeae* or *Chlamydia trachomatis. N. gonorrhoeae* is a **Gram-negative cocci** that causes infection via its **endotoxin** and **pili.** *C. trachomatis* is an **intracellular organism** that exists in various strains (**strains D-K** cause chlamydia and nongonococcal urethritis). Because women are typically asymptomatic during initial infection, the bacteria ascend and cause widespread infection of the pelvic organs. If untreated, **infertility** can result because of scarring of the fallopian tubes. PID typically presents with lower abdominal pain, fever, malaise, vaginal discharge, urinary discomfort, and **adnexal tenderness.** Patients can exhibit the **"chandelier sign"** on physical examination of the cervix and vagina. A cervical swab can detect the presence of *N. gonorrhoeae,* while a cervical scraping is required to detect *C. trachomatis.* Patients infected with gonococcus or chlamydia should have **themselves and their sexual partners treated** for the infection. Also, **coinfection** is common with these two organisms.

Pyelonephritis is caused by an **ascending UTI,** typically resulting from vesicoureteral reflux. Infection may also spread **hematogenously** to the kidney. The causative agent is most commonly *E. coli.* Clinical features include **flank pain, costovertebral angle tenderness,** dysuria, fever, chills, nausea, vomiting, and diarrhea. Urinalysis would reveal bacteriuria, pyuria, and **WBC casts.**

Related Basic Science

Renal failure

Acute renal failure is a rapid, potentially **reversible** decline in renal function resulting in the accumulation of nitrogenous waste in the body. Disorders of the **renal parenchyma** (e.g., nephrotoxicity, acute tubular necrosis) (Table 22-1), **prerenal** conditions [e.g., congestive heart failure [CHF] or GI bleeding 9, and **postrenal** complications (e.g., obstruction) can result in **decreases in glomerular filtration rate (GFR),** resulting in **increased BUN and creatinine levels.** Patients often exhibit urinary volume derangement, and numerous complications can result from lack of treatment or vigorous fluid resuscitation. **Chronic renal failure,** most often caused by **hypertension** or **diabetes mellitus,** is an **irreversible** loss of renal function to less than 20% of normal. Chronic renal failure results in **uremia,** which has systemic manifestations, including CHF, hypotension, lethargy, nausea, and anorexia.

QUICK HIT — Asymptomatic bacteriuria is more likely to advance to pyelonephritis in pregnant women than in non-pregnant women.

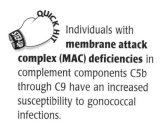

QUICK HIT — Individuals with **membrane attack complex (MAC) deficiencies** in complement components C5b through C9 have an increased susceptibility to gonococcal infections.

QUICK HIT — Infection by strains A-C of chlamydia can result in blindness, while strains L1-L3 can cause lymphogranuloma venereum.

TABLE 22-1	Acute Tubular Necrosis vs. Interstitial Nephritis	
	Acute Tubular Necrosis	**Interstitial Nephritis**
Clinical Features	**Most common cause of acute renal failure**	Acute interstitial renal inflammation leading to acute renal failure
Pathogenesis	• **Renal ischemia** caused by hypotension or shock • Myoglobinuria from crush injuries or intense exercise • Toxic substances such as mercuric chloride, cyclosporine, and IV contrast	• **Drug-induced:** most commonly penicillin derivatives (such as methicillin), NSAIDs, diuretics, captopril, trimethoprim • Autoimmune etiology
Progression	• Reversible if treated • **Fatal if untreated**	Resolves upon withdrawal of offending agent

IV, intravenous; NSAIDs, nonsteroidal anti-inflammatory drugs.

> **QUICK HIT**
> Casts in the urine signify kidney disease. Along with pyelonephritis, **WBC casts** are seen in tubulointerstitial disease. **RBC casts** result from nephritic syndrome, while nephritic syndrome and fat embolism cause **fatty casts** in the urine. Acute tubular necrosis causes **muddy brown casts** and **renal tubular epithelial cell casts.**

Chronic pyelonephritis

Untreated ascending UTIs can lead to **"thyroidization of the kidney,"** which is a histologic description of **chronic pyelonephritis.** When untreated, bacteria (Table 22-2) can result in coarse, asymmetric scarring and deformity of the renal pelvis and calyces. This gross destruction of the kidney can impair renal function.

> **QUICK HIT**
> Fanconi syndrome, a generalized dysfunction in the proximal convoluted tubules, is characterized by impaired resorption of glucose, amino acids, phosphate, and bicarbonate. It can be hereditary or acquired.

TABLE 22-2	Common Infectious Agents of the Urinary Tract	
Agent	**Characteristics**	**Pathogenicity**
Escherichia coli	• **Most common** cause of UTI, resulting from contamination of the genital area with feces • More common in **women** because of the proximity of the anus to the urethra and the short length of the urethra • Can cause cystitis, pyelonephritis, and prostatitis	• Attaches to mucosa via **pili** • **Endotoxin** (LPS) causes inflammation • Host factors include urinary obstructions, sexual intercourse, catheters, diaphragms, and voiding impairment
Staphylococcus saprophyticus	• Causes **"honeymoon cystitis"** (UTI in young sexually active women) • **Gram-positive cocci** arranged in **clusters** • Nonhemolytic, **catalase positive,** and **coagulase negative** • Lacks protein A	Adheres to **uroepithelial cells**
Proteus mirabilis	• Major cause of **nosocomial and community infections** • Gram-negative, motile short rod • Opportunistic infection	• **Urease** positive • Causes stone formation, leading to obstruction
Enterococcus faecalis	• Leading cause of **nosocomial UTIs** • Can cause **septicemia** and **endocarditis** • Normal intestinal and oral flora • Facultative-anaerobic, Gram-positive coccus • Bacitracin resistant	**Resistant to many antibiotics**

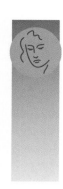

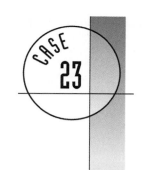
"I'm having difficulty swallowing, and I lost 10 pounds in 1 month."

OBJECTIVES

1. Develop a differential diagnosis and appropriate workup for dysphagia and weight loss
2. Review the innervation and blood supply of the GI tract
3. Understand the physiology associated with esophageal motility
4. Learn the causes, clinical presentation, and diagnosis of Chagas disease
5. Understand the significance of antinuclear antibodies (ANA) and factors that increase ANA levels

HISTORY AND PHYSICAL EXAMINATION

A 38-year-old female complains of recent **difficulty swallowing** both solids and liquids. She has also noticed **substernal pain** after eating and an **unintentional 10-pound loss** in the past month. For the past week, her symptoms have worsened with **regurgitation of food when lying down.** She must therefore elevate the head of her bed and **sleep in a sitting position.** Two weeks ago, she had to miss several days of work because she had **pneumonia.** Physical exam was unremarkable.

APPROPRIATE WORKUP

Barium swallow, esophageal manometry, and CBC panel

DIFFERENTIAL DIAGNOSIS

Hirschsprung disease, GERD, Barrett's esophagus/esophageal carcinoma, achalasia, scleroderma

DIAGNOSTIC LABORATORY TESTS AND STUDIES

Barium swallow:
   Figure 23-1: Barium swallow
Esophageal manometry:
   Increased lower esophageal sphincter (LES) pressure with incomplete LES relaxation in response to swallowing and aperistalsis in lower esophagus
CBC:
   Negative for antinuclear antibodies (ANAs)

FIGURE
23-1   **Barium swallow.**

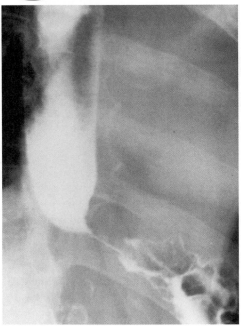

(From Eisenberg RL. Clinical Imaging: An Atlas of
Differential Diagnosis, 4th Ed. Philadelphia: Lippincott
Williams & Wilkins, 2003.)

DIAGNOSIS: ACHALASIA

Achalasia is a motility disorder of the esophagus due to the **loss of the myenteric (Auerbach's) plexus** (nonadrenergic, noncholinergic, inhibitory ganglion cells), causing an imbalance between excitatory and inhibitory neurotransmission. The myenteric plexus mediates receptive relaxation of the LES in response to a food bolus and distal esophageal peristalsis. In achalasia barium swallow shows a **dilated esophagus** with an area of **LES stenosis** or a **hypertensive, nonrelaxed esophageal sphincter.** This is due to failure of the LES to relax and the distal esophagus to undergo peristalsis causing food to accumulate and dilate the lower esophagus. Complications of achalasia include **esophageal squamous cell carcinoma,** diverticula, aspiration pneumonia, and candidal esophagitis. This patient's bout of **pneumonia** is probably due to **aspiration** of undigested esophageal contents perhaps while asleep.

Treatment includes **balloon dilatation** or **botulinum toxin injection**. Since tonic constriction of the LES is due to vagal cholinergic innervation, botulinum toxin inhibits the release of ACh from nerves, reducing the LES tone.

EXPLANATION OF DIFFERENTIAL

Hirschsprung disease is a **congenital megacolon** due to a failure of the **neural crest cells** that form the **myenteric plexus** to migrate in the colon. Therefore, there is a lack of the enteric nervous system on intestinal biopsy. Patients present with **chronic constipation** and the colon proximal to the aganglionic segment is dilated. Figure 23-2 shows a barium enema of a patient with Hirschsprung. This looks similar to the barium swallow with achalasia, but the location is entirely different with Hirschsprung disease in the megacolon while achalasia and GERD affecting the lower esophagus.

GERD is due to abnormal relaxation of the LES in which it is **atonic, or permanently relaxed,** allowing for reflux of acidic or bilious gastric contents into the esophagus.

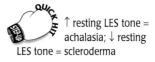
Upper third of the esophagus is **skeletal muscle, middle third** is both **skeletal and smooth muscle,** and lower third is smooth muscle. The **upper third** of the esophagus is innervated by the **vagus nerve** and is the only location in the body where skeletal muscle is not under voluntary control. The **lower third** of the esophagus is innervated by the **splanchnic nerve.**

↑ resting LES tone = achalasia; ↓ resting LES tone = scleroderma

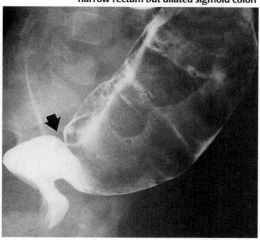

FIGURE 23-2 **Barium enema, Hirschsprung disease.** Barium enema studies in lateral view show transition zone (arrow) with narrow rectum but dilated sigmoid colon

(From Fleisher GR, Ludwig S., Henretig, F., et al. Textbook of Pediatric Emergency Medicine, 5th Ed. Philadelphia: Lippincott Williams & Wilkins, 2006.)

Patients can present with a history of chest discomfort after meals, a substernal burning sensation that is exacerbated upon assuming a supine position.

GERD can also cause **Barrett esophagus** with replacement of nonkeratinized, stratified squamous epithelium with gastric columnar epithelium in the distal esophagus. This is an example of **metaplasia** where one cell type is replaced with another. Barrett esophagus can lead to **esophageal carcinoma.** Other risk factors include **alcohol, smoking, esophageal webs** (i.e., **Plummer-Vinson**), and diverticula (i.e., **Zenker diverticulum**).

Scleroderma is due to excessive **fibrosis and collagen deposition.** It is more prevalent among females and can be diffuse or part of the **CREST syndrome. Diffuse scleroderma** involves the skin with rapid progression and visceral involvement. **Anti-Scl 70 antibody** would have also been present. CREST is a pneumonic for **c**alcinosis, **R**aynaud phenomenon, **e**sophageal dysmotility, **s**clerodactyly, and **t**elangiectasia. There is limited skin involvement with an **elevation in anticentromere antibody.** In this patient, the CBC was unremarkable for antibodies. Moreover, the CREST syndrome would have presented with additional findings besides esophageal dysmotility.

Figure 23-3 is a summary of the differential diagnosis and their respective GI locations.

> **QUICK HIT** Hyperplasia is an increase in the number of cells while dysplasia is an abnormal growth of cells, commonly preneoplastic, with loss of cell shape, size, and orientation.

Related Basic Science

Innervation and Blood Supply of the GI Tract

See Figure 23-4 for innervation and blood supply of the GI tract.

Esophageal Motility

The LES is normally tonically constricted, creating an intraluminal pressure of approximately 30 mm Hg which prevents the reflux of gastric contents into the esophagus. LES pressure and relaxation are regulated by excitatory (ACh and substance P) and inhibitory (NO and VIP) neurotransmitters. As part of the swallowing reflex, the upper esophageal sphincter (UES) relaxes to allow food to enter the esophagus. A peristaltic contraction creates an area of high pressure behind the food bolus propelling the food toward the LES which relaxes as food approaches. This relaxation is vagally mediated with the **neurotransmitter VIP,** which has several major functions. VIP **produces relaxation of GI smooth muscle,** especially the LES. It also **stimulates pancreatic HCO_3^- secretion** and **inhibits gastric H^+ secretion.**

F I G U R E
23-3

Summary of the differential diagnosis (Asset provided by Anatomical Chart Company.)

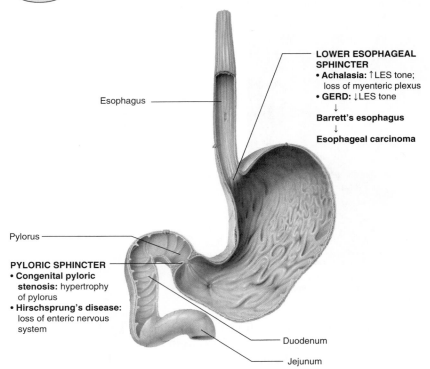

Esophagus

LOWER ESOPHAGEAL SPHINCTER
- **Achalasia:** ↑LES tone; loss of myenteric plexus
- **GERD:** ↓LES tone
  ↓
Barrett's esophagus
  ↓
Esophageal carcinoma

Pylorus

PYLORIC SPHINCTER
- **Congenital pyloric stenosis:** hypertrophy of pylorus
- **Hirschsprung's disease:** loss of enteric nervous system

Duodenum

Jejunum

F I G U R E
23-4

Innervation and blood supply of the GI tract

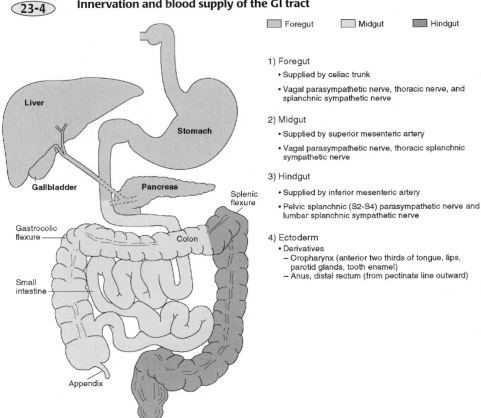

☐ Foregut   ☐ Midgut   ■ Hindgut

Liver

Stomach

Gallbladder

Pancreas

Splenic flexure

Gastrocolic flexure

Colon

Small intestine

Appendix

Rectum

1) Foregut
- Supplied by celiac trunk
- Vagal parasympathetic nerve, thoracic nerve, and splanchnic sympathetic nerve

2) Midgut
- Supplied by superior mesenteric artery
- Vagal parasympathetic nerve, thoracic splanchnic sympathetic nerve

3) Hindgut
- Supplied by inferior mesenteric artery
- Pelvic splanchnic (S2-S4) parasympathetic nerve and lumbar splanchnic sympathetic nerve

4) Ectoderm
- Derivatives
  - Oropharynx (anterior two thirds of tongue, lips, parotid glands, tooth enamel)
  - Anus, distal rectum (from pectinate line outward)

(Reprinted with permission from Mehta S, Milder EA, Mirarchi AJ: Step-Up: A High-Yield, Systems-Based Review for the USMLE Step 1 Examination, 2nd Ed. Philadelphia: Lippincott Williams & Wilkins, 2003, p 111.)

Chagas' disease

Achalasia in Chagas' disease is due to destruction of the **myenteric (Auerbach) plexus** in the esophagus by the protozoan parasite ***Trypanosoma cruzi*** and transmitted by the **reduviid bug.** In Chagas' disease, the myenteric plexus of the colon may be destroyed, causing **toxic megacolon.** In the acute stage, patients can develop either a nodular lesion or furuncle (chagoma) at the site of the bite. Conjunctival contamination with the vector's feces results in unilateral painless palpebral and **periocular swelling (Romaña sign)** and associated lymphadenopathy of nodes draining the lesion. Other symptoms include prolonged fever, tachycardia, fatigue, anemia, weakness, hepatosplenomegaly, lymphadenopathy, and myocarditis. The acute stage lasts 4 to 8 weeks and in rare cases may include myocarditis or meningoencephalitis. Lab findings include anemia, lymphocytosis, thrombocytopenia, and occasional autoimmune abnormalities. Electrocardiograms are abnormal with **A/V blocks** common. **Cardiomyopathy** in Chagas' disease is typically biventricular without pulmonary edema and often has tricuspid incompetence.

Antinuclear Antibodies

Antinuclear antibodies (ANAs) bind to certain structures within the nucleus of cells. They are autoantibodies that are frequently present in people with the following conditions:

- systemic lupus erythematosus
- collagen vascular disease
- myositis
- Sjögren syndrome
- scleroderma
- Hashimoto thyroiditis
- juvenile diabetes mellitus
- vitiligo
- glomerulonephritis
- Addison disease
- pulmonary fibrosis
- chronic liver disease
- pernicious anemia
- rheumatoid arthritis

Medications can also stimulate the production of ANAs, specifically **procainamide,** **hydralazine,** and **phenytoin,** which cause a lupus-like syndrome.

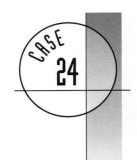

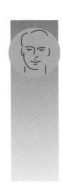

"I have a bump on my neck, and I've lost 20 pounds in 3 months."

OBJECTIVES

1. Develop a differential diagnosis and an appropriate workup for a nontender, enlarged node and unintentional weight loss
2. Learn the three grades of non-Hodgkin lymphomas and their associated clinical presentation
3. Review the histological findings, clinical presentation, and prognosis of cutaneous and adult T-cell lymphomas and Langerhans cell histiocytosis
4. Understand the anatomy and function of the lymphatic system

HISTORY AND PHYSICAL EXAMINATION

A 29-year-old man comes in complaining of **fever, night sweats, weight loss,** and a bump in his neck. He does not complain of a sore throat. He is otherwise healthy, with no significant past medical or surgical history. He has made no change to his diet, and he recalls no trauma to his neck. Physical examination reveals a unilateral **nontender enlarged node** in his cervical chain. The patient believes that it has grown steadily since he first noticed it about 1 month ago. His pharyngeal mucosa appears normal.

APPROPRIATE WORKUP

Blood chemistries, HIV test, and biopsy of lymph node

DIFFERENTIAL DIAGNOSIS

Congenital cyst, HIV infection, Hodgkin disease, infectious mononucleosis (mono), non-Hodgkin lymphoma (NHL), toxoplasmosis

DIAGNOSTIC LABORATORY TESTS AND STUDIES

Blood chemistry:
  Hgb = 10.5 g/dL (L)
  ESR = 25 mm/h (H)
  Lymphocytes = 20% (L)
  Eosinophils = 5% (H)

HIV test:
  Negative results
Biopsy of lymphatic nodule:
  See Figure 24-1 for findings.

FIGURE
24-1 **Classic Reed-Sternberg cell in Hodgkin disease**

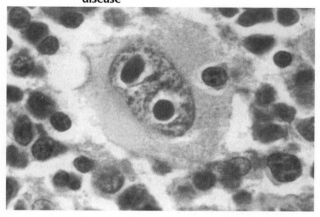

(From Mehta S, Milder EA, Mirarchi AJ. Step-Up: A High-Yield, Systems-Based Review for the USMLE Step 1. Philadelphia: Lippincott Williams & Wilkins, 2000, p 330.)

DIAGNOSIS: HODGKIN DISEASE

Hodgkin disease is a **malignant neoplasm of lymphoid tissue** and one of the most common cancers to affect **young adults.** It affects men more frequently than women. The initial presentation can mimic an inflammatory process (fever, inflammatory infiltrates) or acute infection (fever, leukocytosis, diaphoresis). This patient had a palpable nodule in his cervical lymphatic chain, but this finding is not universal. The neoplasm can arise in mesenteric nodes and cause no symptoms for a long period. It also can affect the mediastinal nodes; in such cases, wheezing and cough may be the presenting symptoms. Mediastinal involvement is especially common in the nodular sclerosis subtype (see below).

According to the Rye classification, the four subtypes of Hodgkin disease, listed from best prognosis to worst, are lymphocyte predominance, nodular sclerosis, mixed cellularity, and lymphocyte depletion. The mixed cellularity subtype is most common overall; the nodular sclerosis subtype is more common in women than men. The **Reed-Sternberg cell** (see Figure 24-1) is found in all subtypes.

The Ann Arbor system (Table 24-1) typically defines the staging of Hodgkin disease. Today, the survival rates for stages I and II approach 100%.

EXPLANATION OF DIFFERENTIAL

A **congenital cyst** in the neck can present as a **slowly enlarging painless mass** or, if infected, an **acutely swollen and tender mass. Branchial cysts,** remnants of the second or third branchial pouches, are located along the anterior border of the sternocleidomastoid muscle. **Thyroglossal duct cysts** appear in the midline anywhere along the path of descent of the thyroglossal duct, which descends from the tongue to form the primordium of the thyroid gland.

QUICK HIT
In general, tumors are staged based on the **TNM** system: local extension of the **T**umor, involvement of lymph **N**odes, and **M**etastases.

TABLE 24-1 Ann Arbor Staging of Hodgkin Disease

Stage I	Single lymph node region involved
Stage II	Two or more lymph node regions on the same side of the diaphragm involved
Stage III	Lymph node regions on both sides of the diaphragm involved
Stage IV	Extralymphatic organs involved

An uninfected cyst can remain asymptomatic, or it may gradually fill with fluid and debris and appear as a slowly growing painless mass in the neck, usually during young adulthood. An infected cyst, which presents acutely as a swollen and painful mass, may occur at any time, including infancy and childhood. This patient's neck mass was solid, not cystic, and located in the cervical lymphatic chain, not in the typical locations of congenital cysts.

HIV infection often causes a **mononucleosis-like syndrome with lymphadenopathy** early in the disease, years before immunodeficiency develops. A patient infected with HIV would have positive ELISA and Western Blot test results, and the node biopsy would show nonspecific follicular hyperplasia of the germinal centers, not Reed-Sternberg cells.

Mono, a lymphoproliferative disease, results from the Epstein-Barr virus. Mono, which typically presents in young adults, is usually benign and self-limited. It can progress to a B-cell lymphoma, however, in immunocompromised patients. Common clinical manifestations of mono include fatigue, **fever,** generalized **lymphadenopathy, sore throat,** and **splenomegaly.** Elevated white blood cell counts with abundant atypical T lymphocytes are common. These two characteristics are not seen in this case.

NHLs can present with generalized painless lymphadenopathy, but without Reed-Sternberg cells. This patient's lymphadenopathy is localized, and the biopsy showed Reed-Sternberg cells, which confirms the diagnosis of Hodgkin disease. The NHLs are discussed and compared with Hodgkin disease below.

Toxoplasma gondii is an **intracellular** parasite that in healthy adults causes toxoplasmosis, a benign mono-like disease with lymphadenopathy, sore throat, and fever. In the **fetus** and **immunocompromised** patients, however, toxoplasmosis can be more severe. The disease is often contracted from eating **raw meat** or handling **cat litter.** Transmission to the fetus occurs transplacentally and can result in fetal CNS damage, abortion, or stillbirth. An infected fetus may be born healthy only to develop chorioretinitis years later, which can lead to blindness. With immune deficiency, a latent infection can reactivate, often in the CNS. Weight loss, night sweats, and Reed-Sternberg cells are not found in toxoplasmosis.

Related Basic Science

Non-Hodgkin lymphomas

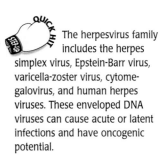

The herpesvirus family includes the herpes simplex virus, Epstein-Barr virus, varicella-zoster virus, cytomegalovirus, and human herpes viruses. These enveloped DNA viruses can cause acute or latent infections and have oncogenic potential.

NHLs are malignant tumors originating from lymphoid tissue. Table 24-2 summarizes the different NHLs; the many types have varying prognoses. The **follicular small-cleaved** type is **most common.** All NHLs defined as follicular are B-cell lymphomas. Most diffuse NHLs are B-cell lymphomas as well, but some are of T-cell origin. Table 24-2 does not show all the working formulation types. Those listed are grouped by grade and common presentation.

Cutaneous T-cell lymphomas

This group includes mycosis fungoides and Sézary syndrome. These **tumors of peripheral T helper cells** (CD4+) usually involve the **skin.** The neoplastic T cells have a characteristic "cerebriform" nucleus with multiple infoldings. Patients with **mycosis fungoides** typically present with an erythematous, eczema-like skin manifestation progressing to formation of plaques. A biopsy of these lesions shows a dermal infiltrate of the characteristic neoplastic T helper cells. **Sézary syndrome** presents with exfoliative erythroderma and circulating T cells, with the characteristic cerebriform nucleus.

Adult T-cell leukemia/lymphoma

This disease is caused by human T-cell leukemia virus type 1 (**HTLV-1**), a **retrovirus** endemic to Japan and the Caribbean. Affected patients present with **generalized lymphadenopathy, skin lesions, hepatosplenomegaly, hypercalcemia,** and an **elevated white cell count.** Characteristic findings of the leukemic cells are elevated IL-2 receptor levels and multilobed "cloverleaf" nuclei. Affected patients have a median survival of 8 months. Some patients, however, follow an indolent course clinically similar to that of the cutaneous T-cell lymphomas.

TABLE 24-2 Non-Hodgkin Lymphomas

Grade	Working Formulation Type	Typical Presentation	Notes
LOW	Small lymphocytic	**Elderly patient with generalized painless lymphadenopathy;** bone marrow, liver, and spleen often involved	Closely resembles chronic lymphocytic leukemia
	Follicular predominantly small cleaved	**Elderly patient with generalized painless lymphadenopathy;** bone marrow the only extranodal site commonly involved; indolent course but refractory to treatment	Associated with **bcl-2** oncogene, an apoptosis inhibitor that results from t(14;18), **most common**
INTERMEDIATE	Diffuse large	**Elderly patient with a rapidly growing extranodal mass** (usually in brain, bone, GI tract, or skin); bone marrow rarely involved; aggressive course but responsive to therapy	Usually of B-cell origin; **wide age range** affected
HIGH	Lymphoblastic lymphoma	**Young man with a mediastinal mass;** closely related to T-cell acute lymphocytic leukemia	Neoplastic cells resemble intrathymic T cells
	Small noncleaved, "Burkitt lymphoma"	**Child with rapidly growing mass in mandible** (African type) **or abdomen** (American type); biopsy shows a **"starry sky" pattern** related to B-cell acute lymphocytic leukemia	Associated with **Epstein-Barr virus** and **c-myc** [a transcriptionalactivator overexpressed by t(8;14)]

Langerhans cell histiocytosis

These diseases stem from tumorous growths of the Langerhans cells of the skin, also called histiocytes. These cells are found in the epidermis, where they act much like macrophages, ingesting foreign material and functioning as antigen-presenting cells. Histopathologically, the lesions show clusters of Langerhans cells with certain typical features: S100 and **CD1** cell markers, indented nuclei, and **Birbeck granules** (which look like tennis rackets on electron microscopy).

In increasing order of severity, the three types of histiocytosis are eosinophilic granuloma, Hand-Schüller-Christian disease, and Letterer-Siwe disease. **Eosinophilic granuloma** usually presents as a **solitary lesion in the skull,** sometimes in the lung. This disease has the best prognosis and sometimes resolves without treatment. **Hand-Schüller-Christian** disease presents with the triad of **diabetes insipidus, skull lesions,** and **exophthalmos.** It usually strikes children younger than 5 years of age. **Letterer-Siwe** disease, an aggressive and often fatal illness, usually affects young children. The widespread signs include lymphadenopathy, pancytopenia, pulmonary involvement, hepatosplenomegaly, and chronic infections.

QUICK HIT Like all antigen-presenting cells, Langerhans cells possess major histocompatibility complex (MHC II) receptors.

QUICK HIT Perhaps the most important tumor drainage pattern is that of **breast cancer.** If a breast tumor has metastasized, the tumor will most likely be found in the ipsilateral **axillary nodes.**

QUICK HIT Nascent chylomicrons have only apoprotein (apo) B-48, but later receive apo E and apo C$_{II}$ from high-density lipoprotein (HDL) to become "mature."

Lymphatic system

The lymphatic system serves several functions, including immune system activity, recirculation of interstitial fluid, and absorption of lipids. It plays a role in many disease processes, especially cancer metastasis. Understanding the pattern of lymph drainage becomes very important when treating malignant tumors. Lymphadenopathy is an important, albeit nonspecific, finding when diagnosing disease.

The lymphatic system starts as blind-ended vessels found in connective tissue, especially under the epithelium and mucous membranes. These vessels are very permeable and absorb fluid, cells, and debris from the interstitial space. All lymph from below the diaphragm enters the **thoracic duct,** which is the largest lymphatic vessel in the body. The thoracic duct and the lymphatics from the left half of the body above the diaphragm drain into the venous system at the point where the subclavian and internal jugular veins meet. At this same point on the right side, all the lymph from the right half of the body above the diaphragm enters the venous blood. In this way, fluid is returned from the interstitial space.

Pathologic states can overwhelm the capacity of the lymphatic system. In certain situations, excessive amounts of fluid are lost from the vascular space to the interstitium. Possible causes include a lack of plasma proteins or decreasing plasma oncotic pressure (nephrotic syndrome, liver disease) and increased hydrostatic pressure in the capillaries and veins (congestive heart failure). The result is fluid accumulation and edema.

The lymphatic system is also necessary for absorption of lipids. The triglycerides synthesized in the intestinal mucosal cells are packaged into **chylomicrons.** The chylomicrons are released into the lymphatic vessel found at the center of the intestinal villus, called the central lacteal. Because of the lymphatic drainage pattern described above, all chylomicrons travel through the thoracic duct and enter the venous blood on the left side.

Lymph nodes act as checkpoints through which the lymph must pass before entering the bloodstream. Here, dendritic cells ingest foreign substances and present them to lymphocytes. Antigenic substances initiate an immune response. Figure 24-2 shows the general architecture of a lymph node.

FIGURE 24-2 **(See also Color Plate 24-2.) Blood from the afferent vessels are filtered through the lymph node before being recollected and exiting via the efferent vessel**

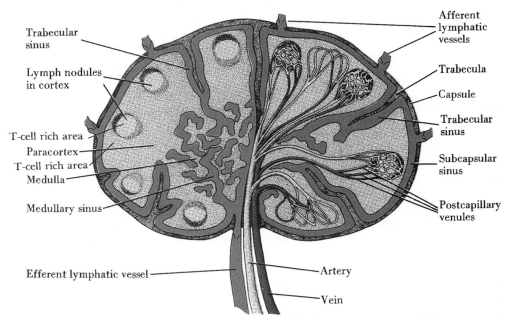

Trabecular sinus

Lymph nodules in cortex

T-cell rich area
Paracortex
T-cell rich area
Medulla

Medullary sinus

Efferent lymphatic vessel

Afferent lymphatic vessels

Trabecula

Capsule

Trabecular sinus

Subcapsular sinus

Postcapillary venules

Artery

Vein

(From Ross MH, Romrell LJ, Kaye GI. *Histology: A Text and Atlas, 3rd Ed.* Philadelphia: Lippincott Williams & Wilkins, 1995, p 343. Based on Bloom W, Fawcett DW. A Textbook of Histology, 10th Ed. Philadelphia: WB Saunders, 1975, p 473.)

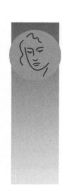

"It hurts when I use the bathroom and I have to go too often! My back also hurts."

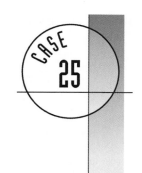
OBJECTIVES

1. Develop a differential diagnosis and appropriate work up for dysuria, frequency of urination, and back pain
2. Review the development of male and female genitalia from common embryological structures
3. Compare and contrast major abdominal hernias
4. Understand the physiology associated with calcium regulation and the role of hormones in calcium homeostasis

HISTORY AND PHYSICAL EXAMINATION

A 33-year-old female presents with complaints of **pain when she urinates, frequent urination,** and a feeling that she **cannot completely void** for the past day. She has also noticed severe **lower back pain** that radiates to the lower abdomen and has felt really warm lately. She denies any blood in her urine. Movement does not affect the pain. She does not recall any family history of renal disease. She is taking Tylenol to relieve her symptoms.

On physical exam, her fever is 103°F. There is **suprapubic** and **costovertebral angle (CVA) tenderness**. Pelvic exam was unremarkable.

APPROPRIATE WORKUP

Blood chemistries, urinalysis, abdominal X-ray and ultrasound (US)

DIFFERENTIAL DIAGNOSIS

Diabetes, acute pyelonephritis, acute appendicitis, nephrolithiasis, acute pancreatitis

DIAGNOSTIC LABORATORY TESTS AND STUDIES

Blood chemistry:
Glucose = 90 mg/dL (N)
WBCs = 11,000/mm^3 (N)
BUN = 15 mg/dL (N)
Creatinine = 1.2 mg/dL (N)
Amylase = 60 U/L (N)
Calcium = 9 mg/dL (N)
Parathyroid hormone
    (PTH) = 400 pg/mL (N)

Urinalysis:
WBCs (H)
Bacteria: present
WBC casts: present
Abdominal radiograph:
Normal
Abdominal ultrasound:
Normal

DIAGNOSIS: ACUTE PYELONEPHRITIS

Acute pyelonephritis results from bacterial invasion of the **renal pelvis or parenchyma.** This most often occurs because of ascending infection from the lower urinary tract. The microorganisms that cause acute pyelonephritis are the same as those that cause lower UTI. *Escherichia coli* is the most common etiological organism. In sexually active young women, infection with *Staphylococcus saprophyticus* accounts for the second most common cause. Clinical features include **flank pain radiating to the iliac fossae and suprapubic area,** CVA tenderness, dysuria, fever, chills, nausea, vomiting, and diarrhea. Urinalysis is usually significant for **bacteriuria, pyuria, and WBC casts.** Pyelonephritis is **more common in women** secondary to a shorter urethra which allows for easier ascension of UTIs. **WBC casts** are virtually pathognomic for acute pyelonephritis.

EXPLANATION OF DIFFERENTIAL

Pyelonephritis can be the initial presentation of previously undiagnosed **diabetes.** Patients with diabetes are more likely to have **bacteruria** and **recurrent urinary tract infections**. Blood glucose would have been high on the blood chemistries to confirm this diagnosis.

In **acute appendicitis,** the patient would have presented with **pain centralized around the umbilicus** that would later **shift to the right iliac fossa.** Pain is aggravated by movement, and on abdominal exam patients exhibit **guarding and rebound tenderness** with palpation of **McBurney's point** (one-third the distance from the anterior superior iliac spine to the umbilicus). Patients with this diagnosis have a history of pain for a few hours, not days, as is the case with this patient. Lab tests would reveal **leukocytosis** and an abdominal CT scan would have indicated a **thickened, inflamed appendix.** If untreated, perforation, peritonitis, and abdominal abscess formation are potential complications.

Nephrolithiasis is secondary to **hypercalcemia** that form **calcium stones** and can completely obstruct the ureter or ureteric pelvis. Hydrostatic pressure is increased, decreasing the net filtration pressure in the glomerulus and resulting in a decline in the GFR. Obstruction of urine flow from a kidney can result in **hydronephrosis** with significant **dilation of the renal pelvis** and **calyces** (Figure 25-1). Clinical presentation of obstruction of ureter with a kidney stone includes **unilateral flank pain radiating to the groin,** tender abdomen to palpation, and **gross hematuria with no red or white cell casts.** Microscopy would **reveal calcium oxalate stones;** an **intravenous pyelogram** that is able to visualize the kidneys, ureters, and bladder would confirm the diagnosis. Blood chemistries would also indicate hypercalcemia.

Causes of hypercalcemia include **primary hyperparathyroidism, malignancy-induced hypercalcemia, hypervitaminosis D, and the milk-alkali syndrome** in which excessive

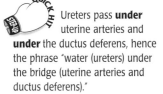 Hypospadias, the abnormal opening of the penile urethra on the ventral (inferior) side of the penis, is due to a failure of the urethral folds to close. Uncorrected, it can lead to UTIs in males.

Dysuria, frequent urination, and urgency in men could suggest prostatic hypertrophy. Urinary retention and stasis of urine can facilitate bacterial overgrowth.

Lactobacillus is part of the normal vaginal flora and functions to maintain a low pH, hence preventing growth of pathogens. Patients taking antibiotics are at increased risk of developing UTIs with *Lactobacilli* suppression and an overgrowth of *C. albicans* (the most common cause of yeast infections).

Pregnant women with normally asymptomatic bacteriuria are at increased risk of developing bacteremia, sepsis, and pyelonephritis with the latter increasing the risk of premature delivery.

Ureters pass **under** uterine arteries and **under** the ductus deferens, hence the phrase "water (ureters) under the bridge (uterine arteries and ductus deferens)."

WBC casts = acute cystitis and pyelonephritis (inflammation in renal interstitium, tubules, and glomeruli)
RBC casts = glomerular inflammation, ischemia, or malignant hypertension
Hyaline casts = normal
Waxy casts = chronic renal failure

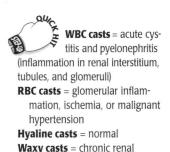

FIGURE 25-1

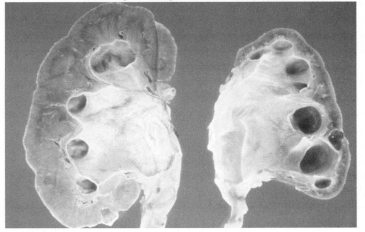

Hydronephrosis. Bilateral urinary tract obstruction has led to conspicuous dilatation of the ureters, pelves, and calyces; The kidney on the right shows severe parenchymal atrophy

(From Rubin E, Farber JL. Pathology, 3rd Ed. Philadelphia: Lippincott Williams & Wilkins, 1999.)

calcium and calcium carbonate (alkali) are ingested. Hyperparathyroidism increases urine calcium concentration to a lesser extent because parathyroid hormone also stimulates renal tubular calcium reabsorption. **Malignancies** can metastasize to bone and cause lysis or secrete a **parathyroid hormone-related peptide (PTHrP).**

Struvite stones, composed of **magnesium ammonium phosphate**, precipitate at a higher pH. *Proteus mirabilis* and *Klebsiella* **produce urease** which hydrolyzes urea, yielding ammonia, bicarbonate, and carbonate, leading to alkaline urine and allowing for crystal formation. Staghorn calculi continue to grow in size, leading to infection, obstruction, or both. Stones cause pain which is **worse on movement.**

Acute pancreatitis is inflammation of the pancreas secondary to **alcohol abuse, mumps, hyperlipidemia, didanosine,** or **gallstones.** Gallstones can lodge in the common bile duct, obstructing the flow of bile into the intestine and backing bile back into the pancreatic duct irritating and inflaming the pancreatic tissue. Patients present with severe **epigastric abdominal pain** radiating to the back, nausea, vomiting, and fever. Lab tests reveal **elevated amylase, lipase,** and **hypocalcemia.** Increased lipases result in **fat necrosis** as pancreatic lipases liquefy fat cell membranes and destroy cells.

Related Basic Sciences

Male and female genital homologues (Figure 25-2)

Abdominal hernias

Diaphragmatic hernias occur when abdominal structures enter the thorax because of a defective development of the **pleuroperitoneal membrane.** The most common diaphragmatic hernia is a protrusion of the stomach through the **esophageal hiatus** of the diaphragm (at T10). A **direct hernia** protrudes through the **inguinal triangle,** medial to the inferior epigastric artery. The inguinal triangle is also known as the **Hasselbalch triangle**

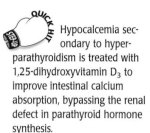

Carcinoid tumors, which secrete **serotonin,** are most common in the appendix. Elevated levels of **5-HIAA** in the urine would confirm the diagnosis.

Hypocalcemia secondary to hyperparathyroidism is treated with 1,25-dihydroxyvitamin D_3 to improve intestinal calcium absorption, bypassing the renal defect in parathyroid hormone synthesis.

Decreased urinary pH increases the concentration of uric acid, facilitating crystallization. Acetazolamide increases urinary pH and hence dissolves uric acid stones.

Chronic pancreatitis can lead to insulin-dependent diabetes as beta cells of the islets of Langerhans are destroyed.

FIGURE 25-2   **Male and female genital homologues**

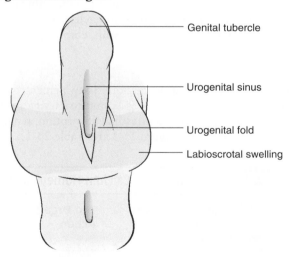

- Genital tubercle
- Urogenital sinus
- Urogenital fold
- Labioscrotal swelling

Male		Female
	Dihydrotestosterone ◄————► Estrogen	
Glans penis	Genital tubercle	Glans clitoris
Corpus spongiosum	Urogenital sinus	Vestibular bulbs
Bulbourethral glands (of Cowper)	Urogenital sinus	Greater vestibular glands (of Bartholin)
Prostate gland	Urogenital sinus	Urethral and paraurethral glands (of Skene)
Ventral shaft of penis (penile urethra)	Urogenital folds	Labia minora
Scrotum	Labioscrotal swelling	Labia minora

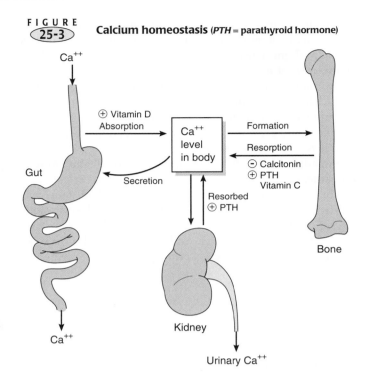

FIGURE 25-3 **Calcium homeostasis** (*PTH* = parathyroid hormone)

QUICK HIT
Salivary and pancreatic amylases are both key to carbohydrate digestion. Salivary amylase starts digestion in the mouth by hydrolyzing α-1,4 linkages. Pancreatic amylase is in the duodenal lumen hydrolyzing starches to oligosaccharides, maltose, and maltotriose.

QUICK HIT
Pancreatic insufficiency can result in malabsorption with steatorrhea. Fat intake must be limited and signs of vitamins A, D, E, and K (fat-soluble vitamin deficiency) should be closely monitored.

QUICK HIT
The femoral nerve is the only structure in "NAVEL" that lies outside of the femoral sheath.

QUICK HIT
A positive calcium balance (in which calcium absorption exceeds urinary excretion) can be seen in growing children, while a negative calcium balance is seen in pregnant women and in women who are breastfeeding.

which is formed by the anatomic borders of the **inguinal ligament, inferior epigastric artery, and lateral aspect of the rectus abdominis muscle.** It is more common in elderly men. **Indirect hernias** are more common in **infants** and occur due to a failure of the **processus vaginalis** to close. They enter the internal inguinal ring lateral to the inferior epigastric artery. Finally, **femoral hernias** result when abdominal structures protrude through the femoral canal, below and lateral to the pubic tubercle. From the superior anterior iliac spine (lateral) to the pubic tubercle (medial), the structures in order are the femoral **n**erve, femoral **a**rtery, femoral **v**ein, **e**mpty space, and **l**ymphatics **(NAVEL).**

Calcium regulation

Calcium is essential to bone formation. Sixty percent of the total calcium in blood is **unbound** (free, ionized), and 40% is bound to plasma proteins. Free calcium is biologically active. Hormones affecting intestinal absorption, renal excretion, and bone remodeling regulate calcium levels (Figure 25-3 and Table 25-1).

TABLE 25-1 The Hormones of Calcium Homeostasis

Hormone	Stimulus for Release	End Organ Action			Effect on Serum Concentration	
		Bone	Kidney tubular resorption	Intestinal absorption	Ca^{2+}	P
PTH	↓ serum Ca^{2+}	↑ resorption	↓ P ↑ Ca^{2+}	↑ Ca^{2+} (via Vit D)	↑	↓
Vitamin D	↓ serum Ca^{2+} ↑ serum PTH ↓ serum P	↑ resorption	↑ P ↑ Ca^{2+}	↑ P ↑ Ca^{2+}	↑	↓
Calcitonin	↑ serum Ca^{2+}	↓ resorption	No change	No change	↓	No change

↑, high; ↓, low; PTH, parathyroid hormone.

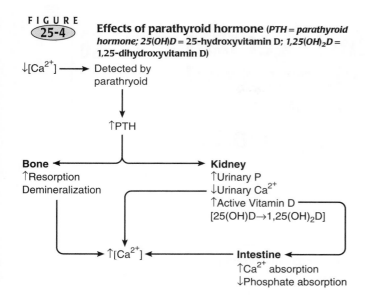

FIGURE 25-4 **Effects of parathyroid hormone** (*PTH = parathyroid hormone; 25(OH)D = 25-hydroxyvitamin D; 1,25(OH)$_2$D = 1,25-dihydroxyvitamin D*)

QUICK HIT
The inferior parathyroid glands develop from the **third pharyngeal pouch.** The **superior parathyroid glands** develop from the **fourth pharyngeal pouch.**

QUICK HIT
DiGeorge syndrome, which is characterized by **thymic and parathyroid aplasia,** results from a lack of development of the **third and fourth pharyngeal pouches.** Children with DiGeorge syndrome are born with hypocalcemia (as a result of absence of PTH) and without T-cell immunity.

QUICK HIT
Bone is predominantly composed of Type I (fibrocartilage) collagen, while cartilage consists of both Type I and Type II (hyaline and elastic) collagen.

Parathyroid hormone (PTH), produced and secreted by **chief cells** in the parathyroid, is the key hormone in calcium regulation (Figure 25-4). Decreases in serum calcium levels stimulate secretion of PTH. PTH raises serum calcium levels by increasing renal calcium absorption in the **distal tubule,** bone resorption, and intestinal calcium absorption via activation of vitamin D in the kidney. PTH inhibits **proximal tubule** resorption of serum phosphate, which acts to bind ionized, free calcium.

The active form of **vitamin D (1,25(OH)$_2$D)** is produced in the liver and kidney in response to decreased serum calcium and phosphate levels and increased serum PTH levels. Vitamin D mainly functions to **increase the intestinal absorption** and **renal resorption** of calcium and phosphate, thereby increasing concentrations of these minerals in the extracellular fluid (ECF).

The thyroid **parafollicular cells** produce and secrete **calcitonin.** An increase in serum calcium stimulates calcitonin secretion, which functions to **inhibit bone resorption.**

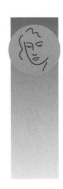

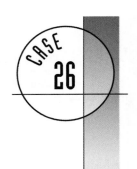

"I sometimes get bad nosebleeds and tend to bleed a lot during my periods."

OBJECTIVES

1. Develop a differential diagnosis and an appropriate workup for excessive bleeding from mucus membranes and menorrhagia
2. Review the common disorders of primary and secondary hemostasis and changes in PT and PTT
3. Learn common characteristics of diseases that increase vascular fragility
4. Differentiate between the microvascular changes associated with primary and secondary hemostasis (coagulation cascade)
5. Learn key features of drugs that control platelet aggregation, inhibit the coagulation cascade, and lyse thrombi

HISTORY AND PHYSICAL EXAMINATION

A 17-year-old girl who goes in for a routine school physical reports excessive menstrual bleeding and nosebleeds (i.e., **epistaxis**) that last up to 10 minutes. There are no ecchymoses and the patient denies any history of hematemesis, hematochezia, or melena. The patient is not taking any medications and denies cocaine abuse or any other external factors that might cause the nosebleeds. The patient's mother and older brother both have a **bleeding disorder.** The physical examination is unremarkable.

APPROPRIATE WORKUP

Blood chemistries

DIFFERENTIAL DIAGNOSIS

Coagulation disorder (e.g., hemophilia A, hemophilia B, vitamin K deficiency), platelet dysfunction (e.g., von Willebrand disease [vWD], chronic autoimmune thrombocytopenic purpura, thrombotic thrombocytopenic purpura, Glanzmann thrombasthenia, Bernard-Soulier syndrome, aspirin intake), increased vascular fragility

DIAGNOSTIC LABORATORY TESTS AND STUDIES

Blood chemistry:
Platelets = 250,000/µL (N)
Prothrombin time (PT) = 13 seconds (N)
Partial thromboplastin time (PTT) = 55 seconds (H)
Bleeding time = 9.2 minutes (H)
Ristocetin assay = No aggregation of platelets

DIAGNOSIS: PLATELET DYSFUNCTION—VON WILLEBRAND DISEASE

vWD is the **most common inherited bleeding disorder.** In 70% of cases, one of the parents is affected and it is inherited as an autosomal dominant disorder. von Willebrand factor (vWF) is synthesized by megakaryocytes and endothelial cells and has several functions. It acts as a bridge between the subendothelium and the platelet glycoprotein Ib; therefore, it is important in the initiation of primary hemostasis. vWF also acts as a factor VIII carrier in the blood. In vWD, there is insufficient synthesis of vWF. Patients usually present with complaints of excessive bleeding from superficial cuts, **bleeding from mucous membranes** (e.g., gums, nasal mucosa), prolonged bleeding after dental work, menorrhagia, and easy bruising. Because vWF acts as a factor VIII carrier in the blood, patients with vWD have a functional or qualitative (not quantitative) deficiency of factor VIII, which leads to a prolonged PTT.

EXPLANATION OF DIFFERENTIAL

Many diseases and drugs can cause excessive bleeding. A careful history and analysis of laboratory values is often necessary to differentiate between these conditions. Three categories of disorders must be considered: platelet dysfunction (i.e., disorders of primary hemostasis), coagulation defects (i.e., disorders of secondary hemostasis), and disorders that increase vascular fragility (i.e., collagen disorders).

A problem with platelet function can be quantitative or qualitative and presents as a deficiency of **primary hemostasis.** Typically, these patients present with small **petechial hemorrhages** on the skin and **mucous membranes.** Blood can ooze externally from the nose and gums, and internal bleeding can occur from the GI mucosa. A **prolonged bleeding time** is diagnostic of primary hemostasis dysfunction. The PT and PTT are normal. Table 26-1 compares some of the different diseases in this category.

Diseases that **increase vascular fragility** present in a manner similar to disorders of primary hemostasis. Bleeding from small vessels can lead to petechial hemorrhages and palpable purpura. With these diseases, however, the **bleeding time is normal.** Table 26-2 lists some of the common diseases that increase vascular fragility.

Secondary hemostasis involves the **coagulation cascade.** Clotting factor deficiencies present as severe bleeding from larger vessels with **hemarthrosis,** large hematomas after trauma, and prolonged wound bleeding. A **prolonged PT or PTT** is diagnostic of a secondary hemostatic dysfunction. The bleeding time is normal. The major disorders of secondary hemostasis are described in Table 26-3.

Related Basic Science

Hemostasis

Hemostasis is the process by which exsanguination due to damage to the vascular system is halted. Thrombosis refers to the same process when it occurs as part of a disease process. **Primary and secondary hemostasis** function together to form a hemostatic plug. Primary hemostasis refers to platelet activity while secondary hemostasis involves the coagulation cascade.

The endothelium itself also plays a key role in hemostasis. Normally, the endothelium has antithrombotic properties. However, after damage, the endothelium becomes a powerful activator of hemostasis. Table 26-4 lists some of the properties of the endothelium and their relation to hemostasis.

Primary hemostasis

Platelets are the functional units of primary hemostasis. After vessel injury, platelets are exposed to the prothrombotic subendothelium and undergo activation. Activation includes adhesion, secretion, and aggregation.

Ristocetin is an antibiotic that causes platelet aggregation in the presence of normal vWF.

Antiphospholipid antibody (lupus anticoagulant) syndrome predisposes to thrombosis and is characterized by normal bleeding time and a normal PT, but a prolonged PTT.

Endothelial cells synthesize factor VIII. The liver makes all of the other clotting factors.

Thrombocytopenia is accompanied by an increase in megakaryocytes in the bone marrow, except in the case of marrow failure.

Bacterial endotoxin causes the endothelium to release tissue factor. This is why Gram-negative sepsis can cause disseminated intravascular coagulation.

TABLE 26-1 **Disorders of Primary Hemostasis**

	Disorder	Characteristics
Quantitative (platelet count below 150,000/µL)	Bone marrow failure	Caused by acute leukemia, megaloblastic or aplastic anemia
	Wiskott-Aldrich syndrome	An immunodeficiency disorder characterized clinically by eczema and thrombocytopenia
	Idiopathic thrombocytopenic purpura	Acute form occurs in children after a viral infection and is self-limited; chronic form occurs most often in young women
	Thrombotic thrombocytopenic purpura	Characterized by thrombocytopenia, microangiopathic hemolytic anemia, fever, renal failure, and transient neurologic signs
	Hemolytic-uremic syndrome	A complication of infection with entero-hemorrhagic *Escherichia coli* (**EHEC O157:H7**); characterized by thrombocytopenia, microangiopathic hemolytic anemia, fever, and renal failure
	Multiple transfusions	Dilutes the blood, lowers platelet count
	HIV	Can involve antiplatelet antibodies and megakaryocyte suppression
	Splenic sequestering	Spleen accumulates platelets, leading to **splenomegaly**
Qualitative (normal platelet count)	von Willebrand disease	vWF is necessary for platelets to bind to exposed subendothelium; involves a functional factor VIII deficiency; **bleeding time and PTT are extended**
	Bernard-Soulier disease	A defect of platelet adhesion; deficiency of glycoprotein **Ib/IX,** the platelet receptor for **vWF**
	Glanzmann thrombasthenia	A defect of platelet aggregation; deficiency of glycoprotein **IIb/IIIa,** which binds **fibrinogen**
	Aspirin	Irreversibly **inhibits cyclooxygenase** and halts production of **TXA_2** for the lifetime of the platelet
	Uremia	Complex pathogenesis

TXA_2, thromboxane A_2; vWF, von Willebrand factor.

TABLE 26-2 **Diseases with Increased Vascular Fragility**

Disease	Characteristics
Scurvy	Caused by **vitamin C deficiency[a]**; characterized by bleeding from the **gums** and petechial lesions in the **skin near hair follicles**
Henoch-Schönlein purpura	A hypersensitivity vasculitis; involves **immune complex-mediated** damage to small vessels; characterized by fever, hemorrhagic urticaria, arthralgia, abdominal pain, and acute glomerulonephritis
Rickettsial and meningococcal infections	Both diseases cause **vasculitis,** leading to a **petechial rash;** meningococcemia can also cause DIC
Ehlers-Danlos syndrome	Inherited abnormalities of collagen and elastin; characterized by hyperextensible joints, stretchable skin, and bleeding from fragile blood vessels
Cushing syndrome	Loss of supportive tissues around vessels leads to increased fragility; leads to **easy bruising** and purple striae

[a]Vitamin C is required for normal collagen synthesis.
DIC, disseminated intravascular coagulation.

TABLE 26-3 Disorders of Secondary Hemostasis

Disorder	PT	PTT	Clotting Factors	Other Characteristics
Hemophilia A	Normal	Prolonged	Factor VIII deficiency	X-linked disease
Hemophilia B (Christmas disease)	Normal	Prolonged	Factor IX deficiency	X-linked disease
Vitamin K deficiency	Prolonged	Prolonged	Factors II, VII, IX, and X effected	Often occurs secondary to fat malabsorption (disease of the pancreas or small bowel)

PT, prothrombin time; PTT, partial thromboplastin time.

Adhesion of platelets to the subendothelium requires vWF. The exposed collagen of the subendothelium is the most powerful activator of hemostasis. **Platelets bind to vWF via glycoprotein Ib/IX, and vWF binds to subendothelial collagen. The platelets are bound to one another through molecules of fibrinogen via glycoprotein IIb/IIIa** (Figure 26-1).

The bound platelets then release stored chemicals from granules. These chemicals include adenosine diphosphate (ADP), an activator of platelet aggregation, and calcium, which is required for the coagulation reactions. Fibrinogen is also released, and thromboxane A_2 (TXA_2) is produced from arachidonic acid by the action of **cyclooxygenase.**

TXA_2 is a potent vasoconstrictor and activator of platelet aggregation. The clump of aggregated platelets is called the primary hemostatic plug. The time it takes for the hemostatic plug to form and stop the loss of blood is the basis of the bleeding time measurement of platelet function. A normal bleeding time is less than 7 minutes.

QUICK HIT Platelets are made by megakaryocytes in the bone marrow. They do not have a nucleus and only survive about 7 days in the circulation.

Secondary hemostasis

Secondary hemostasis involves the **coagulation cascade** and occurs on and around the platelet plug. The clotting factors involved circulate in the blood as inactive zymogens and activate one another in turn by cleavage reactions. These reactions require a **phospholipid complex** on the platelet surface and **calcium,** which is released from platelet granules. Coagulation, therefore, occurs most efficiently in the presence of activated platelets.

The coagulation cascade is divided into two arms: intrinsic and extrinsic. Both of these pathways converge at factor X and conclude with the formation of fibrin from fibrinogen. The fibrin acts as glue between the platelets of the primary hemostatic plug, forming a more solid secondary plug.

The intrinsic arm of the clotting system begins when exposed subendothelial collagen or the surface of an activated platelet initiates the conversion of factor XII to its active form. High-molecular-weight kininogen (HMWK) initially catalyzes this conversion. Activated factor XII then activates more factor XII and converts prekallikrein to kallikrein. Kallikrein then acts to speed the subsequent activation of more factor XII. The reactions of the intrinsic arm then proceed to activate factors XI, IX, VIII, and finally X (Figure 26-2).

TABLE 26-4 Hemostatic Properties of the Endothelium

Prothrombotic Properties	Antithrombotic Properties
Produces von Willebrand factor	Conceals subendothelial collagen
Synthesizes **tissue factor**	Synthesizes **PGI$_2$** and **nitrous oxide**[a]
Has binding sites for factors IX and X	Produces **thrombomodulin**
Secretes t-PA inhibitor	Secretes t-PA

PGI$_2$, prostacyclin; t-PA, tissue plasminogen activator.
[a]Both PGI$_2$ and nitrous oxide are vasodilators and inhibitors of platelet aggregation.

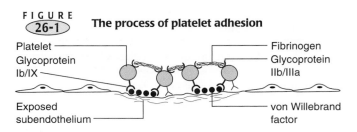

The process of platelet adhesion

FIGURE 26-1

Platelet — Glycoprotein Ib/IX — Exposed subendothelium — Fibrinogen — Glycoprotein IIb/IIIa — von Willebrand factor

PT measures the function of the extrinsic arm of coagulation. PTT is used to assess the intrinsic arm of coagulation.

The extrinsic arm of coagulation begins when tissue factor is released during vascular injury and forms a complex with calcium and factor VII. This activates factor VII, which goes on to activate factor X (see Figure 26-2).

Two major systems are in place to prevent uncontrolled activation of the coagulation cascade. The first is the **thrombomodulin–protein C system.** Thrombomodulin is made by the endothelium. It binds to thrombin and converts it to a protein C activator. Activated protein C then inactivates factors V and VIII. Protein S enhances the effect of protein C. Both **proteins C and S** are made by the liver and are **vitamin K–dependent proteins.** Inherited deficiencies of these proteins lead to a hypercoagulable state. An inherited defect in factor V can make it resistant to the action of protein C (factor V Leiden). Patients with **factor V Leiden** are also at increased risk of thrombosis. The second mechanism of controlling the clotting cascade involves antithrombin III. This large protein is activated by heparin or by natural heparin-like molecules on the endothelial cell membrane. Activated antithrombin III inactivates factors X and II (thrombin). An inherited deficiency of antithrombin III is another example of hypercoagulability.

Drugs that affect hemostasis

Hemostasis can become a pathologic process if it leads to occlusion of a vessel (e.g., myocardial infarction) or if a piece of thrombus breaks free and occludes a distant vessel (e.g., deep venous thrombosis leading to pulmonary embolism). Therefore, a number of drugs are used to inhibit the process of hemostasis.

FIGURE 26-2

The coagulation cascade (*HMW* = high-molecular-weight kininogen; *PK* = prekallikrein)

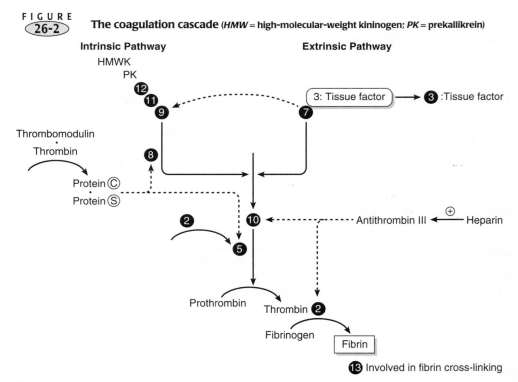

(Adapted from Dudek RW, Fix JD. BRS Embryology, 2nd Ed. Baltimore: Williams & Wilkins, 1998.)

Drugs that control platelet aggregation

Three drugs are used to control platelet aggregation: aspirin, ticlopidine, and clopidogrel. These drugs are advantageous in preventing thrombosis on the arterial side of the circulation. Damaged heart valves, atherosclerotic plaques, and dysrhythmias can all lead to pathologic platelet aggregation and thrombus formation.

Aspirin is the mainstay drug used to prevent platelet aggregation. It is used as prophylaxis in patients at risk for ischemic damage to the brain or heart. Aspirin works by irreversibly acetylating and inhibiting **cyclooxygenase.** Aspirin inhibits the cyclooxygenase in both platelets and endothelial cells, which halts production of **TXA$_2$** and prostacyclin **(PGI$_2$),** respectively. The endothelial cell, which has a nucleus, can synthesize more cyclooxygenase and overcome the inhibition, but the platelet has no nucleus and cannot perform protein synthesis and therefore TXA$_2$ production for the remainder of its life (i.e., about 7 days). PGI$_2$, a powerful vasodilator and inhibitor of platelet aggregation, continues to be produced by the endothelium. Chronic use of aspirin has additional side effects, including GI ulcers, GI bleeding, and hypersensitivity reactions.

Ticlopidine and clopidogrel also inhibit platelet aggregation. They act by inhibiting the activity of ADP, which is released from platelet granules. ADP released from activated platelets is a powerful activator of platelet aggregation. **Ticlopidine and clopidogrel are antagonists at the ADP receptor** and inhibit this effect.

All of these drugs extend the bleeding time. If used in excessive doses, these drugs can cause the petechial rash and mucous membrane bleeding typical of platelet dysfunction.

Drugs that inhibit the coagulation cascade

Stasis on the venous side of circulation is often the impetus for thrombosis and can occur in varicose veins or in the normal veins of immobilized patients. The thrombus can embolize up the inferior vena cava and through the right side of the heart and lodge in a pulmonary artery, causing sudden shortness of breath (e.g., deep venous thrombosis with pulmonary embolism). The classic example is a patient who complains of sudden dyspnea 2 days after orthopedic leg surgery.

Warfarin is a vitamin K antagonist. Factors **II, VII, IX,** and **X** are the vitamin K–dependent clotting factors. Each of these factors undergoes γ-carboxylation by a vitamin K–dependent carboxylase. The vitamin K epoxide generated by the reaction is recycled to the reduced form by vitamin K epoxide reductase. Warfarin inhibits vitamin K epoxide reductase and **prevents the regeneration of reduced vitamin K.** As a result, the vitamin K–dependent clotting factors are produced without the carboxyl group that binds to calcium, and are unable to function properly to aid secondary hemostasis. With the production of these inhibited clotting factors, the probability of thrombosis is decreased.

Warfarin therapy is complicated by many drug interactions and adverse effects. The principal adverse effects are **bleeding and teratogenesis.** Because warfarin only inhibits the regeneration of vitamin K, consumption of large doses of vitamin K can overcome the effect of the drug. Therefore, **vitamin K** is used to treat excessive bleeding associated with warfarin therapy. The onset of action of warfarin takes several days and, without vitamin K supplementation, the effect lasts for several days after therapy is terminated. Warfarin also crosses the placenta and is toxic to the fetus. Because warfarin is metabolized by the **cytochrome P-450 system,** drugs that affect this system (Table 26-5) can increase or decrease the effective concentration.

Unlike warfarin, heparin is given IV and has a rapid onset and short duration of action. **Heparin acts by enhancing the action of antithrombin III,** which inhibits factors II and X (see Figure 26-2). Heparin is used prophylactically after surgery to **prevent deep venous thrombosis** and is used acutely to prevent rethrombosis in an acute myocardial infarction. Heparin is broken down in the reticuloendothelial system and excreted in the urine; therefore, patients with cirrhosis or renal failure should receive lower doses. Prolonged heparin

QUICK HIT Toxic doses of aspirin cause hyperthermia, respiratory depression, and a combination of respiratory and metabolic acidosis.

QUICK HIT Estrogen stimulates increased production of the vitamin K–dependent clotting factors. This is why pregnancy and the use of some oral contraceptives are associated with an increased risk of thrombosis.

QUICK HIT An overdose of heparin is treated with protamine sulfate, with which it forms an inactive complex.

TABLE 26-5 Drugs That Affect Warfarin

Effect on Cytochrome P-450	Drugs	Required Dose Adjustment
Activation	**Phenobarbital** (barbiturate) Phenytoin (antiepileptic) Rifampin (tuberculostatic drug)	Warfarin dose must be increased
Inhibition	**Cimetidine** (histamine blocker) Chloramphenicol (antibiotic) Isoniazid (tuberculostatic drug)	Warfarin dose must be decreased

use can cause **thrombocytopenia** and can increase the risk of bleeding. Hypersensitivity does occur and is characterized by fever, chills, urticaria, and anaphylactic shock. Heparin does not cross the placenta and is therefore safe during pregnancy.

Thrombolytics

All thrombolytic drugs, except urokinase, activate plasminogen to **plasmin,** the body's natural thrombolytic agent. Plasmin hydrolyzes fibrin and lyses thrombi. However, thrombolytic therapy can lead to **bleeding** from previously unseen vascular lesions. Thrombolytics are being used more frequently to treat **pulmonary embolism and myocardial infarction.** Table 26-6 details some of the important properties of these drugs.

> **QUICK HIT**
> Aminocaproic acid is used to treat overdoses of streptokinase.

TABLE 26-6 Thrombolytics

Drug	Mechanism of Action	Considerations
Streptokinase	Forms a complex with plasminogen, which then acts to convert other plasminogen molecules to active plasmin	Hypersensitivity reactions may occur; antistreptokinase antibodies may be present from a previous streptococcal infection, in which case higher doses are needed
Urokinase	Degrades fibrin and fibrinogen directly	Urokinase is not antigenic
Anistreplase (APSAC)	Forms a plasminogen-activating complex with plasminogen that is activated only when it binds to fibrin	Has a mechanism similar to streptokinase, but has a longer half-life and more selectivity for clot lysis
Alteplase (t-PA)	Binds and activates only plasminogen molecules that are bound to fibrin	Has high specificity for clot lysis and a very short half-life

APSAC, acylated plasminogen-streptokinase activator complex; t-PA, tissue plasminogen activator.

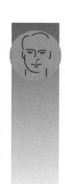

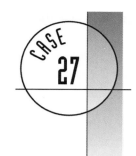

"My stomach pain has worsened, I can't see straight anymore, and it hurts when I urinate.

OBJECTIVES

1. Develop a differential diagnosis and an appropriate workup for decreased visual acuity, diminished abdominal pain with meals, and hematuria
2. Compare and contrast multiple endocrine neoplasms (MEN I, MEN II/IIa, MEN IIb/III)
3. Review key features of autosomal dominant diseases
4. Understand the relationship embryologically and anatomically between the thyroid and parathyroid glands
5. Learn the mechanisms of action of two common second messenger systems (cAMP and IP_3)
6. Describe the four common types of thyroid carcinomas

HISTORY AND PHYSICAL EXAMINATION

A 33-year-old man comes to the primary care physician's office complaining of **chronic abdominal pain.** He states that he has had burning pain in the middle of his stomach over the past 15 years. The pain **diminishes with eating** but has progressively worsened over the past month. Pepto-Bismol used to relieve the pain, but lately it has not worked. The stomach pain wakes him early in the morning, has been spreading over his sides, and now is exacerbated with urination. His urine lately has had an **increased reddish tinge.** The patient also states that he has been having headaches behind his eyes and vision problems. His medical and surgical histories are unremarkable. He states that his mother told him that his father and grandfather both had symptoms like his, but both men died in accidents at young ages. The patient denies alcohol, drug, and tobacco use. His vital signs are stable. On physical examination, the patient exhibits costovertebral angle tenderness, flank pain, epigastric pain on gentle palpation, and **decreased visual acuity** in the peripheral fields.

APPROPRIATE WORKUP

Blood chemistries, urinalysis, abdominal ultrasound, esophagogastroduodenoscopy

DIFFERENTIAL DIAGNOSIS

Appendicitis, diverticulosis, nephrolithiasis, peptic ulcer disease (PUD), Wermer syndrome (multiple endocrine neoplasia [MEN] type 1)

DIAGNOSTIC LABORATORY TESTS AND STUDIES

Blood chemistry:
Ca = 15.0 mg/dL (H)
Gastrin = 1231 pg/mL (H)
Urinalysis:
Ca = 500 mg/24 hours (H)
RBC = (H)

Abdominal ultrasound (US):
Normal appendix
Multiple opaque structures in the renal pelvis bilaterally

Esophagogastroduodenoscopy (EGD):
  Multiple ulcerative lesions of
    duodenum
  Biopsy results negative for
    Helicobacter pylori
CT scan:
  Head = mass lesion in the region of
    the sella turcica compressing
    surrounding structures

Neck = **enlarged parathyroid glands**
Abdomen = mass lesion in the
  body of the pancreas enlarged
  kidneys

DIAGNOSIS: WERMER SYNDROME (MULTIPLE ENDOCRINE NEOPLASIA TYPE I)

Wermer syndrome (MEN Type I) is a combination of neoplasms or hyperplasias found in the **parathyroids, pancreas,** and **pituitary.** Hyperplasia of the parathyroids ultimately leads to the formation of **kidney stones,** the most common manifestation of MEN Type I. Parathyroid hormone (PTH) regulates calcium levels in the body; therefore, excessive PTH secretion by hyperplastic glands leads to increased calcium levels. The kidneys attempt to filter the excess calcium, but are overwhelmed, and kidney stones form. The second most common manifestation is **Zollinger-Ellison syndrome** from a pancreatic adenoma. The pancreatic adenoma releases excess amounts of gastrin, which subsequently causes ulcers and painful chronic diarrhea. Neoplasms of the pituitary, often **prolactinomas,** lead to **visual disturbances** and headaches from pituitary enlargement and compression of the optic chiasm. Occasionally, the pituitary adenoma is nonfunctional. Diagnosis of MEN I is made through CT, which demonstrates mass lesions of the parathyroids, pancreas, and pituitary. MEN I, as well as the other types of MEN, are autosomal dominant.

EXPLANATION OF DIFFERENTIAL

Appendicitis results from a **fecalith obstructing the lumen of the appendix,** leading to bacterial proliferation and eventual rupture from increasing inflammation. Presentation includes **anorexia, nausea,** and **abdominal pain.** The abdominal pain typically starts out diffuse (visceral pain) but can localize to the right lower quadrant as inflammation progresses (somatic pain). An **abdominal US** can identify obstruction and rule out gynecologic causes of abdominal pain.

  Diverticulitis is an **inflammation of diverticula** (pockets of mucosa and submucosa herniating through the muscular layer of the colon). Diverticula are common in **older adults** and can be observed via CT scan or colonoscopy. If inflamed, bloody stools and colicky pain localizing to the lower quadrants are typical manifestations.

  The four most common types of kidney stones include **calcium stones (most common),** uric acid stones, cystine stones, and struvite stones. Kidney stones can present with **colicky flank pain** that may radiate to the groin, **dysuria,** and **hematuria.** The stones typically **form proximally** in the urinary tract and **obstruct distally** at three points along the ureters: the ureteropelvic junction, the ureterovesicular junction, and the point where the ureter crosses the pelvic inlet. Stones **predispose the patient to UTI.** While this patient suffered from **nephrolithiasis** as a result of hyperparathyroidism, nephrolithiasis alone could not explain the constellation of symptoms.

  PUD refers to **chronic ulcers lining the GI tract.** The duodenum is most often affected, but peptic ulcers can occur in the stomach or esophagus. **Peptic ulcers in the stomach** often present with **weight loss** and **pain with meals.** They typically result from **decreased mucosal protection** from gastric acid secondary to nonsteroidal anti-inflammatory drugs (NSAIDs) or *H. pylori* infection. **Duodenal ulcers** present with **weight gain** and **pain that**

QUICK HIT
Gastrin, released by the G cells of the antrum of the stomach, acts on the parietal cells and induces the release of HCl. Gastrin also increases colonic motility.

QUICK HIT
Omeprazole and lansoprazole inhibit the proton pump of the parietal cell by binding to H+/K+–ATPase, thus inhibiting gastric acid secretion.

decreases with meals. Duodenal ulcers typically result from **increased gastric acid production,** which can be idiopathic or secondary to Zollinger-Ellison syndrome. Duodenal ulcers are more common than gastric ulcers, but both cause burning pain that is localized to the epigastric region and that causes **early morning awakening.** Barrett metaplasia is caused by reflux of acidic gastric contents into the esophagus.

Related Basic Science

Multiple endocrine neoplasms

Multiple endocrine neoplasms are groups of neoplasms that commonly occur together. The neoplasms can take the form of hyperplasias, adenomas, or carcinomas and are transmitted in an **autosomal dominant** pattern (Table 27-1).

Autosomal dominant diseases

A dominant gene is one that, if inherited, will be functional regardless of whether the person is only heterozygous for it. Thus, an autosomal dominant gene has a 50% chance of manifesting in the offspring of a couple in which one person is heterozygous for the trait and the other does not have it. Dominant genes are expressed in the heterozygous state. Therefore, when an affected individual has offspring with an unaffected person, 50% of the offspring will be affected (Table 27-2).

The parathyroid and thyroid

The **inferior parathyroid glands** develop from the third pharyngeal pouch and migrate caudally. The **superior parathyroid glands** arise from the fourth pharyngeal arch. A portion of the fourth pharyngeal pouch gives rise to the **parafollicular cells** of the thyroid (calcitonin-producing C cells). The remainder of the thyroid (the follicular cells) develops from the endodermal lining of the foregut (Figure 27-1).

While papillary carcinoma is the most common thyroid cancer, the medullary variant is most often associated with the MEN syndromes (Table 27-3).

Second messenger systems

Endocrine hormones are secreted into the bloodstream and can act at distant sites in the body. These hormones often use second messenger systems, which are the links between the initial signal and the desired cellular response. They are also responsible for **amplification** of the original signal. The two most common types of second messengers are cyclic AMP (**cAMP**) and inositol 1,4,5-triphosphate (**IP$_3$**) (Figures 27-2 and 27-3). Other second messenger systems include cyclic GMP (**cGMP**), **tyrosine kinase,** and nitrous oxide (**NO**).

> **QUICK HIT** The neoplastic cells that form the gastrinoma in Zollinger-Ellison syndrome usually originate from the Δ cells of the pancreas.

> **QUICK HIT** Phentolamine and phenoxybenzamine, α-adrenergic blocking agents, are used for prophylactic treatment of the hypertension seen with pheochromocytoma.

> **QUICK HIT** The severity of Huntington disease can be partly determined by the number of triplet repeats on chromosome 4 (with the number of repeats directly proportional to severity and inversely proportional to age of onset).

> **QUICK HIT** Dysfunction of the parathyroids typically involves hyperplasia rather than neoplastic growth.

> **QUICK HIT** A common cause of hypoparathyroidism is accidental removal of the parathyroid glands during surgical resection of thyroid cancer.

> **QUICK HIT** Psammoma bodies can also be seen in malignant mesothelioma, serous cystadenocarcinoma of the ovaries, and meningiomas.

TABLE 27-1 | Multiple Endocrine Neoplasms

Location of Neoplasm	Result of Neoplastic Lesion	MEN I Wermer Syndrome	MEN II (IIa) Sipple Syndrome	MEN III (IIb) Multiple Mucosal Neoplasm Syndrome
Pituitary	Prolactinoma	×		
Pancreas	Insulinoma	×		
	Gastrinoma			
	Glucagonoma			
Parathyroids	Hyperparathyroidism	×	×	
Adrenal medulla	Pheochromocytoma		×	×
Thyroid	Medullary thyroid carcinoma		×	×
Mucosa	Multiple mucosal neuromas			×

TABLE 27-2 Common Autosomal Dominant Diseases

Disease	Characteristics
Adult polycystic kidney disease	• **Most common renal hereditary disorder** • **Bilateral renal cysts** • **Death by 50 years of age**
Familial hypercholesterolemia	• Low-density lipoprotein receptor defects • **Hypercholesterolemia and atherosclerosis**
Marfan syndrome	• Connective tissue defect resulting from **fibrillin deficiency** • **Hyperextensible joints, long fingers,** tall, **thin** • **Ectopia lentis** • **Proximal aortic aneurysm, mitral valve prolapse**
Neurofibromatosis (von Recklinghausen disease)	• **Multiple neurofibromas** • **Café-au-lait spots** • **Skeletal disorders and increased incidence of tumors**
von Hippel-Lindau disease	• Associated with **renal cell carcinoma** • **Hemangioblastomas of the brain stem, cerebellum, and retina** • **Deletion of short arm of chromosome 3**
Huntington disease	• **Atrophy of the caudate nuclei** • **Progressive dementia and choreiform movements starting** *from* **30 years of age** • **Genetic defect in short arm of chromosome 4**
Familial adenomatous polyposis	• **Numerous adenomatous polyps in the colon** • **100% risk of malignant transformation**
Hereditary spherocytosis	• Deficiency in **spectrin protein,** leading to **osmotic fragility** • **Hemolytic anemia** • **Spheroidal erythrocytes**

FIGURE 27-1 The parathyroid and thyroid

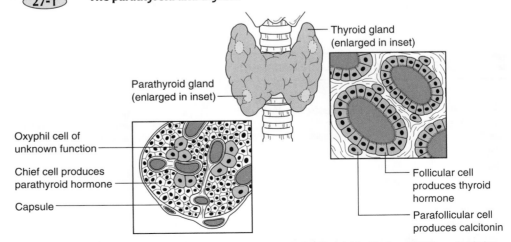

(Adapted from Gartner LP, Hiatt JL. Color Atlas of Histology, 3rd Ed. Philadelphia: Lippincott Williams & Wilkins, 2000, p 209.)

TABLE 27-3 Thyroid Carcinomas

Tumor	Description
Papillary	• **Most common** and **best prognosis** of the thyroid cancers • **3:1 female predominance** • Usually in patients 30 to 50 years of age • "Ground glass" nuclei of neoplastic cells, also called "Orphan Annie eyes" • Possible **psammoma bodies** • Papillary projections covered with cuboidal epithelium within glandular spaces
Follicular	• Worse prognosis than papillary • **3:1 female predominance** • Uniform cuboidal cells lining follicles • Lacks the distinctive nuclear features of papillary carcinoma
Medullary	• Parafollicular cell neoplasm • **Secrete calcitonin** • Associated with MEN IIa and MEN IIb (MEN III)
Hürthle cell	• Anaplastic, undifferentiated neoplasm • Older patients • Rapidly fatal

MEN, multiple endocrine neoplasia.

FIGURE 27-2 **Mechanism of action of cAMP**
(**cAMP** = cyclic adenosine monophosphate)

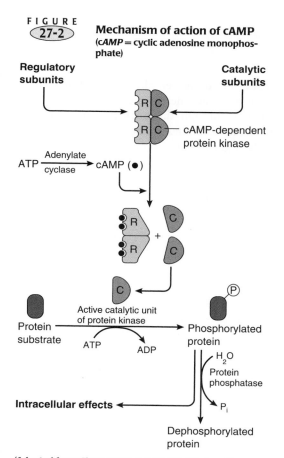

(Adapted from Champe PC, Harvey RA. Lippincott's **Illustrated Reviews in Biochemistry, 2nd Ed. Philadelphia: Lippincott Williams & Wilkins, 1994, p 82.)**

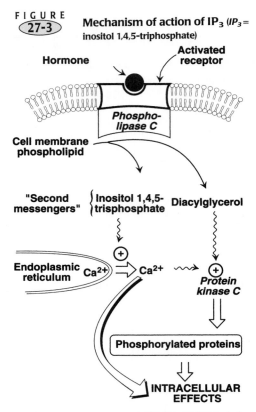

FIGURE
27-3

Mechanism of action of IP₃ $(IP_3 =$ *inositol 1,4,5-triphosphate)*

(From Champe PC, Harvey RA. Lippincott's Illustrated
Reviews in Biochemistry, 2nd Ed. Philadelphia:
Lippincott Williams & Wilkins, 1994, p 83.)

Steroid hormones can also act at distant sites but do not employ a second messenger system. Because steroids are lipophilic, they can penetrate the cell membrane and bind to a **steroid-binding protein,** which then can pass through the nuclear membrane and directly act on DNA and RNA synthesis. The steroid hormones include aldosterone, estrogen, progesterone, testosterone, glucocorticoids, and thyroid hormone.

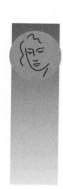

"My girlfriend thinks her neighbors are blow-up dolls and that someone is going to kidnap her."

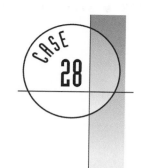

OBJECTIVES

1. Develop a differential diagnosis and appropriate workup for a chief complaint of delusions, anxiety, and normal orientation.
2. Be able to differentiate among the three types of schizophrenia-like disorders and the five types of schizophrenia.
3. Understand the psychological and physical effects associated with the use and withdrawal from stimulant, sedative, opioid, and hallucinogen-related agents.
4. Learn the various types of personality disorders categorized by the DSM-IV-TR.
5. Describe the synthesis and physiologic and therapeutic functions of the neurotransmitter dopamine.
6. Review the mechanisms of action, clinical uses, and side effects associated with typical and atypical antipsychotics.
7. Review the major cellular receptors, the effects if blocked, and associated drugs.
8. Understand the pathophysiology and treatment of Parkinson's disease.

HISTORY AND PHYSICAL EXAMINATION

A man brings his girlfriend, a 26-year-old Caucasian woman, to the psychiatric ED. He states that the patient has recently become **very anxious,** and she keeps repeating that someone has replaced her neighbors with blow-up dolls to trick her. He says that she has felt anxious for about 7 months but became much more confused about 5 days ago. Physical examination reveals **normal vital signs.** The patient appears physically healthy but is poorly groomed. She is **oriented to person, place, and time** but has a **flat and labile affect.** During the interview, she continually wrings her hands, sometimes laughs inappropriately, and appears to **respond to internal stimuli.** Her thoughts are disorganized, and many of her responses are incongruent with the questions asked. She denies drug or alcohol abuse. She admits **hearing voices** that say she will be kidnapped. She denies visual hallucinations. Her cognition and memory are intact.

APPROPRIATE WORKUP

Urinalysis.

> **QUICK HIT STEP-UP** Visual hallucinations are rare in pure psychosis and should always make one think of an organic cause.

DIFFERENTIAL DIAGNOSIS

Psychosis secondary to **mental illness** (schizophrenia, manic episode), psychosis secondary to **organic causes** (delirium, intoxication), personality disorder

DIAGNOSTIC LABORATORY TESTS AND STUDIES

Urinalysis:
Negative drug screen results

DIAGNOSIS: SCHIZOPHRENIA, PARANOID TYPE

Schizophrenia, the most commonly diagnosed psychotic disorder, occurs equally in men and women. It usually is first diagnosed in young adulthood (men between 15 and 25 years of age; women between 25 and 35 years of age). Twin studies have revealed a genetic component to the disease.

The typical patient with schizophrenia has a quiet and uneventful childhood. The "premorbid personality" of schizophrenia describes a child who is shy, quiet, socially withdrawn, and obedient. At the onset of illness, the patient often complains of nonspecific ailments such as headache and diarrhea.

At presentation, the patient with schizophrenia is alert and oriented with **intact memory.** More specifically, long-term memory is intact; however, because patients with acute psychosis cannot concentrate, short-term recall may be impaired. The patient is often anxious but with a **flat or blunted affect.** Emotional expression is often inappropriate and labile. **Thoughts are disorganized and delusional.** The term **"loose associations"** is often used to describe the poor organization of thought manifested by patients with psychosis. For instance, a question about family can prompt an unrelated response about the weather. The **hallucinations** of patients with psychosis are almost always auditory. Certain abnormal speech patterns are also typical of schizophrenia. Among these are neologisms, echolalia, and clang associations.

The symptoms of schizophrenia are often divided into two categories: positive and negative. Positive symptoms include hallucinations, delusions, and loose associations. Flattening of affect, social withdrawal, thought-blocking, and lack of motivation are some prominent negative symptoms.

More than half of all patients with schizophrenia attempt **suicide.** Certain factors such as male sex, high education, unmarried status, and depressed mood are associated with an increased risk of suicide.

Several disorders similar to schizophrenia are listed in Table 28-1.

EXPLANATION OF DIFFERENTIAL

Mania can present very similarly to acute psychosis. Patients with mania have **boundless energy** that manifests in their behavior, speech, and thoughts. They are **excitable** and can become **irritable** and hostile very quickly. **Delusions,** which are not uncommon among these patients, are usually consistent with the manic state. For instance, these patients may believe that they have special powers or abilities. Their **speech is pressured,** meaning that

> **QUICK HIT**
> Broadly defined, psychosis is when a patient's reality differs from the norm.

TABLE 28-1 Schizophrenia-like Disorders	
Disorder	**Description**
Schizophreniform disorder	Identical to schizophrenia, except it **lasts between 1 and 6 months;** true schizophrenia lasts more than 6 months
Schizotypal personality disorder	Unusual personality with magical thinking, ideas of reference, but no overt psychosis
Schizoid personality disorder	**Socially withdrawn,** introverted, isolated, no psychosis

they seem almost unable to get the words out fast enough. Unlike patients with psychosis, however, patients with mania rarely have hallucinations.

Delirium is defined as an **impairment of cognitive functioning accompanied by a general "clouding of consciousness."** Unlike psychosis, delirium occurs secondary to an **organic cause;** common organic causes include meningitis, hypoxia, head trauma, encephalopathy, and the postoperative state. Patients with delirium have **visual hallucinations,** are **not oriented** to place or time, and can be **labile** or even aggressive. The treatment for delirium is to find and treat the underlying medical cause.

Intoxication, a major cause of delirium, can appear much like psychosis. **Alcohol, anticholinergics,** opiates, PCP, **sedatives** (benzodiazepines, barbiturates), and steroids can all cause delirium. A urinalysis drug screen should always be done on a patient suspected to have a psychosis or delirium. **Delirium tremens,** a serious withdrawal reaction from long-term alcohol abuse, is characterized by autonomic instability, sweating, agitation, and vivid hallucinations. (Tables 28-2, 28-3, 28-4, and 28-5).

Personality disorders exhibit a chronic and rigid pattern of relating to society that can result in social and occupational difficulties. Persons with this disorder are often unaware of any problem and are brought to physicians by family or friends. Personality disorders are categorized by the DSM-IV-TR into clusters, summarized in Table 28-6.

> **QUICK HIT** The most serious and life-threatening withdrawal reactions occur with alcohol and barbiturates.

TABLE 28-2 Effects of Use and Withdrawal of Stimulant Agents

Substances	Effects of Use	Effects of Withdrawal
	Psychological	
Caffeine, nicotine	• Increased alertness and attention span • Mild improvement in mood • Agitation and insomnia	• Lethargy • Mild depression of mood
	Physical	
	• Decreased appetite • Increased blood pressure and heart rate (tachycardia) • Increased gastrointestinal activity	• Increased appetite with slight weight gain • Fatigue • Headache
	Psychological	
Amphetamines, cocaine	• Significant elevation of mood (lasting only 1 hour with cocaine) • Increased alertness and attention span • Aggressiveness, impaired judgment • Psychotic symptoms (e.g., paranoid delusions with amphetamines and formication with cocaine) • Agitation and insomnia	• Significant depression of mood • Strong psychological craving (peaking a few days after the last dose) • Irritability
	Physical	
	• Loss of appetite and weight • Pupil dilation • Increased energy • Tachycardia and other cardiovascular effects which can be life-threatening • Seizures (particularly with cocaine) • Reddening (erythema) of the nose due to "snorting" cocaine • Hypersexuality	• Hunger (particularly with amphetamines) • Pupil constriction • Fatigue

Reprinted from Fadem B. BRS Behavioral Sciences, 4th Ed. Philadelphia: Lippincott Williams & Wilkins, 2005.

TABLE 28-3	Effects of Use and Withdrawal of Sedative Agents	
Substances	**Effects of Use**	**Effects of Withdrawal**
	Psychological	
Alcohol Benzodiazepines Barbiturates	• Mild elevation of mood • Decreased anxiety • Somnolence • Behavioral disinhibition	• Mild depression of mood • Increased anxiety • Insomnia • Psychotic symptoms (e.g., delusions and formication) • Disorientation
	Physical	
	• Sedation • Poor coordination • Respiratory depression	• Tremor • Seizures • Cardiovascular symptoms, such as tachycardia and hypertension

Reprinted from Fadem B. BRS Behavioral Sciences, 4th Ed. Philadelphia: Lippincott Williams & Wilkins, 2005.

Related Basic Science

Types of schizophrenia

Five subtypes of schizophrenia are currently defined. The different characteristics of each are outlined in Table 28-7.

Dopamine

Dopamine (DA) is synthesized from amino acids by the same synthetic pathway that produces the two other monoamines: norepinephrine (NEPI) and epinephrine (EPI) (Figure 28-1). DA functions in the CNS as a neurotransmitter. It is also released from sympathetic postganglionic neurons only at the kidney, where it causes vasodilation.

TABLE 28-4	Effects of Use and Withdrawal of Opioid Agents	
Substances	**Effects of Use**	**Effects of Withdrawal**
	Psychological	
Heroin, Methadone Other Opioids	• Elevation of mood • Relaxation • Somnolence	• Depression of mood • Anxiety • Insomnia
	Physical	
	• Sedation • Analgesia • Respiratory depression (overdose may be fatal) • Constipation • Pupil constriction (miosis)	• Sweating, muscle aches, fever • Rhinorrhea (running nose) • Piloerection (goose bumps) • Yawning • Stomach cramps and diarrhea • Pupil dilation (mydriasis)

Reprinted from Fadem B. BRS Behavioral Sciences, 4th Ed. Philadelphia: Lippincott Williams & Wilkins, 2005.

TABLE 28-5 Effects of Use and Withdrawal of Hallucinogens and Related Agents

Substances	Effects of Use	Effects of Withdrawal
Psychological		
Cannabis (marijuana, hashish) Lysergic acid diethylamide (LSD) Phencyclidine (PCP, "angel dust") Psilocybin Mescaline	• Altered perceptual states (auditory and visual hallucinations, alterations of body image, distortions of time and space) • Elevation of mood • Impairment of memory (may be long-term) • Reduced attention span • "Bad trips" (panic reactions that may include psychotic symptoms) • "Flashbacks" (a re-experience of the sensations associated with use in the absence of the drug even months after the last dose)	• Few if any psychological withdrawal symptoms
Physical		
	• Impairment of complex motor activity • Cardiovascular symptoms • Sweating • Tremor • Nystagmus (PCP)	• Few if any physical withdrawal symptoms

Reprinted from Fadem B. BRS Behavioral Sciences, 4th Ed. Philadelphia: Lippincott Williams & Wilkins, 2005.

Therapeutically, the use of DA itself is limited; the most common indication is **shock.** In addition to acting on D_1 and D_2 dopamine receptors, DA acts directly on both α- and β-adrenergic receptors. Acting on the **$β_1$ receptors of the heart,** DA has a positive inotropic and chronotropic effect. Acting on **α receptors in the vasculature,** DA causes vasoconstriction and raises blood pressure. Acting on D_1 and D_2 receptors in the mesenteric and renal vasculature, DA causes vasodilation. This last effect makes DA a better choice than EPI for treating shock. EPI would produce the same effects on the heart and blood vessels, but also would constrict the mesenteric and renal vasculature. In shock, these organs are at risk for ischemic damage. EPI increases that risk, while DA reduces it.

QUICK HIT STEP-UP Most sympathetic post-ganglionic neurons release nor epinephrine. The exceptions are the sympathetics that innervate the sweat glands, which release acetylcholine, and those that innervate the renal vasculature, which release DA.

Antipsychotics: typical

Also called neuroleptics, these drugs are used most commonly to treat schizophrenia. They are also used occasionally to treat the psychotic symptoms that sometimes accompany mania or delirium. Antipsychotics are divided into two classes: typical and atypical. **The typical antipsychotics act by blocking DA (D_2) receptors.** The atypical agents act by a different mechanism and will be discussed later.

The D_2 blocking action of the typical neuroleptics may be responsible for their antipsychotic action. The theory is that overactivity in the dopaminergic mesolimbic pathway causes psychosis and that the neuroleptics relieve psychotic symptoms by blocking D_2 receptors in this pathway.

Because these agents also block D_2 receptors elsewhere, however, certain side effects can develop. Blocking D_2 receptors in the pituitary causes **hyperprolactinemia.** Because hyperprolactinemia suppresses the gonadotropins, amenorrhea develops in women, and

TABLE 28-6	DSM-IV-TR Classification and Characteristics of the Personality Disorders
Personality Disorder	**Characteristics**
CLUSTER A	Avoids social relationships, is "peculiar" but not psychotic
Hallmark: Genetic or familial association:	Psychotic illnesses
Paranoid	• Distrustful, suspicious, litigious • Attributes responsibility for own problems to others • Interprets motives of others as malevolent
Schizoid	• Long-standing pattern of voluntary social withdrawal • Detached; restricted emotions
Schizotypal	• Peculiar appearance • Magical thinking (i.e., believing that one's thoughts can affect the course of events) • Odd thought patterns and behavior without psychosis
CLUSTER B	Dramatic, emotional, inconsistent
Hallmark: Genetic or familial association:	Mood disorders, substance abuse, and somatoform disorders
Histrionic	• Theatrical, extroverted, emotional, sexually provocative, "life of the party" • Shallow, vain • In men, "Don Juan" dress and behavior • Cannot maintain intimate relationships
Narcissistic	• Pompous, with a sense of special entitlement • Lacks empathy for others
Antisocial	• Refuses to conform to social norms and shows no concern for others • Associated with conduct disorder in childhood and criminal behavior in adulthood ("psychopaths" or "sociopaths")
Borderline	• Erratic, impulsive, unstable behavior and mood • Feeling bored, alone, and "empty" • Suicide attempts for relatively trivial reasons • Self-mutilation (cutting or burning oneself) • Often comorbid with mood and eating disorders • Mini-psychotic episodes (i.e., brief periods of loss of contact with reality)
CLUSTER C	Fearful, anxious
Hallmark: Genetic or familial association:	Anxiety disorders
Avoidant	• Sensitive to rejection, socially withdrawn • Feelings of inferiority
Obsessive-compulsive	• Perfectionistic, orderly, inflexible • Stubborn and indecisive • Ultimately inefficient
Dependent	• Allows other people to make decisions and assume responsibility for them • Poor self-confidence, fear of being deserted and alone • May tolerate abuse by domestic partner

Reprinted from Fadem B. BRS Behavioral Sciences, 4th Ed. Philadelphia: Lippincott Williams & Wilkins, 2005.

TABLE 28-7 Types of Schizophrenia

Type	Features
Paranoid	Slightly older age of onset; prominent **delusions of persecution,** grandeur, or both
Disorganized	Slightly younger age of onset; **inappropriate emotions, disorganized thinking,** and poor grooming
Catatonic	Mutism, **"waxy flexibility," motor immobility,** stereotyped movements; has become rare with proper antipsychotic treatment
Undifferentiated	Has characteristics from more than one subtype
Residual	Occurs **following one acute psychotic episode;** flat affect, unusual behavior, disorganized thinking, and social withdrawal; no severe psychotic symptoms such as delusions, hallucinations, or gross disorganization of thought and speech

impotence occurs in men. Excessive prolactin also causes galactorrhea in women. Blocking D_2 receptors in the nigrostriatal pathway causes **movement disorders.** These so-called extrapyramidal side effects are parkinsonism, acute dystonia, acute akathisia, and tardive dyskinesia.

Tremor at rest, muscle rigidity, and bradykinesia characterize neuroleptic-induced **parkinsonism.** Older women are at the greatest risk of developing neuroleptic-induced parkinsonism, which normally manifests early in the course of treatment.

Acute dystonia is involuntary prolonged contractions of muscles, often leading to pain and abnormal postures. These symptoms usually present **early in the course of treatment.** Torticollis, oculogyric crisis, and tongue protrusion are all common manifestations. **Young men** are most commonly affected.

A serious and often misdiagnosed side effect of neuroleptics is **akathisia,** a reaction characterized by severe **restlessness.** Affected patients cannot sit still. They rock back and forth, constantly stand up and sit down, and pace endlessly. This side effect has been known to drive patients to suicide.

Tardive dyskinesia, a serious side effect, usually develops following long-term treatment with high potency antipsychotics. Characteristics are **choreoathetoid movements of the muscles of the mouth,** tongue, and jaw. The cause may be DA receptor upregulation or supersensitivity. In many patients, it is **irreversible.**

The most life-threatening and unpredictable side effect of the antipsychotics is **neuroleptic malignant syndrome,** which can occur at any point during treatment. Affected patients typically present acutely in the ED with severe muscular rigidity, sweating, mutism, tachycardia, hypertension, and agitation. Muscle relaxants (dantrolene) and DA agonists (bromocriptine) are used in treatment.

TABLE 28-8 Cellular Receptors and Their Effects

Receptor Blocked	Effect(s)	Most Noted with
Muscarinic	Dry mouth, urinary retention, constipation, blurred vision, confusion	Thioridazine, chlorpromazine
α-Adrenergic	Orthostatic hypotension	Chlorpromazine
D_2 receptors in the medullary chemo trigger zone	Antiemetic	Haloperidol, fluphenazine, thiothixene
H_1 receptors in the CNS	Sedation	Chlorpromazine, thioridazine

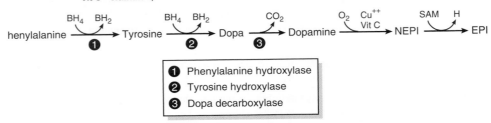

FIGURE 28-1

Dopamine synthesis (*BH₂* = dihydrobiopterin; *BH₄* = tetrahydrobiopterin; *EPI* = epinephrine; *NEPI* = norepinephrine; *SAH* = s-adenosylhomocysteine; *SAM* = s-adenosylmethionine; *vit C* = vitamin C)

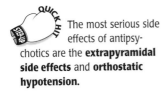

The most serious side effects of antipsychotics are the **extrapyramidal side effects** and **orthostatic hypotension.**

The other side effects of the antipsychotics are related to their interaction with other receptors. Table 28-8 lists these receptors and the resultant side effects.

The side effect profile of a given typical antipsychotic can be predicted with some certainty based on its potency. Figure 28-2 lists some common typical neuroleptics and their relative side effect profiles.

Antipsychotics: atypical

The atypical neuroleptics include **clozapine, risperidone, olanzapine,** and **quetiapine.** Among these, clozapine and risperidone are the most commonly used. Risperidone is an effective drug for schizophrenia and is considered one of the first-line treatments. Clozapine, also effective, is reserved for refractory cases.

Clozapine blocks D_4 and 5-HT$_2$ receptors, not D_2 receptors like the typical antipsychotics. While the typical drugs treat mainly the positive symptoms of schizophrenia, clozapine seems more effective in treating both the positive and negative symptoms. Unfortunately, clozapine does have autonomic and sedating side effects and can cause **agranulocytosis.** Because of this latter adverse effect, patients on clozapine must have their white blood cell count checked regularly.

Risperidone and olanzapine both have some D_2 blocking activity but also block 5-HT$_2$ receptors. Like clozapine, these agents are sedating and have autonomic side effects but tend to cause less orthostatic hypotension.

Parkinson's disease

While schizophrenia is postulated to result from DA overactivity in the mesolimbic pathway, evidence suggests that Parkinson's disease is caused by degeneration of the substantia nigra (Figure 28-3) and the subsequent dysfunction of the nigrostriatal dopaminergic pathway. The treatment of both of these diseases is aimed at restoring normal DA levels.

The typical presentation of parkinsonism is an older patient with **"pill-rolling" hand tremors** at rest, stooped posture, **masked facies, bradykinesia,** and **muscular rigidity.**

FIGURE 28-2

Side effects of the typical antipsychotics

Drug	Potency	Extrapyramidal effects	Sedation, Orthostatic hypotension, Anti-muscarinic effects
Haloperidol Fluphenazine Thiothixine Thioridazine Chlorpromazine	↑	↑	↓

FIGURE 28-3 **Substantia nigra in midbrain**

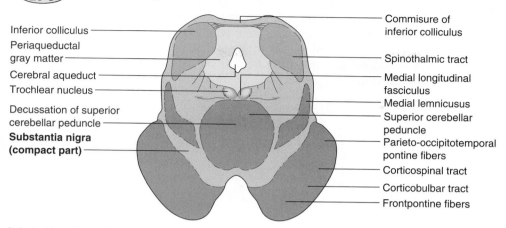

(Adapted from Young PA, Young PH. Basic Clinical Neuroanatomy, Baltimore: Williams & Wilkins, 1997, p 333.)

Most cases of parkinsonism are idiopathic; other etiologies include repeated head trauma, drugs such as antipsychotics and the street drug MPTP, and Shy-Drager syndrome.

The treatment of Parkinson's disease is to **restore DA levels** in the nigrostriatal pathway. An alternative approach is to **lower acetylcholine levels.** The balance between these two neurotransmitters seems as important as absolute DA deficiency in creating the symptoms of Parkinson's disease. The antiparkinson drugs in Table 28-9 are therefore DA agonists and muscarinic antagonists.

TABLE 28-9 **Drugs Used in the Treatment of Parkinson Disease**

Drug	Mechanism of Action	Notes
Drugs That Increase Dopamine in the Striatum		
Levodopa (L-dopa)	DA precursor that can enter the CNS	Can be converted to DA by a plasma decarboxylase; DA causes nausea, hypotension, and dysrhythmia
Bromocriptine	DA receptor agonist	Serious side effect profile including delirium, **hallucinations,** nausea, and orthostatic hypotension
Amantadine	**Anti-influenza drug** that was found to increase DA in the CNS; exact mechanism is unclear; inhibits MAO$_B$	Adverse effects include **hallucinations,** confusion, orthostatic hypotension, acute toxic **psychosis**
Selegiline/Deprenyl		By inhibiting DA breakdown, selegiline administration allows lower doses of L-dopa to be used
Drugs that Decrease Acetylcholine in the Striatum		
Benztropine, trihexyphenidyl	Muscarinic antagonists	Side effects are similar to those of atropine: dry mouth, dry eyes, constipation, urinary retention, confusion

DA, dopamine; MAO$_B$, monoamine oxidase B.

QUICK HIT Because DA itself cannot cross the blood-brain barrier, the precursor L-dopa, which can enter the CNS, is given.

QUICK HIT **Carbidopa,** which is often given along with L-dopa, inhibits the peripheral breakdown of L-dopa to DA by a plasma decarboxylase. Because this allows more L-dopa to enter the CNS, smaller doses can be used, minimizing side effects.

As one might expect, the drugs that increase DA can affect both the nigrostriatal and mesolimbic pathways. Therefore, patients on levodopa (L-dopa) sometimes complain of **involuntary chorea-like movements** (nigrostriatal) and **visual/auditory hallucinations** (mesolimbic). Depression and anxiety also occur with L-dopa therapy.

Anticholinergic agents are used only as adjuvant therapy in Parkinson's disease. These drugs are especially helpful in minimizing tremors but less effective at reducing muscle rigidity. Also, as muscarinic antagonists, they are fraught with side effects.

MAO$_A$ breaks down NEPI and serotonin, while MAO$_B$ breaks down DA.

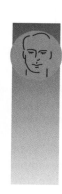

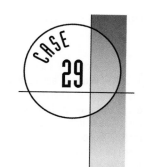

"I get these bad headaches where I feel like I'm having a heart attack and get very dizzy."

OBJECTIVES

1. Develop a differential diagnosis and an appropriate workup for severe headaches with associated chest pain and vertigo
2. Review phenylalanine metabolism and associated pathologies
3. Learn the mechanism of action and clinical use for α_1 antagonists
4. Understand the clinical reasoning behind pheochromocytoma treatment
5. Review the structure and function of the adrenal medulla

HISTORY AND PHYSICAL EXAMINATION

A 25-year-old medical student presents to student health with complaints of intermittent episodes during which he experiences **severe headaches, palpitations, dizziness,** and **diaphoresis.** He also noticed that these attacks are not necessarily related to high stress times (e.g., around exams). He has even had such an attack at an after-exam party and compares these episodes to feeling like he is having a heart attack. He is currently on no medications and **denies any cocaine or amphetamine abuse.** He also denies changes in appetite, heat intolerance, diarrhea, abdominal pain, any relation of his symptoms to meals, or a family history of hypertension. He has noticed an **unintentional 7-pound weight loss** over the past 2 weeks.

On physical exam, his blood pressure was **120/78 mm Hg.** However, **15 minutes later** he developed similar symptoms and his blood pressure rose to **190/120 mm Hg.** Pulse is 100. Funduscopic exam reveals narrowed retinal arterioles. The thyroid is normal in size and consistency. Hands are pale but skin is moist. He also has a mild tremor.

APPROPRIATE WORKUP

Blood chemistries, 24-hour urine sample, abdominal PET scan

DIFFERENTIAL DIAGNOSIS

Graves' disease, carcinoid tumor, pheochromocytoma, and panic disorder

DIAGNOSTIC LABORATORY TESTS AND STUDIES

Blood Chemistry:
Glucose = 350 mg/dL (H)
Creatinine = 1.1 mg/dL (N)
TSH = 1.2 μU/mL (N)
24-hour Urine Sample:
Metanephrine = 0.5 mg (N < 0.1)
Elevated vanillylmandelic acid (VMA)
Drug screen = negative

PET:
Vascular mass above right kidney

DIAGNOSIS: PHEOCHROMOCYTOMA

This patient presents with pheochromocytoma, a tumor that arises from **chromaffin cells of the adrenal medulla.** These cells produce mostly **epinephrine** releasing it into the systemic circulation. The patient's clinical presentation is a manifestation of **high circulating catecholamines.**

Metanephrine, a catecholamine, is a useful diagnostic test if found in the urine. **VMA** is a product of catecholamine metabolism. Therefore, this patient's 24-hour urinary sample indicated elevated levels of catecholamines. The concurrent 24-hour urine creatinine confirms the adequacy of the urine collection. Epinephrine increases glucose levels through several mechanisms. In the liver, it **stimulates glycogenolysis and gluconeogenesis.** In the pancreas, epinephrine **inhibits insulin release** and **stimulates glucagon release**. In fatty tissue, it **stimulates lipolysis**. The liberated fatty acids can be used by tissues as glucose. Finally, in muscle, cellular glucose uptake is inhibited and epinephrine **activates glycolysis** to form lactate and alanine which can be used as precursors in gluconeogenesis.

This patient is experiencing syncope due to **intravascular volume depletion.** The elevated catecholamine levels increase blood pressure. This decreases renin and aldosterone resulting in less sodium and water retention. Patients can also appear pale due to increased vasoconstriction. This patient is also losing weight because he is in a **hypermetabolic state.**

EXPLANATION OF DIFFERENTIAL

Graves' disease is the most common cause of hyperthyroidism. It is an **autoimmune disease** with **TSH receptor antibodies,** stimulating thyroid hormone synthesis. Clinical features include **exophthalmos** (Figures 29-1 and 29-2), diffuse goiter, and pretibial myxedema. The latter is nonpitting edema caused by accumulation of interstitial glycosaminoglycans within the dermis. It is a nonspecific finding and can also be seen in hypothyroidism. Patients with Graves' disease can also experience **weight loss** as thyroid hormones **increase the basal metabolic rate** which also contributes to **heat intolerance.** Lab findings would have revealed **decreased TSH,** and **increased total T_4, free T_4, and T_3 uptake.**

FIGURE 29-1 **Exophthalmos with proptosis and periorbital edema**

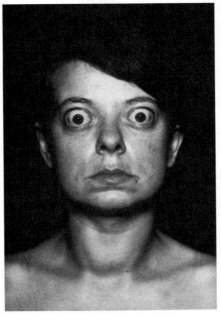

(Reprinted with permission from Rubin E, Farber JL. Pathology, 3rd Ed. Philadelphia: Lippincott Williams & Wilkins, 1999.)

FIGURE 29-2 CT with extraocular muscle enlargement at the orbital apex

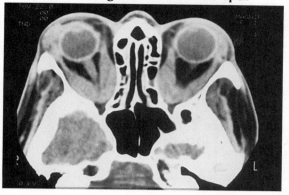

(From Tasman W, Jaeger E. The Wills Eye Hospital Atlas of Clinical Ophthalmology, 2nd Ed. Philadelphia: Lippincott Williams & Wilkins, 2001.)

Carcinoid tumors are derived from **neuroendocrine cells** that metastasize from the small bowel. Urinalysis would have revealed high levels of **serotonin (5-HIAA)**. Clinical presentation would have been concurrent wheezing, diarrhea, and cutaneous flushing. The treatment of choice is **octreotide** which is an analog of somatostatin which is an endogenous inhibitor of growth hormone secretion from the hypothalamus. It is effective in reducing GH levels and hence treating acromegaly (caused by an increase in growth hormone). Somatostatin also has an inhibitory effect on intestinal activity and gastrointestinal motility. Therefore, octreotide is effective in treating diarrhea.

Panic disorder is characterized by **recurrent, unexpected panic attacks** during which symptoms such as diaphoresis, palpitations, chest pain, **fear of losing control,** and nausea are predominant. Urinalysis would reveal no significant findings. The appropriate treatment would be with **selective serotonin reuptake inhibitors (SSRIs)** such as fluoxetine, sertraline, paroxetine, and citalopram. **"Serotonin syndrome"** is a major side effect associated with simultaneously taking SSRIs and MAO inhibitors resulting in hyperthermia, tremor, increased muscle tone, and autonomic instability which can progress to hallucinations and even death.

Related Basic Sciences

Phenylalanine metabolism and associated pathologies (Figure 29-3)

Table 29-1 summarizes the clinical features and biochemistry associated with the diseases in Figure 29-3.

> **QUICK HIT**
> Graves' disease is considered a type II hypersensitivity reaction.

> **QUICK HIT**
> Thyroxine (T_4) is more abundant while triiodothyronine (T_3) is more potent. T_4 is converted to T_3 in the periphery.

> **QUICK HIT**
> Serotonin is decreased in both anxiety and depression. However, norepinephrine is increased in anxiety and decreased in depression.

> **QUICK HIT**
> S-adenosyl methionine (SAM) transfers methyl groups to epinephrine (from norepinephrine), melatonin (from acetyl serotonin) and phosphatidylcholine (from phosphatidylethanolamine). The formation of SAM from ATP and methionine requires vitamin B_{12}.

> **QUICK HIT**
> Epinephrine is a general agonist on α_1, α_2, β_1, and β_2. Norepinephrine is an agonist on α_1, α_2, and β_1 receptors.

FIGURE 29-3 Phenylalanine metabolism and associated pathologies

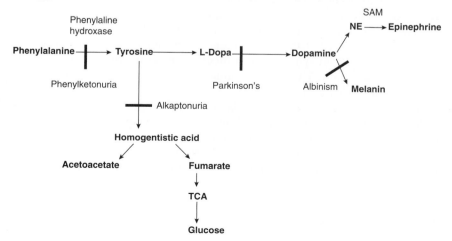

Treat phenylketonuria by minimizing phenylalanine-containing foods (i.e., Nutrasweet) and increasing tyrosine in the diet.

Vitiligo is due to the complete loss of melanocytes that results in depigmented white patches. Albinism is the failure of intact melanocytes to produce pigments.

Parkinson's disease is due to decreased dopamine while schizophrenia is due to increased dopamine.

Parkinson symptoms associated with orthostatic hypotension and autonomic dysfunction is referred to as the Shy-Drager syndrome.

Phenoxybenzamine is the treatment of choice for **phe**ochromocytomas.

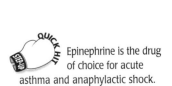

Epinephrine is the drug of choice for acute asthma and anaphylactic shock.

TABLE 29-1 Phenylalanine Associated Diseases		
Disease	**Clinical Presentation**	**Associated Biochemistry**
Phenylketonuria	**Body odor,** mental and growth **retardation,** and eczema	Decreased **phenylalanine hydroxylase** or **tetrahydrobiopterin factor** → excess phenylalanine → phenylketones in urine
Alkaptonuria	Urine **turns black upon standing,** dark connective tissue, and arthralgias	Deficient **homogentisic acid oxidase** which degrades tyrosine → excess alkapton bodies
Parkinson	Pill-rolling **resting tremor,** akinesia, bradykinesia, **masked facies,** and **cogwheel rigidity**	**Decreased dopamine** production
Albinism	Pale skin, white hair, **red eyes,** and increased risk of **skin cancer**	Deficiency in **tyrosinase** which converts tyrosine to melanin; can also result from **lack of migration of neural crest cells**

α₁ ANTAGONISTS

α_1 receptors are located on vascular smooth muscle of the skin and splanchnic regions and **sympathetically constrict blood vessels** in the skin and **dilate blood vessels** in skeletal muscles. Their mechanism of action is via **formation of IP₃** and **increased intracellular Ca²⁺**. **Phenoxybenzamine** and **phentolamine** are **nonselective α blockers.** Because of phenoxybenzamine's irreversible binding of α_1-adrenergic receptors, it is preferred over other α_1 blockers in preoperative preparation for tumor removal. It tends to minimize catecholamine effects during surgery. **Doxazosin, terazosin, and prazosin** are α_1 **selective receptor antagonists.** These selective antagonists are particularly useful for patients who suffer with *both* hypertension and BPH.

Pheochromocytoma treatment

Preoperative **α-adrenergic blockade** with phenoxybenzamine as well as volume expansion is required. **β-blockers** for arrhythmias should only be added after α-blockade. Use of β-blockers without prior α-blockade may worsen hypertension. Nonselective β-blockers antagonize β_1 receptors on the heart and vasodilatory β_2-adrenergic receptors. Therefore, plasma epinephrine can only bind to vasoconstrictor α_1-adrenergic receptors, precipitating a hypertensive crisis.

Adrenal medulla

The adrenal medulla is part of the **sympathetic nervous system,** which tends to act on the body in a coordinated fashion. The parasympathetic system, on the other hand, can activate discrete organ systems (such as stimulating intestinal motility without affecting heart rate). The sympathetic preganglionic cell is **cholinergic,** derived from neuroectoderm, and found in the intermediolateral cell column of the spinal cord at thoracic and upper lumbar levels. This neuron synapses via a **nicotinic receptor** on a postganglionic neuron in the sympathetic chain. The postganglionic cell is **derived from neural crest** and is usually **adrenergic** (releases norepinephrine).

The **chromaffin cells** of the adrenal medulla are modified postganglionic cells. As such, they are derived from neural crest cells and innervated by sympathetic preganglionic nerves that pass through the sympathetic chain and synapse directly on the chromaffin cells. These cells of the adrenal medulla act just like sympathetic postganglionic cells, except they **produce mostly epinephrine** and release it into the systemic circulation.

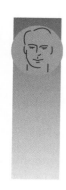

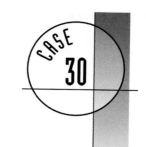

"I'm here for my yearly check-up."

OBJECTIVES

1. Develop a differential diagnosis and an appropriate workup for hypertension at a relatively young age
2. Review the renin–angiotensin–aldosterone system
3. Understand the three types of hypertension
4. Review the mechanisms of actions and side effects of common hypertension medications
5. Review the causes of secondary hypertension

HISTORY AND PHYSICAL EXAMINATION

A **32-year-old African American man** comes in for his yearly checkup. He has no complaints. He states that he is taking no prescription or over-the-counter (OTC) medications. He denies a history of smoking, alcohol, or drug abuse. He is unaware of a family history of hypertension but recalls that his grandfather died of a cerebrovascular accident (CVA) at 50 years of age, and his father died of a myocardial infarction (MI) at 55 years of age. Physical examination reveals that he is apparently healthy and of normal weight; his **blood pressure is 150/98 mm Hg.**

APPROPRIATE WORKUP

Blood chemistries and urinalysis

DIFFERENTIAL DIAGNOSIS

Essential hypertension, secondary hypertension

DIAGNOSTIC LABORATORY TESTS AND STUDIES

Blood chemistry:
  Na = 140 mEq/L (N)
  K = 4 mEq/L (N)
  BUN = 10 mg/dL (N)
  Creatinine = 1.0 mg/dL (N)
  Growth hormone (GH) = (N)
  Free T_4 = 7 mg/dL (N)

Aldosterone = (N)
Glucose = 84 mg/dL
Urinalysis:
  Protein = 0 mg/dL (N)
  RBCs = 0 cells/hpf (N)
  Catecholamines = Minimal (N)

DIAGNOSIS: ESSENTIAL HYPERTENSION

Essential hypertension is a **diagnosis of exclusion,** determined by finding a blood pressure greater than **140 mm Hg systolic, 90 mm Hg diastolic, or both** on **three separate occasions.** Hypertension most commonly presents in the **third to fourth decade of life,**

with a higher incidence in **men;** it is more common and more severe in **African Americans.** Genetic factors may play a role in the etiology of hypertension, as most patients have a family history of the disease. Environmental factors that may contribute to essential hypertension include stress, obesity, cigarette smoking, physical inactivity, and excessive sodium intake.

Hypertension itself is usually **asymptomatic,** although with extremely high pressures headache, retinopathy, and a second aortic sound (A$_2$) may occur. If untreated, long-term hypertension can lead to retinal changes, nephrosclerosis, left ventricular hypertrophy, and cardiac failure. Long-term untreated hypertension is a major predisposing factor for ischemic heart disease and CVA.

EXPLANATION OF DIFFERENTIAL

Because essential hypertension is a diagnosis of exclusion, one must attempt to rule out all causes of **secondary hypertension** before assigning a diagnosis of essential hypertension. The results of this patient's laboratory tests rule out **renal failure** and **endocrine abnormalities,** which are the most likely causes of secondary hypertension. In general, essential hypertension is the diagnosis in 90% of cases, so finding a cause for secondary hypertension is unlikely.

Related Basic Science

Renin–angiotensin–aldosterone system

The juxtaglomerular cells of the kidney release renin in response to a decrease in blood pressure (Figure 30-1). Renin then cleaves angiotensinogen (released from the liver) to angiotensin I. In the lung, **angiotensin-converting enzyme (ACE)** cleaves angiotensin I to **angiotensin II,** which has two major functions. Aldosterone promotes the retention of sodium and water from the distal convoluted tubule, which increases blood volume and subsequently blood pressure (Figure 30-2). Increased blood pressure results in stretching of the atrial wall and subsequent release of atrial natriuretic peptide (ANP) by the atrial

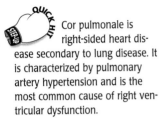

Cor pulmonale is right-sided heart disease secondary to lung disease. It is characterized by pulmonary artery hypertension and is the most common cause of right ventricular dysfunction.

Conn syndrome, also known as hyperaldosteronism, results from an aldosterone-secreting tumor. Characteristics of Conn syndrome include hypertension, hyperkalemia, metabolic alkalosis, and decreased secretion of renin.

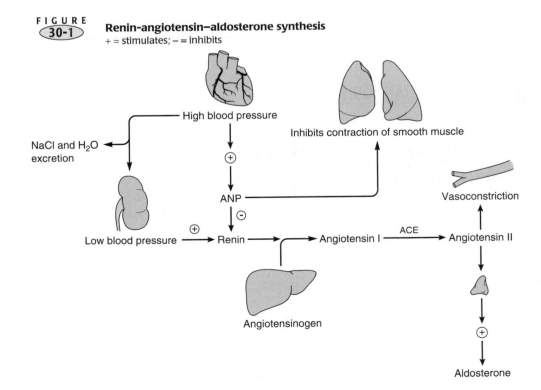

FIGURE 30-1 Renin-angiotensin–aldosterone synthesis
+ = stimulates; – = inhibits

FIGURE
30-2   **Aldosterone synthesis**

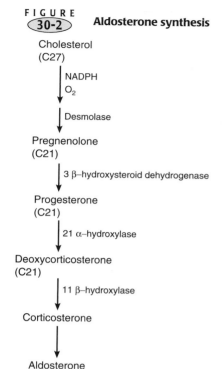

Cholesterol
(C27)
│ NADPH
│ O₂
│ Desmolase
↓
Pregnenolone
(C21)
│ 3 β–hydroxysteroid dehydrogenase
↓
Progesterone
(C21)
│ 21 α–hydroxylase
↓
Deoxycorticosterone
(C21)
│ 11 β–hydroxylase
↓
Corticosterone
│
↓
Aldosterone

myocytes (which raises preload). **ANP acts to lower blood pressure** by increasing excretion of salt and water, which reduces the release of renin and subsequently decreases the contractile effect on smooth muscle.

Hypertension

Three types of hypertension exist: essential, secondary, and malignant (accelerated). **More than 90% of cases of hypertension have no identifiable cause** and are termed essential or primary hypertension (discussed earlier). Secondary hypertension is hypertension that results from an existing disease process. Renal disease is the most common cause of secondary hypertension, but other etiologies also exist (Table 30-1).

Malignant hypertension

Malignant hypertension can be a complication of either essential or secondary hypertension and follows an accelerated clinical course. It most often occurs in **young African American men.** Characteristics of malignant hypertension include a marked **increase in diastolic blood pressure,** focal **retinal hemorrhage** with papilledema, malignant **nephrosclerosis** ("flea-bitten" kidney), left ventricular hypertrophy, and left ventricular failure. Malignant hypertension can result in early death from congestive heart failure (CHF), CVA, or renal failure.

Vascular disease resulting from hypertension

Hypertension can lead to several abnormalities in the vasculature, including atherosclerosis in large arteries, hyaline arteriolosclerosis in small vessels, and proliferative changes and necrosis of arterioles. Arteriolar walls affected by hypertensive changes are weakened and prone to aneurysm and rupture.

Several types of aneurysms can result from long-standing hypertension. **Aortic aneurysms** are characterized by longitudinal intraluminal tears with the formation of a **second lumen within the arterial media.** These aneurysms can rupture, leading swiftly to death. Minute aneurysms, termed Charcot-Bouchard microaneurysms, occur in vessels

QUICK HIT
Angiotensin II stimulates **release of aldosterone** from the zona glomerulosa in the adrenal medulla and also acts as a **potent vasoconstrictor** (low levels act at the renal arterioles; high levels act as a general vasoconstrictor). Physiologically, both actions increase arterial pressure. Increased sodium reabsorption triggered by aldosterone increases blood volume and hence arterial pressure. Vasoconstriction of the arterioles results in increased total peripheral resistance (TPR) and mean arterial pressure.

QUICK HIT
Malignant hypertension is also the most common cause of primary brain parenchymal hemorrhage.

QUICK HIT
Fibromuscular dysplasia, a cause of secondary hypertension, typically occurs in **young women** and shows a "**string of pearls**" appearance on radiograph.

QUICK HIT
Renal artery stenosis, which is more common in women than in men, does not cause hypertension until more than 70% of the lumen is occluded.

TABLE 30-1 Secondary Causes of Hypertension

Pathologic Process	Specific Disease
Renal parenchymal disease	Chronic glomerulonephritis Pyelonephritis Polycystic kidney disease Collagen disease of the kidney
Renovascular disease	**Renal arterial stenosis** caused by **atherosclerosis** **Fibromuscular dysplasia** Emboli Trauma Extrinsic compression by tumors
Endocrine disease	Pheochromocytoma Cushing syndrome Primary aldosteronism Hyperthyroidism Myxedema
Other	Coarctation of the aorta Obstructive uropathy Excessive alcohol intake Oral contraceptives Sympathomimetics Corticosteroids Cocaine Licorice

that are less that 300 micrometers in diameter, most commonly within the basal ganglia. These aneurysms can also rupture, leading to hemorrhagic infarcts.

Treatment

The first line of treatment for mild hypertension is **lifestyle modifications, diet changes (weight loss of 5 to 10%), and avoidance of ethanol, tobacco, and caffeine.** If these measures fail to lower blood pressure, mild hypertension usually is treated with a single drug. More severe hypertension may require a multidrug regimen. Treatment usually begins with either a **diuretic, β-blocker, ACE inhibitor,** or **calcium channel blocker.** If one of these treatments does not control blood pressure, a second drug is added. Usually a β-blocker is added if the initial drug is a diuretic, and vice versa. An ACE inhibitor or calcium channel blocker can be used as a third step for patients who still have high blood pressure following treatment with a two-drug regimen. Alternatively, a vasodilator may be added to the other two drugs.

Thiazide diuretics such as **hydrochlorothiazide** are the most widely used diuretics. The thiazides initially lower blood pressure by increasing excretion of sodium and water. The result is decreased extracellular volume, which also decreases cardiac output and renal blood flow. Thiazide diuretics are also useful in treating hypercalciuria, as they decrease calcium excretion. Side effects include hypokalemic metabolic acidosis as potassium and hydrogen ions are also excreted with sodium and chloride as the flow rate in the early distal tubule increases. Patients can also experience hyperglycemia, hyperlipidemia, hyperuricemia, and hypercalcemia.

Loop diuretics, specifically furosemide, is a sulfonamide that inhibits the cotransport of Na^+, K^+, and $2Cl^-$ in the thick ascending limb of Henle. Given its mechanism of action, it is used to treat edematous states, such as CHF, nephrotic syndrome, pulmonary edema, and cirrhosis. The key difference with thiazide diuretics lies in its treatment of calcium. Loop diuretics *increase* the excretion of calcium, making it suitable for patients with hypercalcemia. Side effects include ototoxicity, hypokalemia, sulfa allergy, and gout. A patient with sulfa allergies and gout can safely take ethacrynic acid instead.

The **β-blockers** reduce blood pressure by decreasing cardiac output and sympathetic outflow from the CNS, thus inhibiting the release of renin from the kidneys and ultimately reducing levels of aldosterone. Propranolol, which acts at β-1 and β-2 receptors, is a prototype β-blocker. Atenolol and metoprolol are selective β-1 blockers and are used when comorbidities such as asthma or diabetes accompany hypertension. β-blockers are more effective in the treatment of Caucasian patients and young adult patients.

ACE inhibitors (captopril, enalapril, and lisinopril) inhibit ACE, reducing levels of angiotensin II and bradykinin (a potent vasodilator). ACE inhibitors increase release of renin because of the loss of feedback inhibition. The most notable side effect of ACE inhibitors is a dry cough. Losartan, a highly selective angiotensin II receptor blocker, produces vasodilation and blocks secretion of aldosterone but lacks the side effects of traditional ACE inhibitors.

Calcium channel blockers (nifedipine, verapamil, and diltiazem) are recommended when the preferred first-line agents are contraindicated or ineffective. They are rarely used as first-line agents; if other drugs fail, then physicians often turn to the calcium channel blockers. These drugs block voltage-dependent calcium channels of smooth and cardiac muscle, which reduces muscle contractility and promotes vasodilation. Nifedipine has the greatest effect on vascular smooth muscle, while verapamil has the greatest effect on the heart.

The **α-adrenergic blocking agents,** such as prazosin, decrease peripheral vascular resistance and reduce arterial blood pressure by relaxing arterial and venous smooth muscle. One of their effects is vasodilation. Therefore, prazosin has been used to treat males with both hypertension and urinary retention in benign prostatic hyperplasia (BPH). Centrally acting adrenergic agents, such as Clonidine and methyldopa, decrease sympathetic outflow from the brain's vasomotor center, decreasing total peripheral resistance and total blood pressure. Clonidine, an α-2 agonist, is mainly used to treat mild to moderate hypertension that has failed to respond to treatment with diuretics alone and is safe to use in patients with hypertension *and* renal disease as blood flow to the kidneys is not compromised. Reserpine and guanethidine are sympathoplegics that deplete neurons of catecholamines.

Hydralazine and minoxidil are two direct vasodilators that function at the arteriolar level, leading to decreased blood pressure but increased cardiac output. Hydralazine can cause a lupus-like syndrome while minoxidil has been used for male-pattern baldness, causing increased growth of body hair.

Excessive use of thiazide diuretics may cause hypokalemia. In contrast, ACE inhibitors may cause hyperkalemia.

Propanolol also can be used to treat panic and anxiety attacks and migraines, but it has been associated with depression in older adults.

ACE inhibitors have been shown to reduce kidney damage in patients with hypertension and diabetes.

Sudden cessation of clonidine by patients can result in severe rebound hypertension.

Biofeedback is a training technique that enables an individual to gain some voluntary control over autonomic body functions and may help decrease blood pressure.

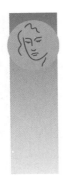

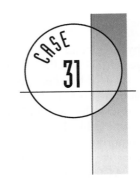

"I think I'm finally pregnant."

OBJECTIVES

1. Develop a differential diagnosis and appropriate workup for possible pregnancy
2. Understand the development, function, and disorders of the placenta
3. Review fetal circulation and associated pediatric cardiology
4. Learn the types, functions, and fluctuations in hormone levels during pregnancy
5. Differentiate between the clinical features associated with preeclampsia and eclampsia
6. Understand how to determine an Apgar score and its significance

HISTORY AND PHYSICAL EXAMINATION

A 28-year-old woman presents to the office desiring a pregnancy test. She and her husband have been trying for 18 months to conceive. Now the patient's menstrual cycle is 1 week late, and she has been nauseous, especially in the morning. The patient took a urine pregnancy test 2 days ago, and the result was positive. Her physical examination is unremarkable.

APPROPRIATE WORKUP

Serum β-hCG test

DIFFERENTIAL DIAGNOSIS

Pregnancy, amenorrhea

> **QUICK HIT**
> The urine pregnancy tests detect hCG, which is produced by the syncytiotrophoblast. Levels of hCG become detectable in the urine by 2 weeks after conception.

DIAGNOSTIC LABORATORY TESTS AND STUDIES

Serum β-human chorionic gonadotropin (hCG) test:
  Positive results

DIAGNOSIS: PREGNANCY

Explanation of Differential

Amenorrhea can be primary or secondary. Primary amenorrhea is when a patient never achieves menarche; the most common cause is Turner syndrome. If a patient's menstrual cycle was normal, but she is now experiencing amenorrhea, that is secondary amenorrhea. Many factors can cause secondary amenorrhea, such as stress, malnutrition (e.g., anorexia nervosa), elevated prolactin levels (e.g., prolactinoma, antipsychotic drug therapy), and pregnancy (the most common cause). Of these causes, only pregnancy is associated with elevated hCG levels.

Related Basic Science

The placenta

The functional endometrium of a pregnant woman is called the decidua and is divided into three parts (Figure 31-1). The decidua basalis is the endometrium found under the placenta. The decidua capsularis is the thin layer covering the implanted blastocyst. The decidua parietalis describes the rest of the endometrium. As the fetus grows, the overlying decidua capsularis expands, fuses with the decidua parietalis, and obliterates the uterine space. The entire decidua is shed following parturition as "afterbirth."

The chorion is formed from both the trophoblast and extra-embryonic mesoderm. The chorion, which completely surrounds the fetus, creates the chorionic cavity. At first, villi cover the entire chorion; however, only those villi in the region of the placenta persist. The chorion therefore becomes divided into "villous chorion" and "smooth chorion." As the fetus grows, the amnion fuses with the smooth chorion, forming the amniochorionic membrane. It is this membrane that ruptures when the "water breaks." Except at the cervical os, the amniochorionic membrane fuses with decidua capsularis, which in turn fuses with the decidua parietalis and essentially disappears.

The placenta, which develops from both the maternal endometrium and embryonic chorion, is the site of maternal-fetal exchange. At implantation, the trophoblast cells begin to invade the endometrium. At about day 10, lacunae appear in the syncytiotrophoblast. These lacunae fill with maternal blood and go on to fuse and form the intervillous space of the placenta. In the fully functioning placenta, maternal blood continually flows in through spiral arteries and bathes the villi. Exchange occurs between the maternal blood in the villous space and fetal blood in vessels within the villi. As the pregnancy progresses, the barrier between the maternal and fetal blood thins, and exchange becomes more efficient to meet the growing demands of the developing fetus.

The placenta has three major functions. The first is transport. The fetus obtains nutrients such as oxygen, proteins, and glucose and rids itself of waste products. The second function is metabolism. The placenta synthesizes glycogen, cholesterol, and fats. The third function is production of hormones, including hCG, human placental lactogen (HPL), progesterone, and estrogen.

The placenta is a selectively permeable barrier that allows several substances to cross to the fetal circulation. A few of these substances are listed in Table 31-1.

Disorders of the placenta include abruptio placenta, placenta accreta, and placenta previa. **Abruptio placenta** describes premature separation of the placenta, which can cause bleeding, fetal death, and disseminated intravascular coagulation (DIC) in the mother.

> **QUICK HIT** The congenital rubella syndrome can include mental retardation, cerebral palsy, deafness, patent ductus arteriosis, cataracts, glaucoma, or fetal death. This occurs when a pregnant woman is infected or immunized with the vaccine, which contains attenuated live virus.

FIGURE 31-1 Relationship of the fetus, uterus, and placenta

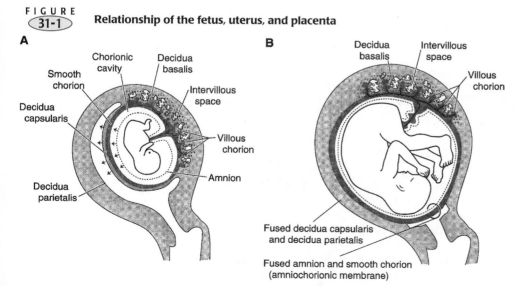

A

Smooth chorion
Chorionic cavity
Decidua basalis
Intervillous space
Decidua capsularis
Villous chorion
Amnion
Decidua parietalis

B

Decidua basalis
Intervillous space
Villous chorion
Fused decidua capsularis and decidua parietalis
Fused amnion and smooth chorion (amniochorionic membrane)

(From Dudek RW, Fix JD. BRS Embryology, 2nd Ed. Philadelphia: Lippincott Williams & Wilkins, 1998, p 67.)

TABLE 31-1	**Substances That Cross the Placenta**
Gases	**Oxygen, Carbon Dioxide, Carbon Monoxide**
Viruses	HIV, CMV, rubella, polio, coxsackie, measles, varicella, variola
Microbes	*Treponema pallidum, Toxoplasma gondii*
Antibodies	IgG
Drugs	Thalidomide, warfarin, phenytoin, cocaine, alcohol, nicotine
	CMV, cytomegalovirus

Placenta accreta is when the placenta is attached directly to the myometrium and not the decidua. This can present at parturition as impaired placental separation and hemorrhage. **Placenta previa** is when the placenta attaches to the lower uterus, over the cervical os. This can cause bleeding during pregnancy.

Fetal circulation

Three shunts characterize the fetal circulation, each of which is designed to bypass organs that are not essential for the fetus. Two of these act to shunt blood past the pulmonary circulation, while the third shunts past the liver. Oxygen-poor and nutrient-poor fetal blood is replenished in the placenta. The blood then returns to the fetus through the umbilical vein. About 50% of this blood passes through the liver; the remainder bypasses the liver and goes through the **ductus venosus** to join the inferior vena cava.

If a pregnant woman's red blood cells are Rh antigen–negative and the red blood cells of her fetus are Rh antigen–positive, there is a risk to the fetus. At any time in the pregnancy, especially with trauma or around the time of delivery, the mother may be exposed to fetal blood. This exposure will first sensitize the mother and cause her to produce anti-Rh antigens. Later in pregnancy, or with future pregnancies, this anti-Rh antibody will cross the placenta and cause hemolysis of the fetal red blood cells. In its worst form, this results in hydrops fetalis. The Coombs test can help determine if such a reaction will take place (Figure 31-2).

The oxygen-rich and nutrient-rich blood mixes with depleted blood from the fetal body. This mixed blood enters the right atrium, where most of it flows through the **foramen ovale** to the left atrium. After mixing with depleted blood from the pulmonary veins, the

FIGURE 31-2   The Coombs' test

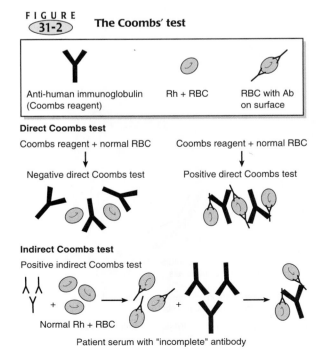

blood is pumped into the aorta. Of the blood that is pumped into the aorta, 50% travels out the umbilical arteries to the placenta.

A small fraction of the blood that enters the right atrium continues to the right ventricle and to the pulmonary trunk. Most of this blood, however, is also shunted to the left side of the heart through the **ductus arteriosus.** Because resistance in the fetal pulmonary circulation is high, blood preferentially travels from the pulmonary trunk through the ductus arteriosis to the aorta, where resistance is much lower.

After birth, circulation in the neonate must quickly change so that the lungs can function normally. One of the first changes is closure of the ductus venosus. This, combined with the closure of the umbilical vessels, causes the central venous pressure to drop. With this drop, the pressure in the left atrium is for the first time higher than that in the right atrium. This pressure difference causes the foramen ovale, a one-way valve, to close. Aeration of the lungs is followed by a drop in resistance in the pulmonary circulation. Blood in the pulmonary trunk now preferentially goes to the lungs and not through the ductus arteriosus. In fact, until the ductus arteriosus closes completely, blood leaks from the high-pressure aorta to the pulmonary trunk. Closure of the ductus arteriosus is complicated. During gestation, prostaglandins produced in response to hypoxia seem to keep the ductus arteriosus open. With the increased oxygen levels that follow respiration, release of bradykinin is involved in closing the ductus arteriosus (Figure 31-3).

QUICK HIT The pulmonary vasculature is unique in that hypoxia causes vasoconstriction, while high oxygen levels cause vasodilation. This relationship tends to maintain V/Q matching.

FIGURE 31-3 **Fetal circulation**

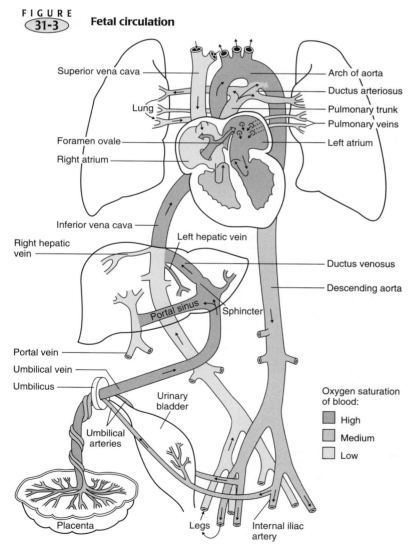

(From Mehta S, Milder EA, Mirarchi AJ. Step-Up: A High-Yield, Systems-Based Review for the USMLE Step 1. Philadelphia: Lippincott Williams & Wilkins, 2000, p 40.)

At birth, the right ventricular wall is thicker than the left because it has been pumping against greater resistance. This reverses within 1 month.

Alprostadil (PGE1) can be used to maintain a patent ductus arteriosus, while **indomethacin,** a nonsteroidal anti-inflammatory drug (NSAID) that inhibits production of cyclooxygenase and prostaglandin, facilitates closing of the ductus arteriosus.

Two major symptoms of elevated prolactin levels in a woman are galactorrhea and amenorrhea.

Up to 20% of healthy pregnant women can have edema of the lower legs, face, and hands.

Hormone levels during pregnancy (Figure 31-4)

Without fertilization, the corpus luteum regresses. If fertilization and implantation are successful, the hCG produced by the placenta maintains the corpus luteum. During the first trimester, the corpus luteum produces estrogen and progesterone, and levels of these hormones steadily rise. In the second and third trimesters, hCG levels have decreased, and the corpus luteum no longer plays a major role. The placenta now produces progesterone. The placenta also produces estrogen by converting dehydroepiandrosterone-sulfate produced in the fetal adrenal gland. The high levels of estrogen and progesterone inhibit secretion of gonadotropin-releasing hormone (GnRH), follicle-stimulating hormone (FSH), and luteinizing hormone (LH). Development of ovarian follicles is therefore inhibited throughout pregnancy.

The high levels of estrogen and progesterone also stimulate the growth and activation of the breasts during pregnancy. Estrogen increases secretion of prolactin, but estrogen and progesterone block the effect of prolactin on the breast. Following parturition, estrogen and progesterone levels fall, and prolactin can stimulate lactation. In a breast-feeding woman, prolactin levels remain high, which shuts down the GnRH/FSH/LH axis. Therefore, the woman will not ovulate until prolactin levels return to normal.

Toxemia of pregnancy

This group of hypertensive disorders is associated with pregnancy. The most serious of these disorders are preeclampsia and eclampsia, both of which usually appear late in pregnancy. **Preeclampsia typically presents with hypertension, edema, and proteinuria.**

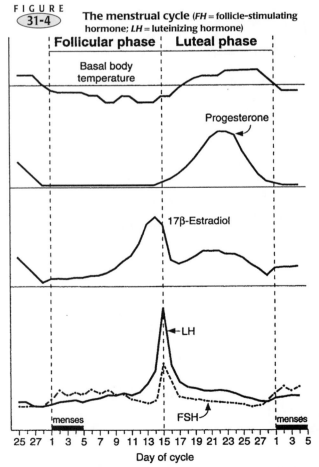

FIGURE 31-4 **The menstrual cycle** (*FH* = follicle-stimulating hormone; *LH* = luteinizing hormone)

(From Costanzo LS. BRS Physiology, 2nd Ed. Philadelphia: Lippincott Williams & Wilkins, 1998, p 278.)

Idiopathic vasospasm causes preeclampsia, and the resultant hypoperfusion can affect many organs. Headache and hyperreflexia can be present in severe forms of preeclampsia. Some risk factors for preeclampsia include young or advanced maternal age, pre-existing hypertension, diabetes mellitus, and nulliparity. The complications and consequences of preeclampsia include abruptio placenta, DIC, hepatic rupture, and eclampsia.

Eclampsia is a more severe form of preeclampsia with CNS involvement and **seizures.** This condition is life-threatening, and the only curative treatment is delivery or termination of the pregnancy.

The Apgar score

The Apgar score (Table 31-2) is used at 1 and 5 minutes after birth to physically assess a neonate. The five categories are each scored from 0 to 2. The highest possible score is 10.

TABLE 31-2 The Apgar Score

Score	Heart Rate	Respiration	Muscle Tone	Reflexes	Color
0	Absent	Absent	Limp	Absent	Pale, blue
1	<100 b/min	Irregular, slow	Flexion of extremities	Grimace	Trunk pink
2	>100 b/min	Strong, crying	Active motion	Vigorous	All pink

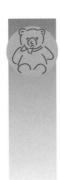

"I've been having bad stomach pains. My belly seems bigger, even though I've lost some weight recently."

OBJECTIVES

1. Develop a differential diagnosis and an appropriate workup for abdominal pain and distension and weight loss
2. Review ovarian structure and function
3. Understand the cause, clinical features, and diagnosis of uterine fibroid and squamous cell carcinoma of the cervix

HISTORY AND PHYSICAL EXAMINATION

A 45-year-old woman presents with an 8-month history of abdominal pain and distension and weight loss. The patient has no GI complaints but admits that she has had to urinate much more frequently lately. She has never been pregnant, and her menstrual periods have always been regular. She has noted no unusual vaginal discharge. She drinks alcohol only occasionally on weekends and does not smoke. Her family history is significant for breast cancer and ovarian cancer in her mother and sisters. Abdominal examination reveals a **mass in the pelvis** and **ascites** in the abdomen.

APPROPRIATE WORKUP

Pelvic US and CT, biopsy of pelvic mass, blood chemistries, and urinalysis

DIFFERENTIAL DIAGNOSIS

Cancer metastasis to ovary, endometrial carcinoma, ovarian neoplasm

DIAGNOSTIC LABORATORY TESTS AND STUDIES

Pelvic US and CT:
    Right ovarian mass, 6 cm in diameter
    Left ovarian mass, 3 cm in diameter
Blood chemistry:
    Elevated serum CA-125

Urinalysis:
    Normal results
Biopsy of masses:
    Serous cystadenocarcinoma

DIAGNOSIS: OVARIAN SEROUS CYSTADENOCARCINOMA

Ovarian cancer is the fifth most common form of cancer in women in the United States. Approximately 20% of ovarian masses are malignant. Because many of these malignancies are detected late in their development, they have a high mortality rate. The most common ovarian neoplasm is the **serous cystadenocarcinoma** (50% of ovarian carcinomas), which is notable in that it is commonly **bilateral.** Risk factors for the development of ovarian cancer include nulliparity and a family history of cancer, especially those cancers associated with the *BRCA1* mutation.

Clinically, ovarian neoplasms present with **lower abdominal pain** and **enlargement, GI complaints, urinary frequency,** and possibly **ascites** from peritoneal metastasis. As with other malignant cancers, ovarian cancer can cause cachexia and weight loss. The tumor marker **CA-125** is elevated in more than 80% of ovarian carcinomas.

EXPLANATION OF DIFFERENTIAL

The most common **metastatic tumors** of the ovary are of müllerian origin (uterus, fallopian tubes, contralateral ovary). Other sources include the breast and GI tract. The **Krukenberg tumor** describes stomach cancer metastasized to the ovaries. The cells of this tumor are shaped like a signet ring and filled with mucin. The biopsy and cytology study would identify this and other types of metastatic cancer.

Endometrial carcinoma, the most common gynecologic malignancy in the United States, often manifests as **vaginal bleeding.** Predisposing factors include unopposed estrogen stimulation, nulliparity, and obesity.

> **QUICK HIT** Unopposed estrogen increases a woman's risk for developing endometrial and breast cancer. For this reason, estrogen hormone replacement therapy usually includes progesterone, which reduces this risk.

Related Basic Science

Ovarian structure and function

The ovaries lie on the posterior aspect of the broad ligament, which is composed of two layers of peritoneum extending from the lateral margin of the uterus to the pelvic wall (Figure 32-1). The **mesovarium** attaches the anterior surface of the ovaries to the posterior surface of the broad ligament. The ovary itself is not peritonealized. The blood supply for the ovaries comes from the ovarian arteries and ovarian veins. The ovarian vessels travel within the **suspensory ligament** of the ovary, which attaches the superior (tubal) pole of the ovary to the pelvic wall. The **ovarian ligament** attaches the inferior (uterine) pole of the ovary to the uterus.

Histologically, the ovary can be divided into a medulla and cortex. The medulla is found on the interior of the ovary and contains the blood vessels, lymphatics, and nerves, which serve the ovary. The functional part of the ovary is the cortex. **The ovarian follicles**

> **QUICK HIT** The left gonadal veins drain into the left renal vein, while the right gonadal veins drain directly into the inferior vena cava.

FIGURE 32-1 Female reproductive organs

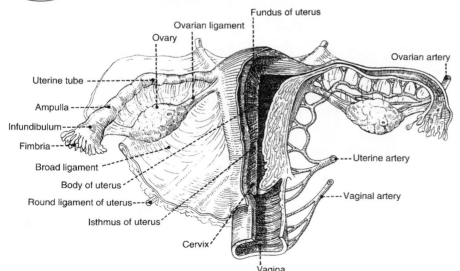

(From Chung KW. BRS Gross Anatomy, 4th Ed. Philadelphia:, Lippincott Williams & Wilkins, 2000, p 243.)

are embedded in the connective tissue of the cortex. A simple cuboidal germinal epithelium forms the outermost layer of the ovary and is continuous with the mesovarian mesothelium. Between the germinal epithelium and the cortex is the **tunica albuginea,** composed of dense connective tissue.

The ovaries have two main functions: gametogenesis and steroid hormone production. The gametes are the oocytes, which migrate from the embryonic yolk sac into the primordial gonad. The oocytes proliferate and reach a peak number of about 5 million at 5 months of fetal life. By birth, atresia (apoptosis) has reduced this number to approximately 1 million. Atresia continues throughout a female human's life, and only 400 gametes reach full maturity.

The process of gamete maturation from oocyte to ovum involves the formation of an ovarian follicle. Gonadotropic hormones **(follicle-stimulating hormone [FSH]** and **luteinizing hormone [LH])** stimulate this process. These hormones are released in response to the pulsatile release on **gonadotropin-releasing hormone (Gn-RH)** that begins at puberty. Follicles in their various stages of development are shown in Figure 32-2. It is the **theca cells** of the follicle, stimulated by LH, that **produce androgens. Granulosa cells,** under the control of FSH, then **convert these androgens to estrogens.** Without conception and successful implantation, the ruptured follicle regresses and forms a **corpus albicans.** If successful implantation occurs, the invading syncytiotrophoblast cells of the embryo produce the β-human chorionic gonadotropin (hCG) that maintains the **corpus luteum.** The corpus luteum continues to be functionally important for approximately the first 8 weeks of pregnancy. After this point, the placenta produces the progesterone necessary to maintain pregnancy.

Other gynecologic neoplasms

Uterine leiomyoma (uterine fibroid) is the most common tumor in women. These benign local proliferations of smooth muscle are found in the myometrium. They occur during the childbearing years, are responsive to estrogen, and regress after menopause.

QUICK HIT

In the testes, LH acts on Leydig cells to stimulate androgen production, while FSH acts on Sertoli cells to maintain spermatogenesis.

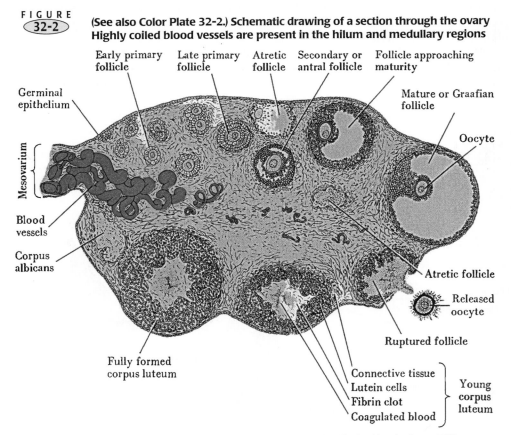

FIGURE 32-2

(See also Color Plate 32-2.) Schematic drawing of a section through the ovary Highly coiled blood vessels are present in the hilum and medullary regions

(From Ross MH, Romrell LJ, Kaye GI. Histology: A Text and Atlas, 3rd Ed. Philadelphia: Lippincott Williams & Wilkins, 1995, p. 680. After C. E. Corliss.)

Some estimate that by 40 years of age, up to 30% of women have fibroids. Of these, most remain asymptomatic. When symptoms do occur, **menorrhagia** is the most common complaint. Large fibroids can cause pelvic pain and urinary problems. Pelvic US diagnoses the tumors, and the definitive treatment is hysterectomy.

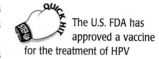

The U.S. FDA has approved a vaccine for the treatment of HPV

Squamous cell carcinoma of the cervix, although rare in the United States, is still a common gynecologic malignancy worldwide. Infection with certain strains of the human papillomavirus (**HPV-16 and HPV-18**) predisposes women to this preventable cancer. This cancer is preventable because cervical intraepithelial neoplasia (CIN), which is detectable by **Papanicolaou test,** precedes it and can be treated. HPV is an STD; therefore, **early sexual activity and multiple sexual partners are risk factors** for the development of cervical cancer. Papanicolaou test results suggestive of CIN are followed by diagnostic testing and, if necessary, surgical removal of affected areas.

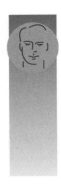

"I'm throwing up a lot of blood!"

OBJECTIVES

1. Develop and explain a differential diagnosis and an appropriate workup for bloody emesis
2. Review the pathophysiology associated with portal hypertension and cirrhosis
3. Review the signs and symptoms of genetic diseases that cause cirrhosis
4. Describe portal blood supply and portacaval anastomoses
5. Discuss social aspects and treatment of alcoholism
6. Review precursors, rate-limiting steps, and end products in gluconeogenesis and fat metabolism

HISTORY AND PHYSICAL EXAMINATION

A 60-year-old man states that he has **vomited large amounts of blood** in the past 24 hours. The patient has an extensive **history of alcoholism,** but denies a history of IV drug abuse. He has recently noted an **increase in the size of his abdomen** and he thinks his eyes have been looking a bit **yellow.** His appetite is unchanged and he denies cough, fever, shortness of breath, or hematochezia. The patient is not taking any medications. Physical examination reveals an emaciated man smelling strongly of alcohol. Chest auscultation is clear. Abdominal examination reveals an abdomen distended by **ascites** but without significant tenderness. There are physical signs of **jaundice, gynecomastia, spider angiomas, caput medusa, ascites, hemorrhoids,** and **testicular atrophy.**

APPROPRIATE WORKUP

Complete blood count, liver function tests, blood chemistries, chest radiograph, abdominal radiograph, CT scan of the chest and abdomen, esophagogastroduodenoscopy, and liver biopsy

DIFFERENTIAL DIAGNOSIS

Acute (erosive) gastritis, bleeding esophageal varices, Boerhaave syndrome, Mallory-Weiss tear, peptic ulcer disease

DIAGNOSTIC LABORATORY TESTS AND STUDIES

Complete blood count:
   Hct = 27% (L)
   Hgb = 9 g/dL (L)

Liver function tests:
   Aspartate amino transferase =
      250 U/L (H)

Alanine amino transferase (ALT)
= 105 U/L (H)

AST:ALT ratio = >2

γ-Glutamyl-transferase (GGT) =
3,000 U/L (H; markedly elevated)

Total bilirubin = 20 mg/dL (H)

Conjugated (direct) bilirubin =
13 mg/dL (H)

Serum albumin = 2.4 g/dL (L)

Blood chemistry:
Prothrombn time = 18 seconds (H)

Chest radiograph:
No pneumothorax

Abdominal radiograph:
No evidence of perforations or free
air under the diaphragm

CT scan of the chest and abdomen:
Esophageal varices

Esophagogastroduodenoscopy (EGD):
Bleeding esophageal varices

Liver biopsy:
Alcoholic cirrhosis (Figure 33-1)

DIAGNOSIS: BLEEDING ESOPHAGEAL VARICES

This patient has bleeding esophageal varices secondary to portal hypertension caused by alcoholic cirrhosis. The physical examination reveals multiple findings of alcoholic cirrhosis (Figure 33-2), including **jaundice, ascites, spider angiomas, gynecomastia,** and **testicular atrophy** (due to inability of the destroyed liver to metabolize estrogen). **Caput medusae, esophageal varices,** and **hemorrhoids** are caused by **venous congestion in the portal system.** Elevated liver enzymes are characteristic of cirrhosis, with AST being approximately two to three times higher than ALT. In cirrhosis, both of these liver enzymes are in the range of 100 to 300 U/L. A markedly elevated GGT is also highly characteristic of alcoholic liver disease. Bleeding esophageal varices must be ligated quickly, usually during EGD, or the patient can die from large amounts of blood loss.

FIGURE 33-1 (See also Color Plate 33-1.) Liver biopsy showing alcoholic cirrhosis

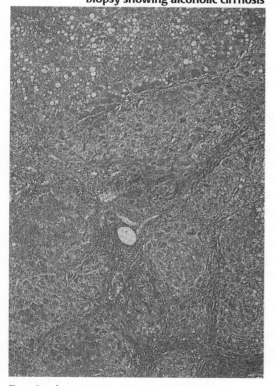

(From Damjanov I. A Color Atlas and Textbook of Histopathology. Philadelphia: Lippincott Williams & Wilkins, 1996, p 225.)

FIGURE
33-2

The major consequences of portal
hypertension in the setting of cirrhosis

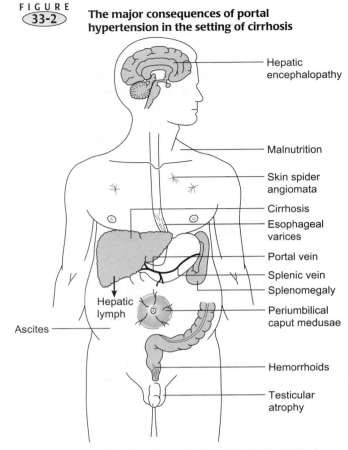

(Adapted with permission from Kumar V, Cotran RS, Robbins SL. Basic
Pathology, 6th Ed. Philadelphia: W.B. Saunders & Co, 1997, p 524.)

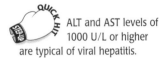

ALT and AST levels of
1000 U/L or higher
are typical of viral hepatitis.

Dupuytren contrac-
tures, which occur as
fibrous proliferation in the palmar
fascia, cause flexion deformities
in the fingers and can be associated with alcoholism.

Chronic gastritis is
characterized by
chronic mucosal
inflammation and atrophy of the
mucous glands. There are two
types: Type A (fundal) is associated
with antibodies to parietal cells
and other autoimmune diseases;
Type B (antral) is associated
with *H. pylori* infection.

EXPLANATION OF DIFFERENTIAL

Acute (erosive) gastritis is a condition in the stomach characterized by **focal mucosal damage,** acute inflammatory changes, necrosis, and **hemorrhage.** This disease is associated with the use of **nonsteroidal anti-inflammatory drugs, chronic alcohol abuse,** curling ulcers (burns), Cushing ulcers (head trauma), and cigarette smoking. Clinically, acute gastritis is characterized by **abdominal pain,** nausea, **hematemesis,** and melena. In this patient, the only way to rule out acute gastritis is EGD.

Boerhaave syndrome is **complete rupture of the esophagus** after severe retching. The rupture is usually located in the **left posterior distal esophagus,** which is a weak area of the esophagus. This location of the rupture causes Boerhaave syndrome to most commonly **present clinically as a left-sided pneumothorax.** Subcutaneous emphysema may also be seen. Although massive bleeding is rare, mortality is quite high. This patient does not complain of retching while vomiting and does not have shortness of breath. His chest radiograph is negative for a pneumothorax, and the EGD confirms that there is no esophageal rupture.

Mallory-Weiss tears are longitudinal, **partial-thickness lacerations of the gastroesophageal junction** usually caused by retching. These lesions are most commonly seen in **alcoholics** and represent approximately 15% of all cases of **massive upper GI bleeding.** This patient does not report any retching, and the EGD shows no evidence of Mallory-Weiss tears.

Ulcers can occur anywhere in the GI tract but primarily affect the **proximal duodenum and the stomach (especially the lesser curvature).** These ulcers are **associated with *Helicobacter pylori* and the use of nonsteroidal anti-inflammatory drugs.** Patients usually **present with abdominal pain.** In this patient, a negative abdominal examination, a negative abdominal radiograph, and an EGD positive for varices points away from the diagnosis of peptic ulcer disease. However, a history of an expanding abdomen may suggest a perforated ulcer that is causing intra-abdominal bleeding, which can be life threatening.

Related Basic Science

Description and blood supply of the liver

The liver is the largest gland and visceral organ in the body. It is surrounded by the peritoneum, except for a bare area superiorly, which lies against the diaphragm. Grossly, the liver appears to be divided into two lobes by the coronary ligament; however, based on hepatic drainage and blood supply, it is really divided into the **right and left lobes** by the gallbladder and inferior vena cava fossae.

The **porta hepatis** is the entryway for the hepatic ducts, proper hepatic artery, and portal vein. The **portal vein** is formed by the union of the superior mesenteric vein and splenic vein. It also receives the left gastric vein, which has esophageal systemic anastomoses. The **common hepatic artery** also carries blood to the liver, but unlike the portal vein, the blood from the hepatic artery is fully oxygenated. The common hepatic artery becomes the **proper hepatic artery,** which proceeds to divide into the **right and left hepatic arteries,** which then enter the liver. The right hepatic artery gives rise to the **cystic artery,** which supplies blood to the gallbladder.

Portacaval anastomoses

Portacaval anastomoses occur when there is venous congestion in the portal system. The blood cannot move forward into the liver and, consequently, is forced to seek other routes. As a result, the following four important portacaval anastomoses are formed:

- Left gastric vein to the esophageal vein (causes **esophageal varices**)
- Superior rectal vein to the middle and inferior rectal veins (may lead to **bleeding hemorrhoids**)
- Paraumbilical veins to the epigastric veins (causes **caput medusae**)
- Retroperitoneal veins to the renal, suprarenal, and gonadal veins

> **QUICK HIT** The epiploic foramen (i.e., foramen of Winslow) lies just posterior to the porta hepatis and is the opening to the lesser sac.

Pathology of the liver

Ascites

Ascites is a collection of serous fluid in the peritoneal cavity and is commonly seen in cirrhosis. It is caused by multiple factors, including sinusoidal hypertension, hypoalbuminemia leading to reduced hydrostatic pressure in blood vessels, leakage of lymph from the thoracic duct, leakage of intestinal fluid caused by portal hypertension, and water retention by the kidneys. Ascites becomes clinically detectable when at least 500 mL of fluid has accumulated in the peritoneum. It is demonstrated in the physical examination by shifting dullness and a fluid wave.

Social aspects and treatment of alcoholism

Alcoholism is a common disease in the United States, with approximately 13% of adults abusing or becoming alcohol dependent. The disorder is characterized by continued drinking despite negative social and medical consequences. Alcoholics develop a tolerance to drinking and may experience delirium tremens and seizures upon withdrawal.

Treatment of alcoholism is based on pharmacotherapy or self-help groups, such as Alcoholics Anonymous (AA), which is a 12-step program that allows alcoholics to organize and deal with their addictions together. AA encourages members to participate and share their experiences with alcohol. For many alcoholics, AA is the only method that can successfully keep them from drinking.

Pharmacotherapy for alcohol addiction is less successful than self-help groups and relies on the negative consequences of drinking while using the medication. Disulfiram is a drug that blocks the actions of aldehyde dehydrogenase in the alcohol breakdown pathway. As a result, acetaldehyde accumulates in the blood, which causes nausea, flushing, and headache every time the patient drinks alcohol.

Genetic diseases that cause cirrhosis

Wilson disease

Wilson disease is an **autosomal recessive** disorder characterized by the accumulation of **toxic levels of copper.** The disease is caused by **defective biliary excretion of copper,** which leads to toxic liver damage. The excess copper causes hemolysis and damage to the liver, brain, eyes, and multiple other organs. Wilson disease presents with **acute or chronic liver disease,** neuropsychiatric changes (i.e., behavior changes, psychosis, Parkinson-like disease), and **Kayser-Fleischer rings** in the eye. Laboratory diagnosis includes a **decrease in serum ceruloplasmin** (a copper-containing liver protein), an increase in hepatic copper content, and markedly **increased urinary excretion of copper.**

Relevant metabolic pathways

Gluconeogenesis

Gluconeogenesis is the process by which the **liver and kidneys synthesize glucose.** The precursors of this process include **lactate and pyruvate** via the Cori cycle, **amino acids** derived from muscle (primarily alanine and glutamine), and **glycerol** released from adipose in lipolysis. While the liver is the primary source of glucose production after a short fast (i.e., overnight), the kidneys contribute more than half of the glucose produced during a long fast. Therefore, occurrences of hypoglycemia are more common in chronic renal failure. The **rate-limiting step** of **gluconeogenesis** involves **pyruvate carboxylase,** which converts pyruvate and carbon dioxide into oxaloacetate.

Fat metabolism

In states of starvation, **glucagon** causes the downstream **phosphorylation** of **hormone-sensitive lipase** in adipose tissue. Upon activation, this enzyme hydrolyzes stored triglycerides to long-chain fatty acids and glycerol. The released **fatty acids** are either broken down to **produce adenosine triphosphate** or are **converted into ketones,** which are used as an energy source, primarily in the CNS. This shift to lipid metabolism is important because it spares protein stores.

QUICK HIT

The antibiotic metronidazole causes a disulfiram-like reaction when patients who are taking it drink alcohol.

QUICK HIT

Asterixis is a flapping tremor of the hands seen in patients with a **metabolic encephalopathy.** It is most commonly associated with **hepatic encephalopathy;** however, it can also be caused by conditions such as uremia and excessive drug ingestion (especially antipsychotics).

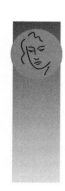

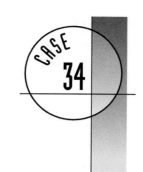

"My abdomen is hurting more and more, and I feel like I'm going to vomit."

OBJECTIVES

1. Develop a differential diagnosis and an appropriate workup for nausea and abdominal pain
2. Differentiate between Crohn disease and ulcerative colitis
3. Review the innervation and blood supply of the GI tract
4. Describe the pathology and clinical presentation of common diseases of the small intestine, large intestine, and rectum

HISTORY AND PHYSICAL EXAMINATION

A 20-year-old woman complains of **crampy pain** of increasing severity in her **right lower abdominal quadrant.** She also reports feeling pain around her umbilicus 12 hours ago. She states that she is **nauseated and has vomited twice** in the past 12 hours, and that she has been unable to defecate normally since the onset of symptoms. She denies a history of chronic bowel symptoms. Upon questioning, she states that she is sexually active and that her last menstrual period was 3 weeks ago. She denies vaginal discharge and abnormal uterine bleeding. Physical examination is remarkable for a temperature of 100.1°F, **guarding and rebound tenderness** in the lower right abdomen, and **positive psoas and obturator signs.** The patient's pain is reproducible with coughing. Pelvic examination is unremarkable.

APPROPRIATE WORKUP

Complete blood count, β-human chorionic gonadotropin (β-hCG), cervical culture, abdominal US, and laparoscopy

DIFFERENTIAL DIAGNOSIS

Acute appendicitis, acute gastroenteritis, ectopic pregnancy, endometriosis, inflammatory bowel disease, Meckel diverticulum, pelvic inflammatory disease (PID), ruptured ovarian cyst

DIAGNOSTIC LABORATORY TESTS AND STUDIES

Complete blood count:
  WBCs = 14,000/μL (H)
β-hCG:
  Negative
Cervical culture:
  Negative
Abdominal ultrasound:
  Inflamed appendix, cannot be compressed
  No gynecologic abnormalities

Laparoscopy:
  Inflamed appendix
  Normal ovaries and fallopian tubes

DIAGNOSIS: ACUTE APPENDICITIS

Acute appendicitis is a potentially serious condition affecting approximately 10% of the population. It occurs when the appendix becomes obstructed by a fecalith, a foreign body, inflammation, or a neoplasm. The obstruction causes increased intraluminal pressure, engorgement, infection, and thrombosis of the vessels in the appendix walls.

Acute appendicitis typically presents initially with **colicky or crampy periumbilical pain** or fullness, which then **migrates to the lower right abdominal quadrant** (i.e., **McBurney point**) within 12 hours. When the patient coughs, the pain is reproduced because of **irritation to the peritoneum. Anorexia, nausea, vomiting, and constipation** are also common presenting symptoms. However, vomiting is usually limited to one or two episodes. The psoas and obturator signs, which are representative of peritoneal irritation, are frequently present in appendicitis. **Moderate leukocytosis** with increased neutrophils and a low-grade fever are also typical.

Acute appendicitis is the **most common reason for surgery** in patients who present with acute abdominal symptoms. If the appendix is not removed, it may become perforated or gangrenous. In addition to removing the appendix, **third-generation cephalosporins** are the preoperative, operative, and postoperative antibiotic of choice.

EXPLANATION OF DIFFERENTIAL

The abdominal pain of **acute gastroenteritis** can be **colicky and may be accompanied by nausea and vomiting.** However, gastroenteritis is also typically **accompanied by diarrhea** and generalized abdominal tenderness that does not localize in the lower right quadrant. The ultrasound finding of an inflamed appendix does not rule out the diagnosis of acute gastroenteritis, but the likelihood of two diseases occurring simultaneously is low.

When a woman of childbearing age presents with abdominal complaints, it is **important to always rule out ectopic pregnancy.** In ectopic pregnancy, lower abdominal peritoneal irritation from the tubal pregnancy can cause **pain and abdominal cramping.** In addition, β-hCG is positive and the **pelvic examination may reveal cervical motion tenderness** and a palpable, tender mass in a fallopian tube. Additionally, a woman with an ectopic pregnancy may present with symptoms and signs of hemorrhage, shock, and uterine bleeding.

Endometriosis is a condition in which endometrial tissue is found outside of the uterus (i.e., in the abdominal cavity). The diagnosis of endometriosis should always be considered in a menstruating woman who presents with abdominal pain.

In endometriosis, the abdominal **pain coincides with menstruation** as the **ectopic endometrial tissue** sloughs. However, as the disease progresses, the pain tends to be less cyclical and may occur at any time during the menstrual cycle. Because this patient's pain is at the appropriate time in her menstrual cycle, endometriosis is a possibility. However, it can be excluded by the abdominal ultrasound, which shows only the inflamed appendix.

Inflammatory bowel disease includes Crohn disease and ulcerative colitis (Table 34-1). Although both Crohn disease and ulcerative colitis have clinical features similar to acute appendicitis, they are less likely in this case because of the lack of diarrhea. Ultrasound and laparoscopy confirm that the inflammation is limited to the appendix.

The signs and symptoms of a **Meckel diverticulum** make it difficult to distinguish from appendicitis. During appendectomy procedures, a small percentage of people are found to have an inflamed Meckel diverticulum instead of an inflamed appendix. Meckel diverticulum is a **remnant of the omphalomesenteric (vitelline) duct** that is usually found within **2 feet of the ileocecal valve.**

The most common causes of **PID** include *Neisseria gonorrhoeae* and *Chlamydia trachomatis*. Risk factors for acute PID include previous PID, multiple sexual partners, use of intrauterine contraceptive devices, history of sexually transmitted diseases, and nulliparity. **Oral contraceptives reduce the risk of developing acute PID.** A woman with PID

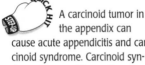

Approximately 10 to 15% of operations for appendicitis reveal a normal appendix. In this situation, the appendix is removed to be sure that when a physician sees the McBurney point scar, she will not falsely assume that the patient does not have an appendix.

A carcinoid tumor in the appendix can cause acute appendicitis and carcinoid syndrome. Carcinoid syndrome is caused by malignant tumor cells that elaborate serotonin, which results in flushing, diarrhea, colic, and malabsorption.

TABLE 34-1 Comparison of Inflammatory Bowel Conditions

	Crohn Disease	Ulcerative Colitis
Typical patient	Young person of Jewish descent Bimodal age distribution: 25–40 years of age and 50–65 years of age Female > male	Person of Jewish descent Recently quit smoking Bimodal age distribution: 20–35 years of age and 65+ years of age Male > female
Clinical findings	Diarrhea Abdominal pain Fever Malabsorption Obstruction	Bloody, mucousy diarrhea Abdominal pain Fever Weight loss Toxic megacolon
Location	Small intestine Colon "Mouth to anus"	Colon Rectum
Histologic findings	Full-thickness inflammation **Granulomas**	Mucosal inflammation **Crypt abscesses**
Gross findings	**Cobblestone appearance** Wall thickening with narrowed lumen **Skipped areas** **Fistulas**	Pseudopolyps Widened lumen Toxic megacolon
Diagnostic evaluation	Colonoscopy Barium enema Upper GI series with small -bowel follow-through	Colonoscopy Barium enema Upper GI series with small-bowel follow-through
Risk of malignancy	Small increase	Large increase
Associated systemic manifestations	Arthritis Eye lesions Erythema nodosum Pyoderma gangrenosum	Arthritis Eye lesions Erythema nodosum Sclerosing cholangitis
Medical treatment	Sulfasalazine Steroids Metronidazole	Sulfasalazine Steroids Metronidazole
Indications for surgery	Obstruction Massive bleeding Perforation Refractory to medical treatment Cancer Toxic megacolon	Toxic megacolon Cancer Massive bleeding Failure to mature Refractory to medical treatment

Reprinted with permission from Mehta S, Milder EA, Mirarchi AJ. Step-Up: A High-Yield, Systems-Based Review for the USMLE Step 1 Examination. Philadelphia: Lippincott Williams & Wilkins, 2000, p 94.

typically presents with lower abdominal pain, fever, vaginal discharge, and abnormal uterine bleeding. The abdominal pain is caused by peritoneal irritation, so **rebound tenderness may be present.** Pelvic examination may reveal **cervical motion tenderness** (cervicitis and salpingitis), adnexal tenderness (oophoritis), and **abnormal cervical or vaginal discharge.** In this patient, the negative pelvic examination and the ultrasound, which does not reveal an inflammatory process in the pelvis, rule out the diagnosis of PID.

A **ruptured ovarian cyst** (i.e., chocolate cyst) is caused by ovarian bleeding during ovulation. The bleeding is contained; however, spontaneous rupture of the cyst causes severe lower abdominal pain. In this patient, the abdominal ultrasound rules out the diagnosis of a ruptured ovarian cyst. Additionally, the pain of a ruptured cyst is more severe and sudden in onset when compared to the pain of acute appendicitis.

Related Basic Science

Innervation and blood supply of the GI tract (Figure 34-1)

Crohn disease versus ulcerative colitis (see Table 34-1)

Common clinical disorders of the small intestine, large intestine, and rectum (Table 34-2)

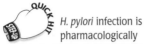 Posterior duodenal ulcers are associated with erosion of the gastroduodenal artery and subsequent hemorrhage.

H. pylori infection is pharmacologically treated with **triple therapy.** The therapeutic regimen typically includes a proton-pump inhibitor (omeprazole) and two of the following antibiotics: clarithromycin, amoxicillin, and metronidazole.

Diverticulosis, the most common cause of bleeding from the lower GI tract, can be differentiated from diverticulitis because, typically, diverticulitis does not cause bleeding.

Small bowel obstructions are usually due to adhesions, while large bowel obstructions are most commonly a result of neoplasms. Ileus, a common cause of temporary small bowel paralysis, commonly occurs postoperatively.

Diverticulitis can be differentiated from appendicitis in terms of location and age. Diverticulitis typically presents as acute abdominal pain in the left lower quadrant in elderly patients. Appendicitis involves acute pain in the right lower quadrant in younger patients.

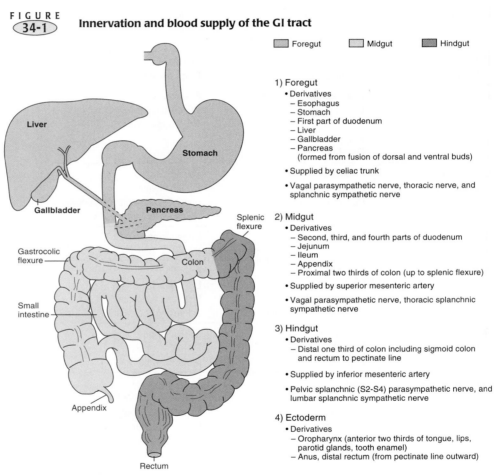

FIGURE 34-1 **Innervation and blood supply of the GI tract**

1) Foregut
 • Derivatives
   – Esophagus
   – Stomach
   – First part of duodenum
   – Liver
   – Gallbladder
   – Pancreas
     (formed from fusion of dorsal and ventral buds)
 • Supplied by celiac trunk
 • Vagal parasympathetic nerve, thoracic nerve, and splanchnic sympathetic nerve

2) Midgut
 • Derivatives
   – Second, third, and fourth parts of duodenum
   – Jejunum
   – Ileum
   – Appendix
   – Proximal two thirds of colon (up to splenic flexure)
 • Supplied by superior mesenteric artery
 • Vagal parasympathetic nerve, thoracic splanchnic sympathetic nerve

3) Hindgut
 • Derivatives
   – Distal one third of colon including sigmoid colon and rectum to pectinate line
 • Supplied by inferior mesenteric artery
 • Pelvic splanchnic (S2-S4) parasympathetic nerve, and lumbar splanchnic sympathetic nerve

4) Ectoderm
 • Derivatives
   – Oropharynx (anterior two thirds of tongue, lips, parotid glands, tooth enamel)
   – Anus, distal rectum (from pectinate line outward)

(Reprinted with permission from Mehta S, Milder EA, Mirarchi AJ. Step-Up: A High-Yield, Systems-Based Review for the USMLE Step 1. Philadelphia: Lippincott Williams & Wilkins, 2000, p 82.)

TABLE 34-2 Common Clinical Disorders of the Small Intestine, Large Intestine, and Rectum

Disorder	Etiology and Pathology	Clinical Features	Notes
Hiatal hernia	Sac-like herniation of stomach through diaphragm	Retrosternal pain (worse in supine position); can lead to **gastroesophageal reflux disease**	Usually occurs in the sliding (versus rolling) form
Duodenal ulcers	***Helicobacter pylori*** (in 90% of cases); hypersecretion of acid; smokers; Zollinger-Ellison syndrome; blood group O; associated with NSAID use	Coffee ground vomitus; **smooth border;** clean base; black stools; pain at night or 2 hr post-prandial; perforation may result in acute pancreatitis	Not precancerous
Ischemic bowel disease	Atherosclerosis of celiac artery or mesenteric artery	Abdominal pain; nausea; vomiting; stool positive for blood	Usually affects watershed areas (splenic flexure or rectosigmoid junction)
Diverticulitis	Outpouchings of the colon obstructed with fecalith leading to inflammation or infection; low-fiber diet	Usually involves the **sigmoid colon;** fever; leukocytosis; colicky pain; usually multiple	False diverticula: pockets of mucosa and submucosa herniated through muscular layer
Appendicitis	Obstruction (usually fecalith or lymphoid hyperplasia); bacterial proliferation and mucosal invasion	Nausea; vomiting; abdominal pain that migrates from epigastrium to right lower quadrant; pain at **McBurney point;** psoas sign or obturator sign; increased WBCs in blood	Differential diagnosis in women includes ectopic pregnancy, ovarian torsion, ruptured ovarian cyst, and PID
Adenocarcinoma of colon and rectum	Chronic inflammatory bowel disease; low-fiber diet; older age; hereditary polyposis or adenomatous disorders	**Increased CEA** (not diagnostic, used to assess treatment); rectosigmoid tumors present in an **annular manner** producing early obstruction and constipation; **right-sided tumors present as blood in stool**	Screen for occult blood in stool; third most common cause of cancer death (after lung and prostate/breast)
Carcinoid tumor	Arise from **neuroendocrine cells** (Kulchitsky cells); release vasoactive peptides such as histamine, serotonin, and prostaglandins	**Increased 5-HIAA in urine;** diarrhea, **flushing;** right-sided heart valve lesions; hypotension; bronchospasm	Most common tumor of the appendix, but also found in the ileum, rectum, and bronchus

CEA, carcinoembryonic antigen; 5-HIAA, 5-hydroxyindoleacetic acid; NSAID, nonsteroidal anti-inflammatory drug; PID, pelvic inflammatory disease.
Reprinted with permission from Mehta S, Milder EA, Mirarchi AJ. Step-Up: A High-Yield, Systems-Based Review for the USMLE Step 1 Examination. Philadelphia: Lippincott Williams & Wilkins, 2000, p 91.

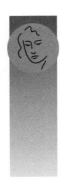

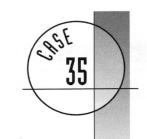

"Who are You? Why am I here?"

OBJECTIVES

1. Develop a differential diagnosis and appropriate work cognitive decline in the elderly
2. Review vitamin functions and their deficiencies
3. Explain a neurologic exam in the aged and recognize normal and abnormal variants
4. Review the effect of disease on neuron structure
5. Differentiate between delirium and dementia
6. Learn the nervous system, somatic, infections and genetic causes of dementia

HISTORY AND PHYSICAL EXAMINATION

A 70-year-old woman is brought to the office by her daughter. The daughter is worried about her mother's memory loss and states that her mother's **memory has become progressively worse over the past 3 years.** The patient has recently become **confused** and is **often agitated** when she **cannot remember how to perform tasks.** She has begun to forget people's names, and a few days ago did not return from the grocery store for 4 hours because she got lost. Yesterday, her daughter reports that her mother forgot to turn off the burner on the gas stove. The patient has no significant past medical history and is not currently taking any medications. She does take one multivitamin daily. According to the daughter, she has no history of alcohol or drug use or depression. The patient has had no weight change or headaches. The physical examination is unremarkable.

APPROPRIATE WORKUP

Thyroid function tests, test for syphilis, thiamine assay, vitamin B_{12} levels, head MRI, and CT scan

DIFFERENTIAL DIAGNOSIS

Alzheimer disease, brain tumor, chronic alcoholism, hypothyroidism, multi-infarct dementia, neurosyphilis, vitamin deficiency, normal aging

DIAGNOSTIC LABORATORY TESTS AND STUDIES

Thyroid function tests:
  Thyroglobulin = 40 ng/mL (N)
  Thyroid-stimulating hormone
    (TSH) = 3.2 μIU/mL (N)
  Thyroxine (T_4) (total) =
    6.2 μg/dL (N)
  T_4 (free) = 1.3 ng/dL (N)
  Triiodothyronine (T_3) =
    87 ng/dL (N)

Venereal Disease Research
  Laboratory test for syphilis:
  Negative
Thiamine assay:
  Within normal limits
Vitamin B_{12} assay:
  468 pg/mL (N)
Head MRI and CT scan:
  Moderate cortical atrophy
  No evidence of hemorrhage, infarct,
    or tumor

DIAGNOSIS: ALZHEIMER DISEASE

Alzheimer disease is a degenerative neurologic disease characterized by **progressive intellectual deterioration and dementia.** The sporadic form presents after 60 years of age. The familial form may present as early as 40 years of age, with a slightly greater incidence in women. A positive family history is found in approximately 50% of cases. Although the cause of Alzheimer disease is unknown, some possible mechanisms include a choline acetyltransferase deficiency or alterations in the nucleus basalis of Meynert, both of which cause a decrease in acetylcholine (Ach) levels. Another theory deals with **abnormal amyloid gene expression** (frequently chromosome 21), which is the most favorable etiologic concept today.

The clinical findings progress over the course of several years and initially include a **loss of recent memory** followed by a **loss of long-term memory and other intellectual functions.** Later in the course of the disease, **motor problems and paralysis may occur.** The morphological changes associated with Alzheimer disease include neurofibrillary tangles, neuritic (senile) plaques, granulovacuolar degeneration, Hirano bodies, and generalized cerebral atrophy with moderate neuronal loss. However, some of these changes are the normal changes associated with aging.

No specific drug therapy is available for halting the disease, and patients tolerate the existing medications poorly. Cholinesterase inhibitors increase the level of ACh, which helps maintain memory. **Donepezil** is the agent of choice, and has replaced **tacrine,** which can cause liver damage. Recent studies have shown that **selegiline** and vitamin E (an antioxidant) may slow the progression of the disease. Nonsteroidal anti-inflammatory drugs and estrogen replacement therapy have also been linked to a lower incidence and slower progression of Alzheimer disease. Antidepressants, antipsychotics, anxiolytics, and behavioral therapy can be used to counteract the psychologic effects of this chronic disease.

> **QUICK HIT**
> Neurofibrillary tangles are also seen in patients with postencephalitic Parkinson disease.

EXPLANATION OF DIFFERENTIAL

Brain tumors can present with neurologic deficits. There can be sensory or motor losses or personality changes. Tumors in the brain can be primary, but are often metastatic (i.e., from the lung). Brain tumors can be visualized with a CT scan.

Chronic alcoholism can cause **Wernicke-Korsakoff syndrome,** which results from a **thiamine deficiency.** Classically, this presents as Wernicke encephalopathy, which includes **psychosis, ophthalmoplegia, and ataxia.** The disease process may progress to Korsakoff syndrome, which is irreversible and **results in memory loss, confabulation, and confusion.** Chronic alcoholism is ruled out in this patient by history and the negative physical examination. If Wernicke encephalopathy were a concern, the patient could be given thiamine to see if the symptoms abate.

Hypothyroidism can be caused by a number of factors, including surgery, radiation, drugs, and autoimmune syndromes. It may also be idiopathic in nature. It is characterized by the syndrome of **myxedema,** which includes **cold intolerance, weight gain, mental and physical slowness, a lowering of the pitch of the voice, thinning hair,** and **edema of the face and hands,** as well as other clinical signs. Hypothyroidism is ruled out by normal thyroid function tests.

Multi-infarct dementia is the **second most common cause of dementia in the elderly.** The multiple infarctions can be caused by arterial occlusion from thrombosis, which is most often caused by **atherosclerosis,** or embolism (less common). Patients with multi-infarct dementia may have other signs of infarction, such as aphasia, motor deficits, and sensory deficits. Infarcts can be ruled out by a CT scan or MRI of the brain.

Neurosyphilis is a form of **tertiary syphilis** that occurs in approximately 8% of untreated cases. It is characterized by **slow inflammatory damage** to organ tissue, small blood vessels, and **nerve cells.** Five common presentations of neurosyphilis exist, including paretic neurosyphilis (general paresis of the insane). General paresis of the insane is a progressive disease of the CNS that leads to **mental deterioration and psychiatric symptoms.** Neurosyphilis is ruled out by a negative Venereal Disease Research Laboratory test.

There are few **vitamin deficiencies** (Table 35-1) that can cause changes in mental status. Thiamine deficiency, which causes Wernicke-Korsakoff syndrome, is one vitamin deficiency

> **QUICK HIT**
> Down syndrome patients frequently develop an Alzheimer-type disease as early as 35 years of age.

> **QUICK HIT**
> Thiamine deficiency also causes beriberi. Dry beriberi is characterized by peripheral neuropathy, especially in the legs. Wet beriberi is characterized by high-output heart failure and peripheral vasodilation.

> **QUICK HIT**
> Hashimoto thyroiditis is an autoimmune disorder characterized by progression from euthyroidism, to hyperthyroidism, to eventual hypothyroidism. It is associated with antithyroglobulin and antimicrosomal antibodies. Histologically, Hashimoto thyroiditis is characterized by dense focal lymphocytic infiltrates in the thyroid.

TABLE 35-1 Vitamin Function and Deficiency

Vitamin	Solubility	Function	Deficiency
Vitamin B$_1$ (thiamine)	Water	Carbohydrate and amino acid metabolism	Beriberi (wet and dry), Wernicke-Korsakoff syndrome
Vitamin B$_2$ (riboflavin)	Water	Component of FAD and FMN, needed for oxidation-reduction reactions	Cheilosis, glossitis, dermatitis, corneal vascularization
Vitamin B$_3$ (niacin, nicotinic acid)	Water	Component of NAD and NADP; needed for glycolysis, TCA cycle, and other oxidation reactions	Pellagra, which is characterized by diarrhea, dermatitis, dementia, and death; requires deficiency of both niacin and tryptophan
Vitamin B$_6$ (pyridoxine)	Water	Needed for transamination, porphyrin synthesis, and synthesis of niacin from tryptophan	Cheilosis, glossitis, anemia, neurologic dysfunction
Vitamin B$_{12}$ (cobalamin)	Water	One-carbon transfers for folate synthesis, conversion of dUMP to dTMP in DNA synthesis	Megaloblastic anemia, neurologic dysfunction
Folic acid	Water	One-carbon transfers, DNA synthesis	Megaloblastic anemia
Vitamin C (ascorbic acid)	Water	Hydroxylation of proline and lysine in collagen synthesis, hydroxylation of dopamine in norepinephrine synthesis	Scurvy, defective formation of osteoid matrix, defective wound healing, hemorrhage
Vitamin A	Fat	Needed for rhodopsin synthesis, glycoprotein synthesis, and epithelial differentiation	Night blindness; squamous metaplasia
Vitamin D (calciferol)	Fat	Promotes intestinal absorption of calcium and phosphorus; stimulates parathyroid hormone release, which promotes resorption of calcium by renal tubules; enhances calcification of bone	Rickets in children, osteomalacia in adults
Vitamin E (α-tocopherol)	Fat	Antioxidant, maintains cell membranes	Possible neurologic dysfunction
Vitamin K	Fat	Needed for carboxylation of glutamyl in synthesis of clotting factors II, VII, IX, X and proteins C and S	Clotting deficiencies, bleeding

dUMP, deoxyuridine monophosphate; dTMP, deoxythymidine monophosphate; FAD, flavin adenine dinucleotide; FMN, flavin mononucleotide; NAD, nicotinamide adenine dinucleotide; NADP, nicotinamide-adenine dinucleotide phosphate; TCA, tricarboxylic acid.
Adapted with permission from Schneider A, Szanto P. BRS Pathology. Philadelphia: Lippincott Williams & Wilkins, 1992, pp 108, 111.

syndrome classically associated with mental status changes. **Vitamin B$_{12}$** deficiency causes megaloblastic anemia and can also result in a prominent **neurologic dysfunction.** Niacin deficiency causes the "four Ds" (i.e., dermatitis, diarrhea, dementia, death). All of these diseases can be ruled out by serum tests for vitamin levels.

Normal aging can often be the cause of many physical findings which can be nonpathologic given a patient's age. It is important to recognize which changes are part of normal aging and which require intervention, such as with geriatric mental status changes, Alzheimer disease, and cranial/motor functions (Tables 35-2 and 35-3).

TABLE 35-2 Changes Associated with Normal Aging and Those Requiring Intervention

Normal Aging	Changes Requiring Intervention
Ability to solve novel problems declines	**Progressive** onset of memory impairment, especially recent memory **plus** at least one of the following cognitive impairments:
Apraxia and agnosia *do not* occur	1. apraxia
Ability to perform ADLs unimpaired	2. delusions and hallucinations
Previously learned material and the ability to use it in solving problems unimpaired	3. agnosia 4. disorientation
Recent memory impairment with sparing of immediate and remote memory	5. impaired problem solving 6. impaired ADLs

Related Basic Science

Effect of disease on neurons

A neuron is the structural and functional unit of the nervous system. Included in a neuron are the perikaryon (cell body), axon, and dendrite. The axon starts as an extension of the cell body called the axon hillock (Figure 35-1).

Neurofibrillary tangles are intracytoplasmic bundles of filaments that occur in neurons, most frequently in the cerebral cortex. Neurofibrillary tangles are **associated with Alzheimer disease** and are made up of microtubules and neurofilaments.

Neuritic (senile) plaques are swollen, eosinophilic nerve cell processes that occur in spherical focal collections and are frequently found in the cerebral cortex and hippocampus. They characteristically have a central amyloid core with a unique peptide structure. The amyloid protein is frequently referred to as A4 amyloid or amyloid β protein.

Acetylcholine (Ach)

Ach is an important **excitatory neurotransmitter.** In the presynaptic terminal, Ach is produced from acetyl coenzyme A and choline by the enzyme choline acetyltransferase. Ach has

TABLE 35-3 Cranial and Motor Function Loss in Alzheimer Disease

Cranial Nerve Function	
I	Smell is almost always impaired
II	Presbyopia; pupils ordinarily smaller; papillary light reflex sluggish; optic discs difficult to see because of small pupils and/or frequent cataracts
III, IV, & VI	Upward gaze often diminished; taste sensation diminished; hearing often impaired—more so with higher frequencies
VII	Taste sensation diminished
VIII	Hearing often impaired, more so with higher frequencies
Motor Function	
1.	Total muscle mass decreases → reduction in strength
2.	Reflex time prolonged
3.	Stretch reflexes slowed
4.	Vibratory sensation diminished or lost, especially in lower extremities
5.	Gait deteriorates with upper extremity coordination preserved relative to the lower extremities → increased numbers of falls among the elderly

*Cranial nerves V, IX, X, XI, and XII are usually intact in the elderly.

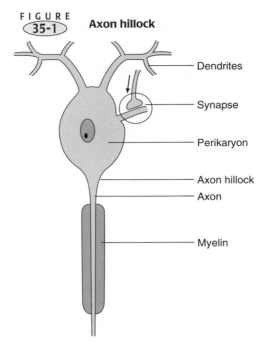

FIGURE
35-1
Axon hillock

- Dendrites
- Synapse
- Perikaryon
- Axon hillock
- Axon
- Myelin

been shown to play a role in **learning and memory.** If the level of choline acetyltransferase is decreased, the amount of Ach is lower, which is one theory behind the pathogenesis of the clinical manifestations of Alzheimer disease.

Other causes of dementia (Table 35-4)

Additional conditions that may cause dementia are listed in Table 35-4. **Rabies** can be another potential cause of dementia. It is transmitted by the **rhabdovirus** (Figure 35-2) and the **Negri body** is pathognomonic for it (Figure 35-3).

Behavioral science: delirium versus dementia (Table 35-5)

Genetic diseases that cause dementia

Huntington disease is an **autosomal dominant** disease. It results in progressive degeneration and **atrophy of the caudate nucleus, putamen, and frontal cortex** with neuronal degeneration and gliosis, ultimately leading to death. Dementia is common during the final stages of the disease.

> **QUICK HIT**
>
> Pick disease also causes dementia. It is characterized by swollen neurons, Pick bodies (i.e., round, intracytoplasmic inclusions of neurofilaments), and marked cortical atrophy, generally in the temporal and frontal lobes.

TABLE 35-4 Causes of Dementia

Nervous System Causes	Somatic Causes	Infectious Causes
Alzheimer disease	Cardiovascular disease	AIDS
Vascular dementia	Endocrine disorder	Creutzfeldt-Jakob disease
Brain trauma	Nutritional deficiency	Cryptococcal meningitis
Cerebral hypoxia	Liver disease	Fungal meningitis
Huntington disease	Normal-pressure hydrocephalus	Neurosyphilis
Intracranial tumor	Renal disease	Tuberculosis
Multiple sclerosis	Respiratory disease	Viral encephalitis
Parkinson disease	Sarcoidosis	Rabies
Pick disease		

AIDS, acquired immunodeficiency syndrome.
Adapted with permission from Fadem B. High-Yield Behavioral Science. Philadelphia: Lippincott Williams & Wilkins, 1996, p 50.

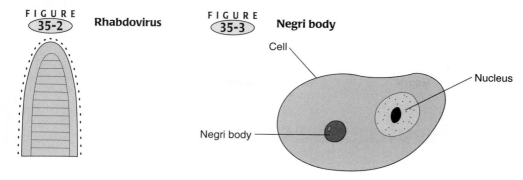

FIGURE 35-2 Rhabdovirus

FIGURE 35-3 Negri body

Cell

Nucleus

Negri body

Krabbe disease is an **autosomal recessive, lysosomal storage disease** that is caused by a lack of **galactosylceramidase** and leads to the **accumulation of galactocerebroside** in the brain. Krabbe disease is characterized by optic atrophy, spasticity, and early death. Pathologically, globoid bodies, which are large, multinucleated, histiocytic cells, are seen in the white matter.

Metachromatic leukodystrophy is another **autosomal recessive, lysosomal storage disease** that results in **demyelination and progressive dementia.** This disease is caused by a deficiency of **arylsulfatase A** and the buildup of sulfatide in the brain, kidneys, liver, and peripheral nerves.

TABLE 35-5 Delirium & Dementia

Delirium	Dementia
Hallmark: impaired consciousness	**Hallmark:** loss of memory and intellectual ability
Consciousness impaired or clouded	Consciousness not impaired
Develops quickly	Develops slowly
Stupor or agitation	Normal level of arousal
Illusions or hallucinations, often visual	No illusions or hallucinations
Associated primarily with anxiety	Associated primarily with depression
Autonomic dysfunction	Little autonomic dysfunction
Diurnal variability (worse at night [i.e., "sundowners"])	Little diurnal variability
Frequently reversible (remove the cause and it resolves)	Only 15% of cases reversible (no effective treatment, pharmacotherapy for associated psychiatric symptoms)

From Fadem B. High-Yield Behavioral Science. Philadelphia: Lippincott Williams & Wilkins, 1996, p 51.

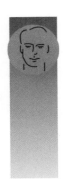

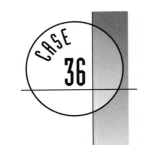

"I'm having chest pain."

OBJECTIVES

1. Develop a differential diagnosis and appropriate workup for sudden onset of chest pain
2. Compare and contrast cardiac diseases in terms of EKG tracings, cardiac enzyme elevations, and clinical presentations
3. Review cardiac conduction and the five phases of conduction of the heart
4. Relate physiological changes with a cardiac cycle
5. Review the cranial nerve distribution for pain sensation

HISTORY AND PHYSICAL EXAMINATION

A **55-year-old** man presents to the ED with chest pain that has lasted for **7 hours.** The patient describes the pain as a **heaviness** and tightness in his chest that **radiates to his left shoulder** and **down his left arm.** He claims to have had some lightheadedness, weakness, **nausea,** and **vomiting.** The patient states that nothing has made the pain better or worse, and that he has never had symptoms this severe. The patient has a history of **hypercholesterolemia** and **hypertension** as well as a **family history** of coronary heart disease. He has a 30 pack-year history of **smoking** and leads a **sedentary** lifestyle. The patient reports no history of drug use. On physical examination, the patient is tachycardic, diaphoretic, and in acute distress.

APPROPRIATE WORKUP

Blood chemistries, EKG, and chest X-ray

DIFFERENTIAL DIAGNOSIS

Acute myocardial infarction (MI), angina pectoris, aortic dissection, esophageal spasm, pancreatitis and biliary tract disease, pericarditis, pulmonary embolism

DIAGNOSTIC LABORATORY TESTS AND STUDIES

Blood chemistry:
  Potassium = 4.0 mEq/L (N)
  Creatinine = 1.0 mg/dL (N)
  BUN = 10 mg/dL (N)
  WBCs = 13,000/μL (H)
  Amylase = 50 U/L (N)
  Lipase = 70 mIU/mL (N)
  Alkaline phosphatase = 35 U/L (N)

Troponin I = 4 ng/mL (H)
CK-MB = 5 U/L (H)
EKG:
  Leads V_4, V_5, V_6 = ST-segment **elevation**
Chest radiograph:
  No active disease

DIAGNOSIS: ACUTE MYOCARDIAL INFARCTION

MI is the most frequent cause of morbidity from ischemic heart disease. It can be characterized by two distinct patterns of myocardial necrosis: **transmural** and **subendocardial.** Transmural infarction is necrosis that traverses the **entire ventricular wall.** Most transmural infarctions are associated with occlusion of a coronary artery by a thrombus. Immediate EKG changes show **elevation** of the ST segment. **Q waves** are permanent evidence of a transmural MI, and rarely disappear over time. Subendocardial infarction is necrosis limited to the **interior one third** of the ventricular wall. Immediate EKG changes show **ST-segment depression,** and there are **no Q waves.**

Laboratory studies consistent with an MI are an elevated troponin I (i.e., greater than 0.4 ng/mL). A rise in the MB (muscle-brain) fraction of CK is also characteristic of MI. However, evaluation of the CK-MB is quickly being replaced by troponin I, which rises more quickly than the CK-MB (Figure 36-1).

Complications of MI include arrhythmias, myocardial rupture, ruptured papillary muscles, mural thrombi, and ventricular aneurysms. **Arrhythmias** are the **most common cause of death** in the first few hours after infarction. Rupture of the myocardium usually occurs within the first 4 to 10 days and can result in **cardiac tamponade,** which is compression of the heart due to hemorrhage into the pericardial sac. Mural thrombi form on the endocardium overlying the infarct and may embolize with resultant cerebrovascular accident or other end-organ ischemia. The diagnosis of an acute MI can be made in this patient because his history is consistent with MI, EKG changes exist, and troponin I and CK-MB are elevated.

EXPLANATION OF DIFFERENTIAL

Angina pectoris is a symptom that results from a mismatch between the supply and demand of myocardial oxygen that is often triggered by physical exertion. It is characterized by sudden chest pain. Although angina can precede MI, more often it is a **discrete event that**

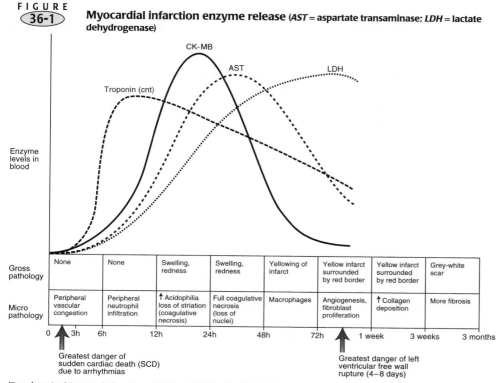

FIGURE 36-1 Myocardial infarction enzyme release (*AST* = aspartate transaminase; *LDH* = lactate dehydrogenase)

(Reprinted with permission from Mehta S, Milder EA, Mirarchi AJ. Step-Up: A High-Yield, Systems-Based Review for the USMLE Step 1 Examination. Philadelphia: Lippincott Williams & Wilkins, 2000, p 53.)

causes short-term chest pain (usually a few minutes) that is relieved by rest or sublingual nitroglycerin. Angina pain that does not relieve with rest or sublingual nitroglycerin may be considered unstable angina pectoris. This unstable pattern represents deterioration in the normal "stable" pattern of angina and must be evaluated immediately. In this patient, the history of pain for 7 hours rules out unstable angina as the final diagnosis; however, unstable angina could be part of the inciting event that caused the MI.

Aortic dissection is a tear in the intima of the aorta. As the intimal tear elongates along the length of the aorta, a false lumen is produced. Aortic dissection is characterized by an **abrupt onset** of **tearing chest or back pain.** It can be diagnosed by performing an aortogram, which will reveal a double lumen (i.e., the original lumen and the false lumen). Although not as specific as an aortogram, aortic dissection may also produce a widened mediastinum on a chest radiograph and can usually be confirmed by a contrast chest CT scan. Predisposing factors include hypertension and cystic medial degeneration such as in Marfan's syndrome. In this patient's situation, aortic dissection can be ruled out by a normal chest radiograph, elevated cardiac enzymes, and EKG changes showing ST-segment elevation.

Esophageal spasm is characterized by retching, chest pain, dysphagia, and regurgitation associated with esophageal motor dysfunction. It is usually progressive and intermittent in its course. Esophageal spasm is ruled out by the changes in cardiac enzymes and EKG changes, which are characteristic for an MI. Patients can have relief of esophageal spasm with sublingual nitroglycerin given for angina, often delaying diagnosis.

Pancreatitis and biliary tract disease can be ruled out by normal levels of amylase, lipase, and alkaline phosphatase. A history of alcoholism or gallstones would raise these diseases higher on the list of differentials.

Pericarditis is the clinical manifestation of a disease process involving irritation and inflammation of the pericardial sac. It presents with sharp, retrosternal chest pain that is frequently sudden in onset and radiates to the trapezoid region. The pain is partially relieved by leaning forward or sitting up and is made worse with inspiration or movement. Pericarditis is associated with infection, connective tissue disorders (e.g., systemic lupus erythematosus), metabolic disorders, trauma, MI, and certain drugs. Pericarditis frequently demonstrates a leukocytosis. In this case, leukocytosis is present, so an echocardiogram could be performed to rule out this disease.

Pulmonary embolism most frequently presents with tachycardia, pleuritic chest pain, and dyspnea. If pulmonary embolism is suspected, a V/Q lung scan or chest CT scan is performed. Patients with deep venous thrombosis (DVT) in the lower extremities are at risk for developing a pulmonary embolism. Virchow's triad of venous stasis or thrombosis, endothelial injury, and hypercoagulability places patients at high risk for developing a DVT. A DVT may produce emboli that pass through the right side of the heart and wedge in the pulmonary vasculature, causing a pulmonary embolism. In this patient's case, pulmonary embolism is not likely because it usually occurs in bedridden or immobile people; however, it should be considered until the results of the EKG and cardiac enzymes are known.

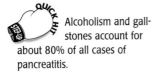

Alcoholism and gallstones account for about 80% of all cases of pancreatitis.

Related Basic Science

Pain sensation

Pain of visceral origin is usually vaguely localized and can be felt in a surface area far from the true source, a phenomenon known as referred pain. This occurs because the neurons that supply the skin, where the pain is felt, enter the same segment of the spinal cord as the neurons that conduct the pain stimuli from the visceral organ. For example, the pain of an **MI** can be felt in the chest wall, left axilla, or down the left arm, because spinal cord segments C4 and C5 receive sensory fibers from the skin areas of the left upper extremity and shoulder as well as from the heart. All of these sensory fibers synapse with the same group of neurons in the spinal cord, which can result in misinterpretation of the origin of the pain.

FIGURE
36-2 **The heart**

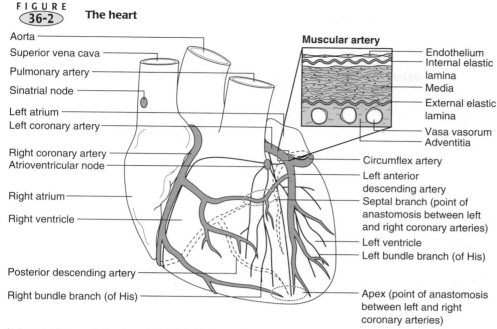

(Adapted with permission from Mehta S, Milder EA, Mirarchi AJ. Step-Up: A High-Yield, Systems-Based Review for the USMLE Step 1 Examination. Philadelphia: Lippincott Williams & Wilkins, 2000, p 43.)

Cardiac conduction

The cardiac conduction system is made up of specialized cells that initiate the heartbeat and electrically coordinate contraction of the heart chambers (Figure 36-2). The **sinoatrial (SA) node,** located in the wall of the right atrium, normally initiates contraction of the heart; therefore, it is known as the "pacemaker." The atrioventricular (AV) node is located at the interatrial septum and is the next step in the conducting system after the SA node. Distal to the AV node, the impulses travel through the bundle of His in the interventricular septum. The bundle of His separates into the right and left bundle branches, and then into the Purkinje fibers. The electrical impulses travel to the left and then the right bundle branch, to the Purkinje fibers, and finally cause the ventricular myocytes to contract. The **AV node** and the **His-Purkinje** system are termed "latent pacemakers" because they only express automaticity if the **SA node is suppressed.**

Electrical excitation of the heart is controlled by SA and AV nodal ("pacemaker") cells. The SA and AV nodal cells possess a "slow response" morphology with an action potential that has three phases (0, 3, and 4) (Figure 36-3). **Phase 0** is the **upstroke** and is caused by an increase in calcium conductance, causing inward calcium current. **Phase 3** is **repolarization** caused by an increase in potassium conductance and an outward potassium current. **Phase 4,** known as slow repolarization, **accounts for the pacemaker activity of the SA node.** Phase 4 is caused by an increase in sodium conductance and an inward sodium current, also known as the **funny current.** This current is turned on by repolarization of the membrane potential from the preceding action potential. The intrinsic rate of phase 4 depolarization is fastest in the SA node and slowest in the His-Purkinje system.

True contraction of the heart is performed by the cells of the ventricles, atria, and Purkinje system. These cells possess a "fast response" morphology with an action potential that has five phases (0, 1, 2, 3, 4) (Figure 36-4). Phase 0 is the upstroke of the action potential and is caused by an increase in sodium conductance. This increase in conductance causes sodium to move into the cell and cause depolarization. Phase 1 is a brief period of initial repolarization caused by the movement of potassium ions out of the cell and a decrease in sodium conductance. Phase 2 is the plateau caused by a transient increase in

QUICK HIT Referred pain occurs in diseases other than MI. For example, in the case of biliary disease or a suprahepatic abscess, pain can be referred to the right shoulder.

QUICK HIT An acute MI can also present with no pain at all (silent MI).

QUICK HIT Heart block is an impairment of the normal electrical conduction between the atria and ventricles. First-degree heart block is characterized by an elongated PR interval, so the time between atrial and ventricular contraction is longer than normal. In second-degree heart block, not all the electrical pulses reach the ventricles, so some ventricular beats do not occur. In third-degree heart block, no electrical impulses reach the ventricles, so the atria and ventricles beat independently.

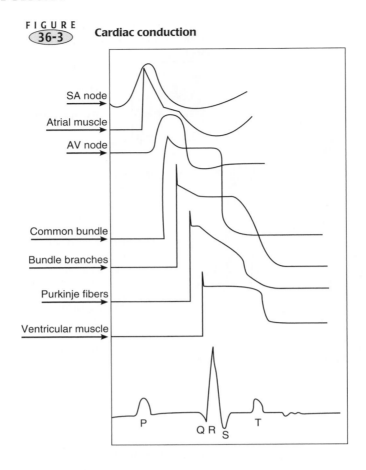

FIGURE
36-3   **Cardiac conduction**

calcium conductance, causing calcium to move into the cell, and an increase in potassium conductance, causing potassium to move out of the cell. In phase 2, these two currents are balanced and the membrane potential remains stable. Phase 3 is the repolarization phase, during which the potassium conductance is greater than the calcium conductance, resulting in a large flow of potassium out of the cell. Phase 4 is the resting membrane potential and is the time when inward and outward currents are equal.

Each heartbeat is represented on the EKG by three major deflections that record the sequence of the electrical propagation through the heart. The **P wave represents atrial depolarization.** The PR interval, which starts at the beginning of the P wave and ends at the beginning of the Q wave, varies inversely with the conduction velocity through the AV node. For example, when the heart rate increases, the PR interval decreases. **The QRS complex represents depolarization of the ventricles.** The QT interval, which begins at the beginning of the Q wave and ends at the end of the T wave, represents the entire depolarization and repolarization of the ventricles. The ST segment, which begins at the end of the S wave and ends

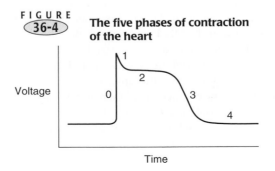

FIGURE
36-4   **The five phases of contraction
of the heart**

at the beginning of the T wave, is isoelectric and is the period when the ventricles are depolarized. The **T wave itself represents ventricular repolarization** (see Figure 36-3).

Atherosclerosis

Atherosclerosis is characterized by fibrous plaques or atheromas in the intima of the arteries. The plaques have a central core of cholesterol and cholesterol esters and contain lipid-laden macrophages (foam cells), calcium, and necrotic debris. The central core is covered by a subendothelial, fibrous cap consisting of smooth muscle cells, foam cells, fibrin, and other coagulation proteins as well as other extracellular matrix material. **The most significant consequence of atherosclerosis is ischemic heart disease and MI,** which is the most common cause of death in the United States.

The most common theory on the pathogenesis of atherosclerosis is the **reaction to injury theory,** in which the primary event in the initiation of atherosclerosis is injury to the arterial endothelium. This injury may be produced by a variety of agents, but more importantly it is perpetuated by hyperlipidemia. Hyperlipidemia is thought to promote foam cell formation, act as a chemotactic factor for monocytes, inhibit macrophage motility, and injure smooth muscle cells. This leads to platelet adhesion, platelet aggregation, and platelet-derived growth factor release, all of which induce the proliferation and migration of smooth muscle cells into the intima. The local inflammatory response to endothelial injury causes monocytes to enter the subendothelium, engulf lipids, and be converted into lipid-laden foam cells.

Common EKG Tracings

FIGURE
36-5   **ECGs of important arrhythmias**

Normal ECG

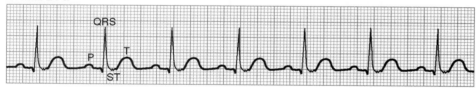

- P wave is atrial depolarization (atrial repolarization usually occurs during the QRS and remains unseen in ECG)
- PR interval (.12–.2 seconds) measures time between atrial and ventricular depolarization
- QRS interval (normally less than .1 second) reflects the duration of ventricular depolarization
- T wave is ventricular repolarization

Sustained ventricular tachycardia

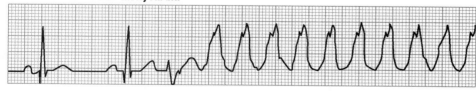

- Constant QRS morphology and fairly regular cycle length
- Initiating beat morphology may differ from ongoing VT
- AV dissociation a hallmark but not always present, nor easy to identify when present

Ventricular fibrillation

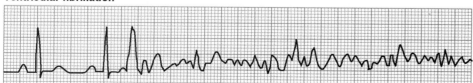

- Undulating baseline, no organized electrical activity
- Incompatible with life
- Atria may be dissociated, still in sinus rhythm

F I G U R E
36-5   **(Continued)**

Atrial flutter

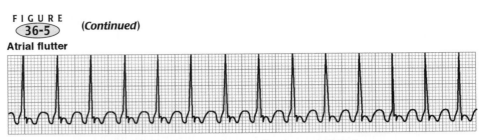

- A regular, saw-toothed pattern of atrial activity, usually very near 300/min
- Discrete, organized atrial activity on intracardiac electrograms
- Usually even-numbered AV conduction ratio (2:1, 4:1)

Atrial fibrillation

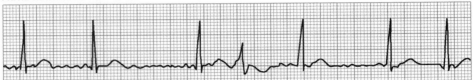

- Undulating, low amplitude atrial activity on ECG
- Intracardiac electrogram shows chaotic rapid spikes
- Variable conduction pattern as AV node is constantly bombarded with impulses; "long-short" sequences yield wide QRS complexes (aberrant, "Ashman" beats)

Wolff-Parkinson-White syndrome

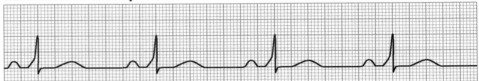

- Accessory atrioventricular conductions
- Anterograde or retrograde conduction
- Tachyarrhythmias
- Blurred QRS (referred to as δ-wave)

Cardiovascular therapeutics

Nitroglycerin

Nitroglycerin is an organic nitrate that is usually used in sublingual form for the **quick relief of an attack of angina** exacerbated by exercise or emotional stress. In the cells of vascular smooth muscle, nitroglycerin is converted to nitric oxide, which activates guanylate cyclase and increases cyclic guanosine monophosphate. Elevated cyclic guanosine monophosphate leads to dephosphorylation of the myosin light chain, causing the relaxation of vascular smooth muscle.

In addition to relaxation of vascular smooth muscle, nitroglycerin has **two major effects: dilation of large veins and dilation of coronary vasculature.** The dilation of large veins results in the pooling of blood in these veins and a subsequent decrease in the venous return to the heart, thereby reducing the work of the heart. Dilation of the coronary vasculature provides increased blood supply to the heart. When combined, these two effects cause a decrease in the heart's myocardial oxygen consumption because of decreased cardiac work.

Antiarrhythmic drugs (Figure 36-6)

Antiarrhythmic drugs, used when patients with an MI develop arrhythmias, are classified according to their primary effects on the action potential of cardiac muscle. Many antiarrhythmic drugs, however, have actions that place them in more than one class or have an

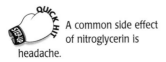

Aspirin, which inhibits platelet aggregation, is the first medication that should be given to a patient suspected of having an MI.

A common side effect of nitroglycerin is headache.

FIGURE
36-6 **Antiarrhythmic drugs**

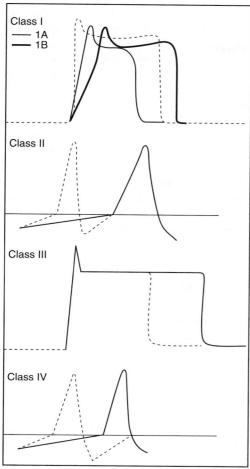

active metabolite that has a different action on the heart. These drugs have many toxicities, the most important being that they cause other arrhythmias to occur. In general, Classes IA and III affect the fast-response cells (atria, ventricles, His-Purkinje system) and are used for both atrial and ventricular arrhythmias. Classes II and IV affect the slow-response cells (SA and AV node) and are used in supraventricular arrhythmias to slow the rate of conduction through the AV node.

Class I antiarrhythmic drugs block voltage-sensitive sodium channels. The decreased rate of sodium entry slows down the rate of rise of phase 0 of the action potential. Therefore, these drugs cause a decrease in excitability and conduction velocity. Class I itself is broken down into three categories (IA, IB, and IC) according to effect on the duration of the action potential.

Class IA agents **(quinidine, procainamide, disopyramide),** beyond slowing phase 0 depolarization, also prolong phase 3 of the action potential, thus increasing the ventricular effective refractory period and prolonging the action potential. On EKG, these drugs cause an increase in the QT interval and QRS complex, but no change in the PR interval. Class IA agents affect both atrial and ventricular arrhythmias.

Class IB agents **(lidocaine, mexiletine, tocainide)** shorten phase 3 repolarization, therefore decreasing the action potential duration. On EKG, there may be no change in the PR interval or QRS complex or a decrease in the QT interval. Class IB agents are used in acute ventricular arrhythmias, especially ventricular fibrillation due to MI, and in digitalis-induced arrhythmias. Lidocaine is the drug of choice for emergency treatment of ventricular fibrillation and tachycardia.

QUICK HIT
STEP-UP

Torsades de pointes (twisting of the points) is a form of ventricular tachycardia characterized by differing amplitudes of the QRS complex, as if they are twisting about the baseline. It is most commonly found in patients with prolonged QT intervals and is frequently caused by various antiarrhythmic drugs.

Class IC agents (**flecainide, encainide, propafenone**) markedly slow phase 0 depolarization, but have no effect on action potential duration. On EKG, there is no change in the QT interval, an increase in the QRS complex (more so than Class IA), and an increase in the PR interval. Because of the toxicities associated with Class IC agents, they are used as a last result in refractory tachyarrhythmias.

Class II antiarrhythmics (**propranolol, esmolol, metoprolol, atenolol, timolol**) are β-adrenergic antagonists. These drugs suppress phase 4 depolarization, therefore suppressing automaticity, prolonging AV conduction, and decreasing heart rate and contractility. These agents act by decreasing cyclic adenosine monophosphate, thus decreasing calcium currents. On EKG, these drugs increase the PR interval, but show no change in the QT interval or the QRS complex. Class II antiarrhythmics are used for supraventricular arrhythmias and for controlling the rate of depolarization of the ventricles in atrial fibrillation and atrial flutter.

Class III antiarrhythmics (**amiodarone, sotalol, bretylium**) act by blocking potassium channels. Consequently, there is decreased outward potassium current during repolarization of cardiac cells and prolonged phase 3 repolarization. This prolongs the effective refractory period, which increases the duration of the action potential without effecting phase 0 depolarization. On EKG, the QT interval is markedly increased, and there is no change in the PR interval or the QRS complex. Class III agents are used for atrial and ventricular arrhythmias.

Class IV antiarrhythmics (**nifedipine, verapamil, diltiazem**) are the calcium channel blockers. These drugs shorten the action potential by decreasing the inward calcium current, resulting in a decrease in the rate of phase 4 spontaneous depolarization. This, in turn, slows conduction in tissues that are dependent on calcium currents, such as the SA and AV nodes. EKG changes include an increased PR interval, but no change in the QT interval or QRS complex. Class IV agents are useful in nodal arrhythmias and supraventricular arrhythmias.

Digoxin and **adenosine** are two antiarrhythmic drugs that do not fall under a specific category. Digoxin is only used in atrial fibrillation and atrial flutter to decrease the ventricular response. However, digoxin is used conservatively because it can induce arrhythmias (ventricular tachycardia or fibrillation). Adenosine inhibits cyclic adenosine monophosphate–induced calcium influx (decreasing automaticity) and directly inhibits AV nodal conduction. It is the drug of choice for treating acute supraventricular tachycardia.

Calcium channel blockers

Calcium channel blockers **inhibit the inward movement of calcium** into the L-type calcium channels of the myocytes and the smooth muscle of coronary and peripheral vasculature. There are three main drugs in this class: nifedipine, verapamil, and diltiazem. **Verapamil** has its most pronounced effects on the heart, and acts as a negative inotrope. It is used to treat **angina, supraventricular arrhythmias,** and **migraine headaches.** Diltiazem has a less pronounced negative inotropic effect on the heart than verapamil, but has a more favorable side effect profile. **Nifedipine,** on the other hand, has a more pronounced affinity for vascular calcium channels than for calcium channels in the heart; therefore, it is used more frequently than the other two drugs for **hypertension.**

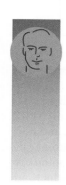

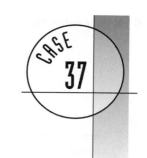

"My left side really hurts, and my urine is red."

OBJECTIVES

1. Develop a differential diagnosis and appropriate workup for unilateral abdominal pain and hematuria
2. Review renal embryology
3. Learn the key features associated with Wilm's tumor, transitional cell cancer, and polycythemia
4. Understand the timeline and distinguishing features for transplant rejections (i.e., immediate versus long term)
5. Review the mechanisms of action and side effects for common immunosuppressants

HISTORY AND PHYSICAL EXAMINATION

A 35-year-old man presents with blood in his urine and pain on his left side. He states that he never before experienced this pain, but has occasionally had blood in his urine. He denies a history of drinking, tobacco, or drug use but does take several antihypertensive medications. His past medical history is significant for recurrent **UTIs, nocturia, hypertension,** and intermittent **abdominal pain.** He has a **family history of kidney disease;** both his father and grandfather died young from "some kind of kidney failure." Further family history reveals that his brother died at 45 years of age of a **subarachnoid hemorrhage.** On physical examination, his blood pressure is **150/95 mm Hg,** and palpation reveals significant left flank pain. On abdominal examination, his kidneys are palpable bilaterally and more tender on the left side.

APPROPRIATE WORKUP

Blood chemistries, urinalysis, renal US, and urography

DIFFERENTIAL DIAGNOSIS

Adult polycystic kidney disease (APKD), juvenile polycystic kidney disease (JPKD), medullary sponge kidney, nephronophthisis (medullary cystic disease), renal cell carcinoma (RCC)

DIAGNOSTIC LABORATORY TESTS AND STUDIES

Blood chemistry:
    Creatinine = 2.5 mg/dL (H)
    BUN = 40 mg/dL (H)
    Hgb = 15 g/dL (N)
    ALT = 10 U/L (N)
    AST = 12 U/L (N)
Urinalysis:
    Protein = 3 + (H)
    RBCs = 2 + (H)

Renal US:
    Enlarged kidneys bilaterally
    Multiple cysts (>5) in the renal cortex and medulla
Retrograde urography:
    Cystic indentations within calyces of kidney

DIAGNOSIS: ADULT POLYCYSTIC KIDNEY DISEASE

APKD is an **autosomal-dominant** disease, with the defect on chromosome **16.** The dominant characteristic of APKD is multiple fluid-filled cysts lining **both kidneys.** These cysts infiltrate the kidney parenchyma and lead to end-stage renal failure in 10% of cases. APKD usually presents in the third to fourth decade of life with **flank pain, hematuria,** and **nocturia.** Other notable findings include **hypertension, palpable kidneys,** hepatomegaly, headache, and increased urinary frequency. Patients are at increased risk of developing urinary tract infections which can ascend into the kidney. The multiple cysts, which are essentially pools of urine that do not drain, make treatment extremely difficult. Asymptomatic cysts can also be found in the liver, stomach, lungs, spleen, and pancreas. There is a strong association between APKD and berry aneurysms. APKD has no definitive treatment, and patients progressing to renal failure may require bilateral nephrectomies with subsequent renal transplantation.

EXPLANATION OF DIFFERENTIAL

JPKD is an **autosomal-recessive** disorder marked by closed renal cysts. This **fatal** disease causes death during early infancy.

Medullary sponge kidney is characterized by small medullary cysts and **impaired tubular function.** This disease has a bimodal distribution in the population, with peaks in adolescence and the third to fourth decades of life. Often, affected patients present with symptomatic renal calculi, infection, or hematuria. Medullary sponge kidney **does not lead to renal failure.** Diagnosis can be made by retrograde urography. In this patient, medullary sponge kidney could be suspected upon presentation. The palpable kidneys, US findings, and ultimately the retrograde urography findings differentiate this disease from APKD.

Nephronophthisis (medullary cystic disease) is a kidney disease affecting **older children.** Characteristic manifestations include scarred and **shrunken kidneys** with **cysts in the medulla.** Patients often progress to renal failure and require kidney transplantation. This diagnosis is unlikely in this patient, given his age and the enlarged size of his kidneys.

RCC is the most **common renal cancer** and usually occurs in men in the sixth and seventh decades of life (Figure 37-1). Classical presentation includes **hematuria, a palpable mass, and flank pain;** fever, increased production of erythropoietin (EPO), and ectopic hormone elaboration can also occur. Increased EPO can lead to an increased RBC mass and **secondary polycythemia.** Ectopically produced hormones include corticotropin, prolactin, growth hormone (GH), parathyroid-like hormone, and renin. Histologically, RCC is characterized by **clear cuboidal cells** arranged into tubules. RCC is associated with **cigarette smoking** and von Hippel-Lindau disease. In this patient, RCC is a possible diagnosis, because he has hematuria and flank pain with a palpable mass. He is relatively young for RCC, however, and bilateral masses coupled with the US findings of cystic kidneys exclude RCC as the final diagnosis.

Related Basic Science

Renal development

The intermediate mesoderm forms the urogenital ridges, which lead to formation of the **nephrogenic cord.** The nephrogenic cord is responsible for the formation of the **pronephros, mesonephros,** and **metanephros** (Table 37-1). The urogenital sinus forms the **bladder;** together, the urogenital sinus and endoderm form the urethra. The most distal part of the urethra derives from **ectoderm.**

Other renal diseases

Renal diseases can result from physical or metabolic disturbances of the kidney, ureters, or bladder. They can occur during any part of the life cycle (Table 37-2).

A **berry aneurysm** is a saccular lesion that occurs most often in the **circle of Willis,** especially in areas of bifurcation. The most common site is the bifurcation of the anterior communicating artery. A rupture of the aneurysm can lead to a **subarachnoid hemorrhage.**

Recessive polycystic kidney disease (RPKD) is a pediatric renal disease with survival beyond infancy and development of hepatic fibrosis.

Tuberous sclerosis is an autosomal-dominant disease characterized by CNS abnormalities (i.e., seizures, mental retardation). Multiple cysts also form on kidneys.

Simple renal cysts are typically **asymptomatic** and must be distinguished from tumors. They are usually discovered incidentally or postmortem.

von Hippel-Lindau disease is characterized by **hemangioblastomas** or **cavernous hemangiomas** of the cerebellum, brain stem, or retina, as well as adenomas and **cysts** in the kidneys, adrenal glands, and other major organs. von Hippel-Lindau disease is associated with a defect on chromosome 3 and can cause **RCC.**

EPO, a glycoprotein produced in the kidney, causes proliferation and differentiation of RBCs in the bone marrow. Pathologically elevated levels can be found in various renal diseases. EPO is also created recombinantly and used to stimulate erythrocyte production in patients with anemia.

FIGURE 37-1 (See also Color Plate 37-1.) Renal cell carcinoma

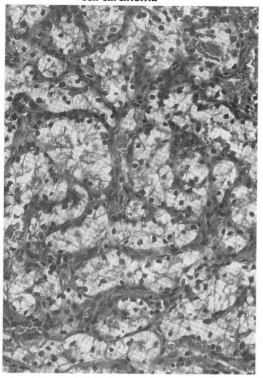

(From Damjanov I. Histopathology: A Color Atlas and Textbook. Philadelphia: Lippincott Williams & Wilkins, 1996, p 291.)

Immunosuppression

Renal cancers, especially **Wilms tumors,** respond quite well to **chemotherapy.** Some chemotherapeutic agents used to combat renal tumors can also be used as immunosuppressive agents after kidney transplantation to prevent rejection of the donated kidney (Figure 37-2).

These agents, however, have significant side effects (Table 37-3).

The most common cause of UTIs in men is aberrant anatomy. UTIs in men warrant further work-up for cause.

TABLE 37-1	Comparison of Embryologic Kidneys
Pronephros	• Forms in the 4th week of gestation • Immediately regresses • **Has no apparent function**
Mesonephros	• Forms in the 4th week of gestation • Functions as the fetal kidney until the permanent kidney is functional (9th week of gestation) • Forms the **ductus deferens, epididymis, ejaculatory duct,** and **seminal vesicle** • Forms the **ureteric bud** (responsible for formation of the **ureter, renal pelvis, calyces,** and **collecting tubes**)
Metanephros	• Creates the **adult kidney** in the 5th week of gestation (in conjunction with the ureteric bud) • Becomes functional in the 9th week of gestation • **Forms nephrons from its mesoderm**

TABLE 37-2 Pathology Associated with the Renal System

Disease	Description
Wilms tumor	• Most **common kidney tumor in children,** occurs between 2 and 5 years of age • Presents as a large, solitary well-circumscribed mass that is often palpable • Is associated with a defect in chromosome 11 and WAGR **(Wilms tumor, aniridia, genitourinary malformations,** and **mental retardation)** • **Has a good prognosis**
Transitional cell cancer	• Is the most common tumor of the urinary collecting system (renal calyces, ureters, and bladder) • Manifests as a **hematuria** • Is associated with exposure to **cigarette smoking, benzidine or aniline dye,** phenacetin abuse, and long-term treatment with cyclophosphamide
Polycythemia	• Is also called erythrocytosis • Increases the concentration of erythrocytes and level of Hct • Causes such symptoms as headaches, tinnitus, vertigo, blurred vision, epistaxis, increased blood viscosity, pruritus, plethora, bone pain, and hepatosplenomegaly Categories: ***Primary*** Polycythemia vera: Abnormal proliferation of myeloid stem cells with normal to low EPO levels ***Secondary*** **Appropriate** (decreased tissue oxygenation with compensatory EPO rise): Lung disease, high altitude, heart disease **Inappropriate** (normal tissue oxygenation with elevated EPO): RCC, von Hippel-Lindau disease, APKD ***Relative*** Hemoconcentration from decreased plasma volume (poor fluid intake or increased fluid output from urine, sweat, or insensible losses)

APKD, adult polycystic kidney disease; EPO, erythropoietin; RCC, renal cell carcinoma.

FIGURE 37-2 Transplant rejection timeline

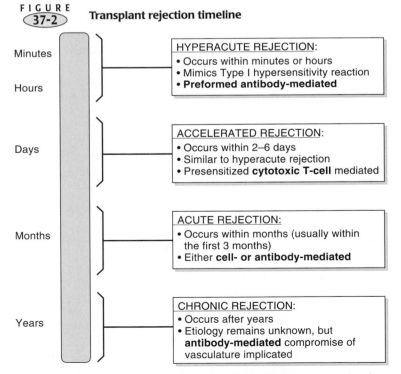

HYPERACUTE REJECTION:
• Occurs within minutes or hours
• Mimics Type I hypersensitivity reaction
• **Preformed antibody-mediated**

ACCELERATED REJECTION:
• Occurs within 2–6 days
• Similar to hyperacute rejection
• Presensitized **cytotoxic T-cell** mediated

ACUTE REJECTION:
• Occurs within months (usually within the first 3 months)
• Either **cell- or antibody-mediated**

CHRONIC REJECTION:
• Occurs after years
• Etiology remains unknown, but **antibody-mediated** compromise of vasculature implicated

(From Mehta S, Milder EA, Mirarchi AJ. Step-Up: A High-Yield, Systems-Based Review for the USMLE Step 1. Philadelphia: Lippincott Williams & Wilkins, 2000, p 213.)

TABLE 37-3 Immunosuppressive Pharmacotherapy

Immunosuppressant	Mechanism of Action	Adverse Effects
Azathioprine	• Is a purine antagonist • Inhibits nucleic acid metabolism • Blocks both **cell-mediated** and **humoral responses** • Is metabolized by **xanthine oxidase**	• Bone marrow depression • Rash • Fevers • Nausea and vomiting
Muromonab (OKT3)	**Acts as an antibody to CD3 on T-lymphocytes**	• **Anaphylactic reaction** • Fever • Seizures • Encephalopathy • Cerebral edema • Aseptic meningitis
Cyclosporine	• **Inhibits T-helper cell activity** • Blocks IL-2, IL-3, and INF-γ formation	• **Nephrotoxicity** • Hepatotoxicity • Hypertension • Anaphylactic reactions
Tacrolimus (FK506) (Prograf)	Blocks activation of T-cell transcription factors	• **Hyperglycemia** • Nephrotoxicity • Neurotoxicity
Cyclophosphamide	• Destroys proliferating lymphocytes • Alkylates resting cells	• **Hemorrhagic cystitis** • GI and bone marrow toxicity

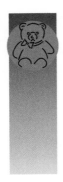

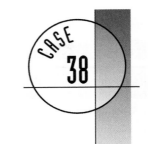

"I can't breathe when I'm running."

OBJECTIVES

1. Develop a differential diagnosis and an appropriate workup for the clinical presentation of wheezing, chest tightness, and dyspnea
2. Review lung volumes
3. Determine the causes of increased and decreased lung compliance
4. Understand the physiologic control of breathing
5. Review the types of chronic obstructive pulmonary diseases and their differentiating characteristics
6. Describe the mechanisms of action and uses of adrenergic and cholinergic drugs

HISTORY AND PHYSICAL EXAMINATION

An 8-year-old boy presents with complaints of a nonproductive cough, **dyspnea,** chest tightness, and **expiratory wheezing.** His mother states that she first noticed these symptoms 2 weeks ago when the boy began soccer practice. She has noticed **prior episodes** with exercise or "just spontaneously" but has never taken her son for treatment. **Both parents smoke** in the home; there are no pets, new furniture, or new carpeting. The patient takes no medications but has **several allergies.** Physical examination is significant for tachycardia and tachypnea with prolonged expirations. **Intercostal retractions** are noted as well as nasal flaring. Auscultation of the lungs reveals diffuse, high-pitched expiratory wheezes.

APPROPRIATE WORKUP

Blood chemistries, chest X-ray, and pulmonary function tests

DIFFERENTIAL DIAGNOSIS

Asthma, pneumonia (bacterial, mycoplasmic, or viral)

DIAGNOSTIC LABORATORY TESTS AND STUDIES

Blood chemistry:
WBCs = 13,000/mm^3 (H)
Eosinophils = 6% (H)
Chest radiograph:
Overinflation
No increased anterior-posterior
(A-P) diameter (Figure 38-1)
Pulmonary function tests:
Forced vital capacity
(FVC) = Decreased

Forced expiratory volume in 1 second
(FEV1)/FVC = Decreased
FEV1/FVC with bronchodilator
(albuterol) = Improved from
baseline, but still below normal

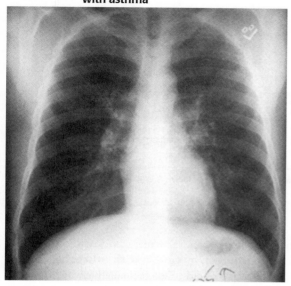

FIGURE 38-1 Chest radiograph of a patient with asthma

(From Brant WE, Helms CA. Fundamentals of Diagnostic Radiology, 2nd Ed. Philadelphia: Lippincott Williams & Wilkins, 1999, p 446.)

DIAGNOSIS: ASTHMA

Asthma is a **reversible airway obstruction** characterized by constriction of airway smooth muscle, hypersecretion of mucus, inflammatory cell infiltration of the airway mucosa, and thickening of the pulmonary epithelial basement membrane. In patients with asthma, **certain inhaled substances** and other stimuli will cause an "asthma attack." Microscopically, the **lungs are edematous with inflammatory infiltrate** consisting of eosinophils in the bronchial walls. Hypertrophy of both the bronchial wall musculature and submucosal mucous glands is noted along with whorled mucous plugs (Curschmann spirals) and elongated double-pyramid crystals (Charcot-Leyden crystals).

Asthma is divided into two types: **allergic** and **intrinsic.** The allergic type is a **Type 1 hypersensitivity reaction** and is **most common in childhood.** The intrinsic type shows **no immediate hypersensitivity** and **occurs in adults.**

In this patient, the diagnosis of asthma is based on the characteristic history of wheezing that is **relieved by a bronchodilator, overinflation of the lungs on chest radiograph** (Figure 38-1), and **leukocytosis with eosinophilia.** Exacerbation of asthma during exercise can result from either an inciting substance in the air or the exercise itself. The family history of smoking in the house is contributory, as **cigarette smoke** irritates the lungs and can **exacerbate asthma.**

Treatment is based on pharmacologic dilation of the bronchial tree. Both **albuterol** (β2 agonist) and **ipratropium** (antimuscarinic) are **bronchodilators** used for acute exacerbations of asthma. **Inhaled corticosteroids** are the next line of treatment in those with moderate to severe asthma. **Cromolyn** limits mast-cell degranulation to prevent asthma reactions but is not useful in managing an acute asthmatic attack. The antileukotriene drugs, **zileuton** (an inhibitor of 5-lipoxygenase) and **zafirlukast** (a leukotriene-receptor antagonist), are also effective in the prophylactic treatment of asthma. **Theophylline** is a bronchodilator that relieves airflow obstruction and decreases symptoms in chronic asthma.

EXPLANATION OF DIFFERENTIAL

Pneumonia is an infection of the lung parenchyma that involves both the **alveolar space and interstitial tissue.** It is classically a bacterial disease (usually *Streptococcus pneumoniae*); however, viruses and mycoplasma are common causes as well. Symptoms, which typically

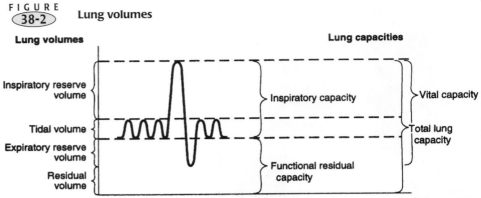

FIGURE
38-2   Lung volumes

(From Costanzo LS. BRS Physiology, 2nd Ed. Philadelphia: Lippincott Williams & Wilkins, 1998, p 123.)

include **cough productive for sputum and fever,** can vary according to the infectious organism and be as **nonspecific as a nonproductive cough with wheezing.** In this patient, the symptoms of coughing and wheezing related to exercise lead toward the diagnosis of asthma, especially when the family and social history is considered.

Related Basic Science

Lung volumes (Figure 38-2)

Compliance of the lungs and chest wall is **inversely related to elasticity.** Therefore, decreased elasticity in the lung tissue increases lung compliance and vice versa. Many processes can alter lung compliance (Table 38-1). Compliance is greatest in the middle range of pressures; as the pressures increase, compliance decreases. Compliance can also be expressed as the slope of a pressure-volume curve. The tendencies of the lungs to collapse and the chest wall to expand maintain the pressure within the pleural cavity at a negative value. When inspiration is desired, the diaphragm contracts and flattens, which lowers the pressure within the pleural cavity, and the lungs expand. Expiration is done by relaxing the breathing muscles and allowing the lungs to collapse. Inflation and deflation of the lungs on a pressure-volume graph follow different curves, a phenomenon known as **hysteresis** (Figure 38-3).

Control of breathing

The brainstem, which coordinates the sensory information and controls the muscles of respiration, regulates breathing. Input is via the **vagus** and glossopharyngeal nerves. The vagus relays information from the **peripheral chemoreceptors** and **mechanoreceptors** in the lung, while the glossopharyngeal relays information from only the peripheral

TABLE 38-1	Causes of Increased and Decreased Lung Compliance
Causes of ↓ Lung Compliance	**Causes of ↑ Lung Compliance**
High expanding pressures	Emphysema (↓ elastic fibers)
↑ pulmonary venous pressure	Age
Fibrosis (deposition of collagen)	
Lack of surfactant	

From Costanzo LS: BRS Physiology, 2nd Ed. Philadelphia: Lippincott Williams & Wilkins, 1998, p 127.

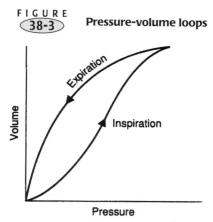

FIGURE 38-3 Pressure-volume loops

(From Costanzo LS. *BRS Physiology*, 2nd Ed. Philadelphia: Lippincott Williams & Wilkins, 1998, p 126.)

chemoreceptors. The dorsal respiratory group of the **medullary respiratory center** controls inspiration and generates the rhythm of breathing. Output from this area travels to the diaphragm via the **phrenic nerve (cervical roots C3, C4, C5).** The ventral respiratory group is also located in the medullary respiratory center and is responsible for the forceful expiration required during exercise. Other control centers include the apneustic center, which stimulates inspiration; the pneumotaxic center, which inhibits inspiration; and the cerebral cortex, which allows breathing to be under voluntary control. Chemoreceptors for carbon dioxide, hydrogen, and oxygen include the **central chemoreceptors** in the medulla and peripheral chemoreceptors in the carotid and aortic bodies (Table 38-2). Lung stretch receptors, irritant receptors, juxtacapillary receptors, and joint and muscle receptors relay information about lung condition to the brain for processing.

The V/Q ratio is the **ratio of the alveolar ventilation to pulmonary blood flow.** It is **normally 0.8,** which equates to ventilation and perfusion that achieve the ideal exchange of oxygen and carbon dioxide. If blood flow to the lung is blocked, then the **V/Q ratio is infinite,** and no gas exchange occurs. If the airways are completely blocked, then ventilation is zero, and therefore V/Q is zero. Because there is no gas exchange, the oxygen and carbon dioxide of the pulmonary capillary blood approach their values in the mixed venous blood. This is termed a **shunt,** and the oxygen and carbon dioxide of alveolar gas will approach the values of inspired air.

Chronic obstructive pulmonary disease

Asthma, emphysema, chronic bronchitis, and bronchiectasis are all chronic obstructive pulmonary diseases (COPDs). An increased resistance to airflow characterizes COPD. **Emphysema** presents with dyspnea, is **strongly associated with smoking,** and is characterized

QUICK HIT Patients with COPD have a chronically elevated CO_2 level and a chronically depressed O_2 level. For this reason, their O_2 level stimulates their drive to breathe instead. CO_2 level (as in healthy patients). If patients with COPD receive O_2 to raise the oxygen saturation in their blood, their drive to breathe is eliminated, and breathing may stop.

TABLE 38-2 Comparison of Central and Peripheral Chemoreceptors

	Location	Stimuli that Increase Breathing Rate
Central chemoreceptors	Medulla	↓ **pH** (↑ Pco_2)
Peripheral chemoreceptors	Carotid and aortic bodies	↓ **Po₂** (if < 60 mm Hg) ↑ Pco_2 ↓ pH

From Costanzo LS. BRS Physiology, 2nd Ed. Philadelphia: Lippincott Williams & Wilkins, 1998, p 144.

TABLE 38-3	Types of Emphysema
Type	**Description**
Centroacinar	Central or proximal parts of the acinus
Panacinar	Uniform destruction of the acinus
Paraseptal	Involves the distal acinus, usually sparing the proximal portions

by enlargement of distal air spaces with alveolar wall destruction to the terminal bronchioles. Emphysema is classified according to the anatomy of the lesion (Table 38-3). **Chronic bronchitis** is defined clinically by a persistent cough with sputum production for at least 3 months in at least 2 consecutive years. It is characterized pathophysiologically by mucous gland hyperplasia and hypersecretion in the bronchi. It is **typically attributed to tobacco smoke** and air pollution. **Bronchiectasis** occurs when there is airway dilation and scarring of the bronchi caused by **persistent or severe infections.** It can present with cough, purulent sputum, and fever.

Drugs affecting the adrenergic and cholinergic receptors

The **adrenergic drugs** affect α **and** β **receptors** usually activated by norepinephrine (NEPI) or epinephrine (EPI).

Sympathomimetics act directly on the adrenergic receptors.

- EPI interacts with both α **and** β **receptors**. At **low doses**, it mainly affects β **receptors**, causing **vasodilation**. At **high doses**, it mainly affects α **receptors**, causing **vasoconstriction.** EPI is the primary drug used in bronchospasm, such as to treat acute asthma and anaphylactic shock.
- The major effects of NEPI are on the α-**adrenergic receptors.** NEPI is **mainly used to treat shock** because it increases vascular resistance and therefore pressure. A notable side effect is reduced blood flow to the kidney. NEPI is never used to treat asthma.
- Dopamine (DA) can activate α-**adrenergic and** β-**adrenergic** receptors as well as **D-1 and D-2 dopaminergic** receptors. DA is the drug of choice for **shock,** because it **increases blood pressure and perfusion to the kidney** and splanchnic areas.

Indirect sympathomimetics stimulate sympathetic receptors via activity on the **presynaptic terminal.**

- Amphetamine increases release of NEPI into the synaptic cleft, thus causing repetitive stimulation of the postsynaptic receptors. It can be used for **attention deficit hyperactivity disorder** in children, appetite control, and narcolepsy.
- Cocaine **blocks reuptake of NEPI, serotonin (5-HT), and DA** into the presynaptic terminal, causing intense euphoria.

Mixed action adrenergic agonists induce release of NEPI from the presynaptic terminal and activate postsynaptic adrenergic receptors.

- Ephedrine raises systolic and diastolic blood pressures by **vasoconstriction and cardiac stimulation** and produces **bronchodilation.** It can be used prophylactically to prevent asthma attacks.

Nonspecific β *agonists (B1/B2):*

- Isoproterenol stimulates **both** β-**1 and** β-**2 receptors** and can be used to provide cardiac stimulation in emergencies. This drug is rarely used as a bronchodilator because of its effects on the heart.

β-1 agonists:

- Dobutamine is used to **increase cardiac output** in heart failure.

β-2 agonists are used for symptomatic relief of bronchospasm in asthma.

- Metaproterenol produces **dilation of the bronchioles** and improves airway function; thus, it is used as a bronchodilator to treat asthma by reversing bronchospasm.
- Terbutaline is more specific than metaproterenol and has a longer duration of action. It is used as a **bronchodilator** and also to **relieve premature contractions** in labor.
- Albuterol is most widely used in its inhaled form to **relieve bronchospasm** and is very similar to terbutaline.

α-1 agonists:

- Phenylephrine is a **vasoconstrictor** that raises systolic and diastolic blood pressures and acts as a nasal decongestant.
- Methoxamine raises blood pressure by causing **vasoconstriction of the arterioles,** thus increasing total peripheral resistance.

α-2 agonists: Drugs binding to **α-2 receptors, which are presynaptic receptors,** *inhibit release of NEPI from the presynaptic terminal.*

- Clonidine acts centrally to produce inhibition of sympathetic vasomotor centers, therefore **lowering blood pressure.**

Adrenergic antagonists inhibit sympathetic receptors by either reversible or irreversible mechanisms, thus preventing endogenous catecholamines from binding to the receptors.

Nonspecific α antagonists reduce the sympathetic tone of blood vessels, **decreasing vascular resistance and blood pressure** *and subsequently causing reflex tachycardia.*

- Phenoxybenzamine is an irreversible, noncompetitive drug used to treat the symptoms of a **pheochromocytoma.**
- Phentolamine produces a competitive blockade and is also used to treat the symptoms of a **pheochromocytoma.**

α-1 selective antagonists:

- Prazosin, terazosin, and doxazosin are competitive blockers used to treat **hypertension.**

Nonspecific β-adrenergic antagonists:

- Propranolol, the prototype β antagonist, is used to treat **hypertension** by **decreasing cardiac output.** It is also used to treat glaucoma, migraine, angina, myocardial infarction (MI), and hyperthyroidism.
- Timolol and nadolol are more potent than propranolol. Timolol reduces production of aqueous humor in the eye, and is therefore used for chronic open angle glaucoma. Nadolol has a very long duration of action.

β-1 selective antagonists:

- Acebutolol, atenolol, metoprolol, and esmolol are **cardioselective** and do not affect the bronchial tree. Thus, these drugs are used in **patients with hypertension and impaired pulmonary function.**
- Labetalol is both an **α and a β blocker.** It produces peripheral vasodilation, therefore reducing blood pressure. It is used to treat elderly or Black patients with hypertension, for whom increased peripheral vascular resistance is undesirable.

Drugs affecting neurotransmitter uptake or release:

- Reserpine blocks the transport of neurotransmitters into storage vesicles in the adrenergic nerves of all body tissues and causes an overall decrease in sympathetic function.
- Guanethidine blocks the release of stored NEPI, resulting in gradual decreased blood pressure in patients with hypertension and decreased heart rate.

The **cholinergic agents** act on receptors that are activated by acetylcholine (ACh), namely muscarinic and nicotinic receptors.

Direct acting muscarinic agonists:

- Bethanechol increases intestinal motility and tone and expulsion of urine. It is used to stimulate **atonic bladder,** generally in postoperative, nonobstructed urinary retention.

- Carbachol has a high potency and long duration of action. Thus, it is used only in the eye as a miotic agent and to decrease intraocular pressure in patients with **glaucoma.**
- Pilocarpine is a drug of choice in the emergency lowering of intraocular pressure in both **narrow angle and wide angle glaucoma.**

Indirect-acting cholinergic agonists: Reversible anticholinesterases inhibit acetyl-cholinesterase (AChE), an enzyme that specifically breaks down ACh in the synapse. Consequently, these drugs promote a high level of ACh in the synapse.

- Physostigmine inhibits AChE both peripherally and centrally in both muscarinic and nicotinic synapses. It increases intestinal and bladder motility, produces miosis, and decreases intraocular pressure in glaucoma. It can also be used to **treat toxic overdoses of anticholinergic drugs** because of its entry into the CNS.
- Neostigmine does not enter the CNS like physostigmine but has a greater effect on skeletal muscle, and is therefore used in the symptomatic treatment of **myasthenia gravis.** It is also used to stimulate the bladder and GI tract.
- Pyridostigmine is used in the chronic management of **myasthenia gravis.**
- Edrophonium has actions similar to that of neostigmine but is more rapidly absorbed and has a shorter duration of action. This drug is used in the **diagnosis of myasthenia gravis.**

Irreversible anticholinesterases inhibit AChE and cause a long-lasting increase in ACh. Reactivation of AChE can be accomplished only if the **antidote** (i.e., **pralidoxime**) is given before "aging" of the irreversible anticholinesterase to the enzyme.

- Sarin has extremely rapid aging and is therefore essentially irreversible. It is the classic **"nerve gas"** used in war.
- Echothiophate
- Malathion

Cholinergic antagonists block the actions of the cholinergic agonists.
*Antimuscarinic agents **block the effects of parasympathetic innervation** and therefore leave the sympathetic innervation unopposed.*

- Atropine is the **classic muscarinic blocker.** It blocks all cholinergic activity in the eyes, causing mydriasis and cycloplegia which lead to inability to focus and blurry vision. Atropine is also used as an antispasmodic agent to relax the GI tract and bladder, as an antidote for cholinergic agonists, and occasionally as an antisecretory agent to block upper and lower respiratory secretions before surgery.
- Scopolamine has a greater action on the CNS and a longer duration of action than atropine and is one of the most effective drugs available for **motion sickness.** Scopolamine is much more effective prophylactically than it is as treatment. Interestingly, this drug also blocks short-term memory.
- Ipratropium is used to **treat asthma** and COPD.

QUICK HIT
STEP-UP

Atropine has five classic side effects, which can be remembered by the mnemonic "Red as a beet, blind as a bat, dry as a bone, hot as a hare, and mad as a hatter." These correlate with the side effects of (1) cutaneous flushing, (2) blurry vision from mydriasis and cyclo-plegia, (3) anhydrosis (inability to sweat), (4) unopposed sympathetic activity on the hypothalamus, and (5) psychosis.

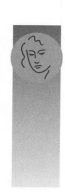

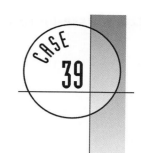
"I feel really tired and confused. I've also lost 5 pounds in 2 weeks!"

OBJECTIVES

1. Develop a differential diagnosis and an appropriate workup for unintentional weight loss and feelings of fatigue and confusion
2. Compare and contrast the serum antidiuretic hormone (ADH) levels, plasma osmolarity, and urine osmolarity for syndrome of inappropriate antidiuretic hormone (SIADH), central diabetes insipidus, nephrogenic diabetes insipidus, and psychogenic polydipsia
3. Understand the physiology associated with ADH
4. Review the types, mechanisms of action, and properties of diuretics
5. Compare and contrast small cell versus squamous cell carcinoma of the lung
6. Learn the causes and clinical presentation of the superior vena cava syndrome

HISTORY AND PHYSICAL EXAMINATION

A 50-year-old female is admitted to the hospital for an elective procedure. She complains of **general malaise, confusion,** and a 5-pound **weight loss** over the past 2 weeks. She denies any recent bouts of diarrhea or vomiting and is not on any medications. She has no signs of heart failure and recalls no past medical history of cardiovascular problems or liver disease.

On physical exam, her vital signs and physical exam were normal.

APPROPRIATE WORKUP

Blood chemistries, urinalysis, chest X-ray, CT scan of the head

DIFFERENTIAL DIAGNOSIS

SIADH, central diabetes insipidus, nephrogenic diabetes insipidus, psychogenic polydipsia

DIAGNOSTIC LABORATORY TESTS AND STUDIES

Blood Chemistry:
Glucose = 80 mg/dL (N)
Ketone bodies = (N)
Na^+ = 115 mEq/L (L)
K^+ = 4.0 mmol/L (N)
Cl^- = 90 (L)
pH = 7.4
Anion gap = 12 (N)
Plasma osmolality = **250 (L)**

Urinalysis:
Osmolality = **290 mOsm/kg (H)**
Na^+ = 46 mmol/L (H)
Glucose = negative
Chest radiograph:
Unilateral hilar enlargement
CT scan, head:
Normal

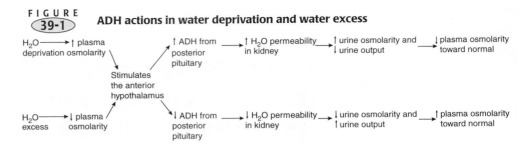

FIGURE 39-1 ADH actions in water deprivation and water excess

DIAGNOSIS: SIADH

This patient presents with a **syndrome of inappropriate antidiuretic hormone** (SIADH). **ADH** is secreted by the **posterior pituitary** and acts on **renal V$_2$ receptors** (mechanism: **adenylate cyclase**) to **increase water permeability** of the late distal tubule and collecting duct principal cells. ADH also acts on arterial **V$_1$ receptors** (mechanism: **Ca^{2+}–IP$_3$**) and **vaso-constricts arterioles**. Figure 39-1 explains the functions of ADH as it relates to water deprivation and excess.

An excess of ADH causes water reabsorption which increases plasma osmolarity, resulting in this patient's hyponatremia. This results in a fluid shift from the extracellular compartment to the intracellular compartment. In the brain, this shift can cause **cerebral edema** and **neurologic effects**, such as **confusion** in this patient. If this condition is not corrected, this patient can develop severe coma and convulsions.

In assessing patients who may potentially have SIADH, it is important to rule out other causes. This patient reported no history of vomiting, diarrhea, or diuretic use, all of which can cause sodium wasting and result in hyponatremia. However, with significant fluid losses, this patient would have *hypovolumic* hyponatremia, as opposed to **hypervolumic** hyponatremia. This patient was also questioned about any cardiovascular conditions or liver disease because both can cause fluid retention and hyponatremia resulting in *hypervolumic* hyponatremia.

The urine osmolarity increases because water is reabsorbed from the late distal tubule and collecting duct without a proportionate solute absorption. Therefore, the diagnosis of SIADH is established in this patient based on her lab findings of **low sodium (hyponatremia), decreased plasma osmolality increased urine sodium, and increased urine osmolality.**

SIADH is usually secondary to **small cell carcinoma of the lung** with excess ADH secretion. However, lesions or tumors of the hypothalamus or pituitary can also cause SIADH.

Urine osmolarity serves as a guide to selection of fluid for replacement. When urine osmolality is less than 300 mOsm/L, correct with isotonic saline; if urine osmolality is greater than 300 mOsm/L, consider hypertonic saline. **Furosemide** can also be used in conjunction with isotonic or hypertonic saline as it helps maintain urine output and blocks secretion of ADH. **Demeclocycline** interferes with the action of ADH at the renal collecting duct by impairing generation and action of cyclic AMP.

EXPLANATION OF DIFFERENTIAL

Central diabetes insipidus (DI) is the excretion of large amounts of **very dilute urine** because of a **lack of secretion of ADH** or **insensitivity to ADH** in the kidney. Central DI is a result of a lack of hypothalamic ADH secretion. Central DI can be due to a pituitary tumor, head trauma, or surgery.

Nephrogenic diabetes insipidus results when **the kidneys are unable to respond** to ADH. ADH levels are not necessarily low. The kidneys' response to ADH is impaired. Common causes include lithium toxicity, demeclocycline, and secondary hypercalcemia. Both central and nephrogenic DI results in plasma osmolarity that is high secondary to renal excretion of water over sodium.

Psychogenic polydipsia is due to **intentional intake of excessive water.** The kidneys are functioning normally and work to remove excessive ingested water resulting in a max-imally dilute urine of approximately 50 mOsm. Table 39-1 summarizes these trends in plasma ADH levels, plasma osmolarity, and urine osmolarity.

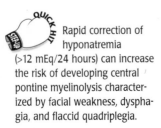

Rapid correction of hyponatremia (>12 mEq/24 hours) can increase the risk of developing central pontine myelinolysis characterized by facial weakness, dyspha-gia, and flaccid quadriplegia.

TABLE 39-1	Lab Findings in SIADH, Central and Nephrogenic DI, and Psychogenic Polydipsia		
Disease	**Serum ADH**	**Plasma Osmolarity**	**Urine Osmolarity**
SIADH	↑	↓	↑
Central DI	↓	↑	↓
Nephrogenic DI	↑	↑	↓
Psychogenic polydipsia	↓	↓	↓

Related Basic Sciences

Antidiuretic hormone

ADH is released from the posterior pituitary. It is secreted in response to an **increased plasma osmolarity** and reduces the osmolarity by increasing water reabsorption in the collecting ducts of the kidneys. This is achieved by the **insertion of aquaporins** which serve as water channels into the luminal membranes of the **collecting ducts**. Figure 39-2 summarizes the effects of ADH along the nephron.

ADH is also secreted in **response to low blood pressure** and acts to **increase water reabsorption** in the kidney and hence expand extracellular fluid. ADH also causes **arterial vasoconstriction,** restoring normal blood pressure. ADH is effective in the regulation of blood pressure in response to **major blood loss,** such as hemorrhage, but not in the minute-to-minute regulation of normal blood pressure.

The overall response of ADH to decreased blood pressure is summarized in Figure 39-3.

QUICK HIT

ADH **vasoconstricts** by binding to V_1 **receptors** on arterioles and increases total peripheral resistance. ADH **reabsorbs water** by activating V_2 **receptors** on the renal collecting ducts.

FIGURE 39-2

Effect of ADH along the nephron

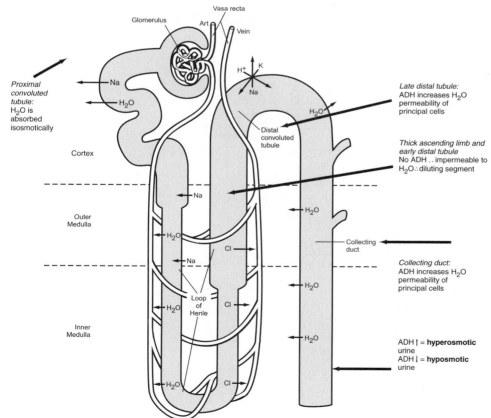

(Modified from McClatchey KD. Clinical Laboratory Medicine, 2 Ed. Philadelphia: Lippincott Williams & Wilkins, 2002.)

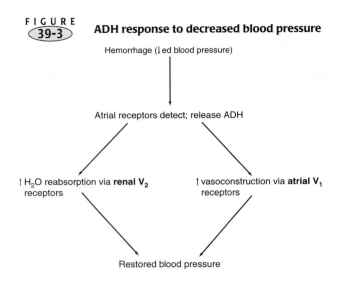

FIGURE
39-3 **ADH response to decreased blood pressure**

Hemorrhage (↓ed blood pressure)

↓

Atrial receptors detect; release ADH

↑ H_2O reabsorption via **renal V_2** receptors

↑ vasoconstriction via **atrial V_1** receptors

Restored blood pressure

Desmopressin is an ADH synthetic analog that has the same renal effects as ADH with significantly less vasoconstriction. It is used to treat **central diabetes insipidus** when the pituitary does not secrete ADH.

Diuretics

Diuretics **increase urine formation**. The degree to which solute and water excretion is increased depends on the site and mechanism of action. The **strongest diuretics (loop diuretics)** act in a segment where a large percent of filtered Na^+ is reabsorbed. Conversely, the **weakest diuretics (K-sparing diuretics)** act in a segment where a small percent of filtered Na^+ is reabsorbed. Figure 39-4 summarizes their locations while Table 39-2 summarizes their mechanisms of action, clinical uses, and side effects of key diuretics.

Small cell versus squamous cell carcinoma of the lung (Figures 39-5 and 39-6 and Table 39-3)

FIGURE
39-4 **Diuretics effects on the nephron**

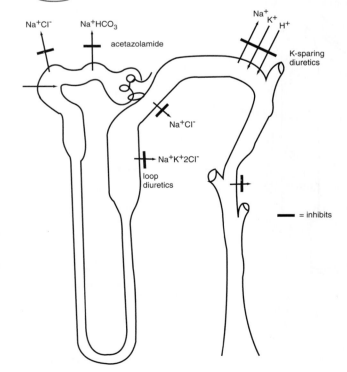

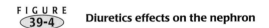

QUICK HIT Ethacrynic acid has the same mechanism of action as furosemide but is not a sulfonamide. It can be used in patients with sulfa allergies and can also be used in patients who also suffer with hyperuricemia.

QUICK HIT Carcinoid tumors are metastatic tumors to the lung from the small bowel that secrete increased levels of serotonin. Clinical presentation includes diarrhea, salivation, wheezing, and cutaneous flushing. Diagnosis is made with increased levels of 5-HIAA in the urine. Treatment: octreotide.

QUICK HIT Peripheral lung tumors include adenocarcinoma, bronchioalveolar carcinoma, and large cell carcinoma.

TABLE 39-2 Diuretics

Diuretic	Mechanism of Action	Electrolytes Lost in Urine	Properties
Acetazolamide	Inhibits carbonic anhydrase in **PCT** and prevents HCO_3^-, reabsorption	Na^+, HCO_3^-, K^+	Results in **metabolic acidosis** Causes decreased secretion of HCO_3^- in aqueous humor Used to treat **glaucoma**
Loop diuretics (furosemide)	Prevents cotransport of Na^+, K^+, Cl^- in the **thick ascending limb**	Na^+, Cl^-, Ca^{2+}, K^+	Has rapid onset and short duration of action, which is ideal for relieving acute edema Produces side effects such as **hypokalemic metabolic alkalosis** and ototoxicity
Thiazides	Inhibits transport of Na^+ and Cl^- into cells of **DCT**	Na^+, Cl^-, K^+	Causes decreased Ca^{2+} excretion; can lead to K^+ wasting with chronic therapy Results in **increased glucose and lipid levels** in some patients
K^+-sparing diuretics	Binds to intracellular aldosterone steroid receptors in **collecting tubules** Blocks induction of Na^+ channels and Na^+/ATPase synthesis	Na^+, Cl^-	Results in decreased secretion of K^+ and H^+, which can lead to **hyperkalemic metabolic acidosis** Can cause **gynecomastia**

ATPase, adenosine triphosphatase; Ca^{2+}, calcium; Cl^-, chloride; DCT, distal convoluted tubule; K^+, potassium; Na^+, sodium; PCT, proximal convoluted tubule.
Modified from Mehta S, Milder EA, Mirarchi AJ. Step-Up: A High-Yield, Systems-Based Review for the USMLE Step 1 Examination, 2 Ed. Philadelphia: Lippincott Williams & Wilkins, 2003, p 156.

FIGURE 39-5 (See also color plate) Classic appearance of small cell carcinoma, with sheets of small cells, slightly spindled shape, finely granular chromatin, and very scant cytoplasm.

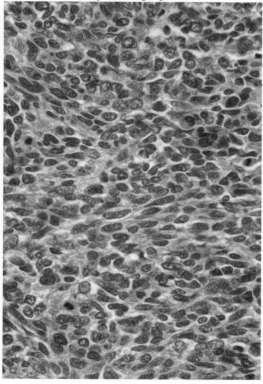

(From Cagle PT, MD. Color Atlas and Text of Pulmonary Pathology. Philadelphia: Lippincott Williams & Wilkins, 2005.)

F I G U R E
39-6
(See also color plate) Malignant squamous cells forming a keratin pearl, with adjacent small cell carcinoma cells in a combined tumor.

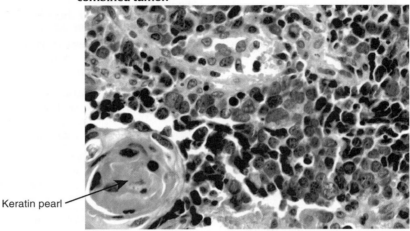

Keratin pearl

(From Cagle PT, MD. Color Atlas and Text of Pulmonary Pathology. Philadelphia: Lippincott Williams & Wilkins, 2005.)

Superior vena cava syndrome

Superior vena cava (SVC) syndrome involves **obstruction of the superior vena cava**, resulting in **swelling** and **neurologic symptoms**. **Dyspnea** is the most common presenting symptom with **facial and upper extremity edema.** The SVC syndrome is often associated with **small cell cancer** but can also be associated with TB. A common finding to support small cell carcinoma as the primary cause of SVC is the **Horner syndrome** with ptosis, miosis, and anhidrosis.

TABLE 39-3 Small versus Squamous Cell Carcinoma of the Lung

	Small Cell (Oat Cell)	Squamous Cell
Location	Central	Central
Histology	Undifferentiated; most aggressive, **small, dark blue cells** (Figure 39-5)	Cavitation; **keratin pearls** (Figure 39-6)
Ectopic secretion	**ACTH** (causing Cushing syndrome) and **ADH** (causing SIADH)	**PTH-like peptide** (causing hypercalcemia)
Clinical presentation	Cough, hemoptysis, airway obstruction, weight loss, and history of smoking	

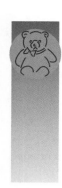

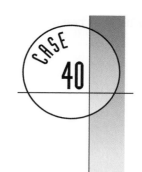

"My child has been very irritable and has been holding his ear."

OBJECTIVES

1. Develop a differential diagnosis and appropriate workup for ear inflammation and irritation of the ear
2. Review the embryology and anatomy of the ear
3. Learn the auditory pathway and vestibular system
4. Differentiate between the facial (VII) and vestibulocochlear nerves in terms of function and associated pathologies
5. Review three common genetic diseases that increase susceptibility to infection

HISTORY AND PHYSICAL EXAMINATION

A woman brings her 3-year-old son to the office. According to her, the boy has had a **fever** and has been **irritable** and **holding on to his right ear** for the past day and a half. She states that the patient had a **cold about 1 week ago** and is still coughing occasionally. On physical examination, palpation of the maxillary and frontal sinuses is unremarkable; the right **tympanic membrane looks red, opaque,** and **bulging.** The membrane appears to be **moving poorly with insufflation.** Findings of the contralateral ear examination are normal.

APPROPRIATE WORKUP

Vital signs and audiogram

DIFFERENTIAL DIAGNOSIS

Otitis externa, otitis media, sinusitis

DIAGNOSTIC LABORATORY TESTS AND STUDIES

Vital signs:	**Audiogram:**
Temperature = 101.9°F (H)	Decreased hearing acuity in right ear

DIAGNOSIS: OTITIS MEDIA

Otitis media, or **middle ear infection,** is most common in children **younger than 3 years, with incidence decreasing with age.** It results when the eustachian tube, which drains fluid from the middle ear, becomes blocked. Trapped fluid in the middle ear becomes a culture medium for bacteria. In children, the most common causative organisms of acute otitis media are *Streptococcus pneumoniae, Haemophilus influenzae,* and *Moraxella catarrhalis.* Viral or fungal organisms are other possible causes. The most common causes of chronic otitis media are *Pseudomonas aeruginosa, Staphylococcus aureus,* or a fungus.

Viral infections usually produce serous exudates, while bacterial infections produce suppurative exudates. Clinically, a **viral URI** often **precedes** otitis media, which then presents with **ear pain, fever,** and **decreased hearing acuity.**

EXPLANATION OF DIFFERENTIAL

Otitis externa is an infection of the outer ear canal. Characteristics include **tenderness of the ear canal** and an **inflamed external canal,** often covered by friable cerumen. Patients present with a **pruritic and painful ear with a red swollen canal.** The most common organisms infecting the external auditory canal are *P. aeruginosa, S. aureus,* and streptococci. In this patient, the outer ear was normal and nontender, which excludes otitis externa as the diagnosis.

Clinically, **sinusitis** presents with **malaise, headache,** and **tenderness** over the affected sinuses. The paranasal, maxillary, ethmoid, frontal, and sphenoid sinuses are aerated cavities in the facial bones. They are lined with respiratory epithelium that includes mucus-secreting goblet cells. Blockage of the ostia that drain the sinuses or delayed movement of the mucus can lead to infection of the sinuses. A **viral infection is a common precursor** of sinusitis and promotes the actual infection, which most often is caused by *S. pneumoniae, H. influenzae, or* staphylococci. In this patient, sinusitis is ruled out because ear pain usually is not a complaint in sinusitis. Moreover, the patient has no tenderness to palpation over the sinuses.

Related Basic Science

Development of the ear

The **internal part of the ear develops from the otic placode** that is part of the surface ectoderm. The **external part of the ear develops from first pharyngeal groove** (Table 40-1).

Anatomy of the ear

The external ear consists of the following elements:

- **auricle**—cartilage connected to the skull by ligaments and muscles
- **external acoustic meatus**—outer one-third is cartilage, and inner two-thirds is bone
- **tympanic membrane**—contains the **cone of light** (reflection of light in the anterior–inferior quadrant) and **umbo** (most depressed center point of the concavity)

The **middle ear** consists of the following elements:

- **tympanic cavity**—the space internal to the tympanic membrane
- **ossicles**—**malleus** (touches the tympanic membrane), **incus,** and **stapes**
- **muscles**—stapedius muscle inserts on the stapes and prevents excessive oscillation during a loud noise; tensor tympani muscle inserts on the malleus and draws it medially, thus making the tympanic membrane taut

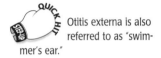

Otitis externa is also referred to as "swimmer's ear."

TABLE 40-1 Pharyngeal Arch and Pouch Derivatives

Arch	Pouch	Muscle	Nerve
Arch I	Tubotympanic recess Eustachian tube	Muscles of mastication	Trigeminal (V) (mandibular branch)
Arch II	Palatine Tonsils	Muscles of facial expression	Facial (VII)
Arch III	**Inferior parathyroids** Thymus	Stylopharyngeus	Glossopharyngeal (IX)
Arches IV–VI	**Superior parathyroids** Ultimobranchial body	Intrinsic muscles of the larynx	Vagus (X)

The **inner ear** consists of the following elements:

- **bony labyrinth**—a hollow bony structure filled with **perilymph** in which the membranous labyrinth is suspended; parts include the **vestibule, semicircular canals**, and **cochlea**
- **membranous labyrinth**—a membranous "bag" suspended in perilymph and **filled with endolymph**; includes the **utricle** and **saccule** in the vestibule, **semicircular ducts**, and **cochlear duct**, containing the **spiral organ of Corti**

Auditory pathway (Figure 40-1)

The **cochlea** houses the structures that **receive and convert sound energy into neural signals.** The cochlea is a unique structure in that it contains a "tube within a tube," separated by the tectorial membrane. The outer tube contains perilymph, while the inner tube contains endolymph and the hair cells. The hair cells are **auditory receptor cells** that transduce sound energy into electrical potentials. They are located **on the basilar membrane,** are **bathed in endolymph,** and have stereocilia that extend out and attach to the tectorial membrane. The **basilar membrane** separates the cochlear duct from the scala tympani. The basilar membrane has an important function in **pitch localization,** with 20 Hz being localized at the apex of the cochlea, and 20,000 Hz being localized at the base. Vibration of the basilar membrane by sound is transduced via the stereocilia to hair cells that convert the vibration into a neural impulse that travels centrally via the **cochlear nerve (cranial nerve VIII).**

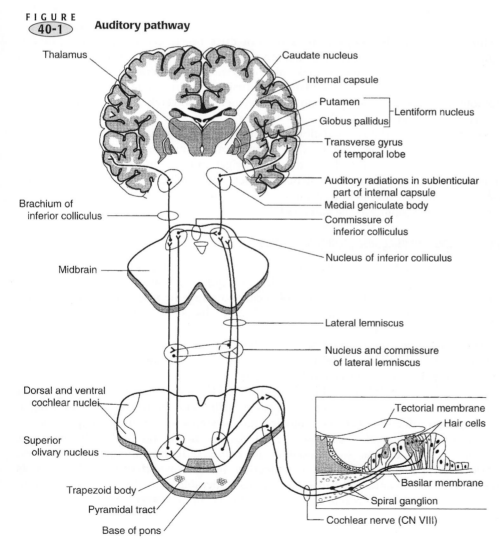

FIGURE 40-1 **Auditory pathway**

(From Fix JD. BRS Neuroanatomy, 2nd Ed. Baltimore: Williams & Wilkins, 1994, p 178.)

Facial nerve (cranial nerve VII)

The facial nerve mediates **facial movements, taste, salivation,** and **lacrimation.** It originates in the pons, runs through the internal auditory meatus and facial canal proximal to the internal ear structures, and **exits the skull via the stylomastoid foramen.** After exiting, the facial nerve travels through the parotid gland superficially. Lesions of the facial nerve cause **Bell palsy** (lower motor neuron [LMN] lesion resulting in ipsilateral paralysis of all muscles of facial expression); **central facial palsy** (upper motor neuron [UMN] lesion resulting in paralysis of the contralateral lower facial muscles); **hyperacusis** (paralysis of the stapedius muscle), **loss of corneal reflex** (cranial nerve VII is the efferent limb; cranial nerve V is the afferent limb); and **loss of taste** (anterior two-thirds of the tongue).

Vestibulocochlear nerve (cranial nerve VIII)

The vestibulocochlear nerve mediates **balance** and **hearing.** It originates in the pons, enters the internal auditory meatus, and remains in the temporal bone. The nerve consists of two divisions: the **vestibular nerve** and the **cochlear nerve.** Lesions of the vestibular nerve cause vertigo and nystagmus. Lesions of the cochlear nerve may cause hearing loss (sensorineural deafness) or tinnitus.

Vestibular system

The vestibular system, located in the bony labyrinths of the inner ear, consists of two units: the **semicircular canals** and the **otolithic apparatus (utricle** and **saccule).** The function of the **semicircular canals is to transduce angular acceleration,** while the function of the **otolithic apparatus is to transduce linear acceleration** and **gravitational forces.** Both units convey information to the vestibular nuclei of the brain stem via cranial nerve VIII. The vestibular nuclei project to the nuclei of cranial nerves III, IV, and VI (control eye movement); the spinal cord (provides postural stability); cerebral cortex (promotes awareness of body position and movement); and cerebellum (maintains visual stability during head movement).

    Nystagmus, a rhythmic oscillation of the eyes, occurs normally from vestibular and visual stimuli. Nystagmus not related to these normal stimuli occurs for many reasons (e.g., alcohol intoxication). Cold or hot water irrigation of the external auditory meatus stimulates the hair cells in the semicircular ducts, thus inducing nystagmus. Normally, cold-water irrigation results in nystagmus to the **opposite side,** while warm-water irrigation results in nystagmus to the **same side.**

Genetic diseases increasing susceptibility to infection

Bruton disease is an X-linked agammaglobulinemia characterized by a **B-cell deficiency.** It is caused by an X-linked recessive defect, resulting in **low levels of all types of immunoglobulins.** Patients are at **risk of recurrent pyogenic infections,** usually beginning after 6 months of age. Histologically, Bruton disease is characterized by poorly defined germinal centers.

    Severe combined immunodeficiency (SCID) is an autosomal-recessive disorder characterized by **B-cell** and **T-cell deficiency.** A deficiency in **adenosine deaminase (ADA)** causes a **defect in early stem-cell differentiation** and ultimate lack of T and B cells. SCID can also have other etiologies including an autosomal-recessive tyrosine kinase defect, or an X-linked IL-2 receptor defect. Patients present with **recurrent bacterial, viral, fungal, and protozoal infections because their immune systems are severely compromised.**

    Wiskott-Aldrich syndrome is also characterized by **B-cell** and **T-cell deficiency.** The main defect in this disease is a **weakened IgM response to capsular polysaccharides.** Consequently, patients are at risk of **infection by encapsulated bacteria such as** *Streptococcus pneumoniae.* The disease becomes noticeable in the first year of life; clinical manifestations include eczema, thrombocytopenia, and **recurrent infections.**

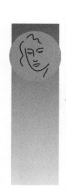

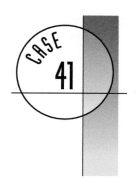

"My knuckles hurt. The pain has gotten worse in the past several months."

OBJECTIVES

1. Develop a differential diagnosis and an appropriate workup for pain in bilateral metacarpophalangeal joints
2. Compare and contrast clinical features of osteoarthritis and rheumatoid arthritis
3. Learn distinctive features of selected arthritides and related disorders
4. Review the function of synovium
5. Learn the anatomy and innervation of the facial nerve
6. Understand key clinical features and associations of osteomyelitis
7. Differentiate among seronegative arthritides, specifically ankylosing spondylitis, Reiter syndrome, and psoriatic arthritis
8. Learn the pharmacologic management of rheumatoid arthritis

HISTORY AND PHYSICAL EXAMINATION

A 35-year-old White woman complains of **bilateral metacarpophalangeal** joint swelling and tenderness of several months' duration. She has noticed "decreased flexibility" in her hands, and complains of generalized **morning stiffness.** She has no allergies, takes no medications, and denies a history of recent illness. She is married and states that neither she nor her husband has had any additional sexual partners. She states that she has not been camping or in grassy or wooded areas recently. On physical examination, she is noted to have **radial deviation of the wrist, ulnar deviation of the fingers,** and flexion–hyperextension abnormalities of the fingers (i.e., **swan-neck and boutonnière deformities**). Her elbows are notable for **subcutaneous nodules** over the olecranon processes.

APPROPRIATE WORKUP

Vitals, blood chemistries, serology, and hand radiograph

DIFFERENTIAL DIAGNOSIS

Lyme disease, osteoarthritis, rheumatoid arthritis, septic arthritis

DIAGNOSTIC LABORATORY TESTS AND STUDIES

Vitals:
    Temperature = 99°F (N)
Blood chemistry:
    WBCs = 8000/μL (N)
    Hgb = 11.0 g/dL (L)
    Mean corpuscular volume = 90 μm^3 (N)
Serology
    Rheumatoid factor = Positive
    ESR = 40 mm/hr (H)

ELISA for *Borrelia burgdorferi* = Negative
Hand radiograph (Figure 41-1):
    Localized erosion and decalcification of bones proximal to joints
    Swan-neck and boutonnière deformities present

FIGURE
41-1   **Radiographic representation of bony deformities of the hand**

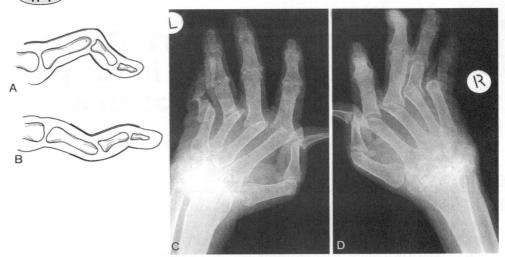

(Reprinted with permission from Yochum TR, Rowe LJ. Essentials of Skeletal Radiology, 2nd Ed. Baltimore: Williams & Wilkins, 1995, p 863.)

DIAGNOSIS: RHEUMATOID ARTHRITIS

Rheumatoid arthritis is a chronic, systemic, inflammatory disease that may affect almost any part of the body, but most prominently the joints. The hallmark of the disease is a **proliferative synovitis** that results in the destruction and eventual fusion of joints. The incidence of rheumatoid arthritis is approximately 1% in the population, and it is **three times more common in women** than in men. Peak onset is between 20 and 40 years of age.

Rheumatoid arthritis is a **clinical diagnosis** made using the criteria of the American Rheumatism Association. Three of the following seven criteria must be present to make the diagnosis of rheumatoid arthritis:

1. Morning stiffness
2. Arthritis of three or more joints
3. Arthritis of the hand joints
4. Symmetrical arthritis
5. Rheumatoid nodules
6. Serum rheumatoid factor
7. Roentgenographic/radiographic changes

In this patient, the findings of bilateral metacarpophalangeal joint swelling and tenderness, subcutaneous rheumatoid nodules, swan-neck and boutonnière deformities with bone erosion, normocytic anemia (characteristic of many chronic diseases), elevated ESR, and positive serum rheumatoid factor make rheumatoid arthritis a clear diagnosis.

EXPLANATION OF DIFFERENTIAL (TABLE 41-1)

Lyme disease is caused by the **spirochete B. burgdorferi** and is spread by the bite of the tick *Ixodes dammini.* **Erythema chronicum migrans** and general malaise are notable symptoms. The disease can cause chronic neurologic and cardiac symptoms as well as asymmetric oligoarthritis. Lyme disease is characterized by three stages:

1. Erythema chronicum migrans (i.e., a red rash with central clearing)
2. Neurologic and cardiac disease
3. Autoimmune migratory polyarthritis

Diagnosis of Lyme disease is based on ELISA, but must be confirmed with a Western blot test. In this patient, a diagnosis of Lyme disease can be ruled out based on the

TABLE 41-1 Distinctive Features of Selected Arthritides and Related Disorders

Type	Etiology	Incidence	Most Frequent Site	Notable Features
Rheumatoid arthritis	Autoimmune	Women ages 20–50	Joints of hands, knees, and feet; proximal interphalangeal and metacarpophalangeal joints	Subcutaneous nodules; rheumatoid factor (anti-IgG)
Ankylosing spondylitis	Probably autoimmune; may have genetic component	Young men	Spine and sacroiliac joints	Vast majority of patients positive for HLA-B27 antigen
Osteoarthritis (degenerative joint disease)	Mechanical injury ("wear-and-tear"); may have a genetic component	After age 50; somewhat more frequent in women	Weight-bearing joints; distal and proximal interphalangeal joints	Osteophytes; Heberden and Bouchard nodes; joint mice
Gout	Hyperuricemia with deposition of urate crystals in multiple sites	Men older than age 30	Metatarsophalangeal joint of great toe	Tophi; kidney damage; urate nephrolithiasis
Gonococcal arthritis	Infection with *Neisseria gonorrhoeae*	Variable	Knee, wrist, small joints of hands	Often monoarticular
Hypertrophic osteoarthropathy	Secondary manifestation of chronic lung disease, cyanotic heart disease, and various non-pulmonary systemic disorders	Variable, depending on primary disorder	Fingers, radius, and ulna	Clubbing of fingers; periostitis

Reprinted with permission from Schneider AS, Szanto PA: BRS Pathology. Baltimore, Williams & Wilkins, 1993, p 345.

negative history of exposure to wooded areas and grassy fields, the lack of erythema chronicum migrans, and, more specifically, the negative ELISA.

Osteoarthritis is the **most common form of arthritis.** It is caused by **mechanical injury ("wear and tear"),** is most often seen in **weight-bearing joints,** and is usually found in the older population. It is characterized by destruction of articular cartilage with **narrowing of the joint space, sclerotic joint changes, subchondral cyst formation,** and **formation of bone spurs.** Bone spurs that form at the perimeter of the articular surface are called osteophytes, of which there are several types. Osteophytes at the distal interphalangeal joints are called Heberden nodes, osteophytes at the proximal interphalangeal joints are called Bouchard nodes, and osteophytes that break off and float free in the joint space are called joint mice. Unlike rheumatoid arthritis, osteoarthritis is considered a **noninflammatory disorder,** with only a small amount of inflammatory cells seen in the joint space. In this patient, the constellation of findings point away from osteoarthritis, especially given the patient's young age.

Septic arthritis is a form of arthritis caused by **hematogenous spread** of bacteria into the joint space or **direct trauma** to the joint. It is **most often caused by *Staphylococcus aureus*** (Gram-positive, coagulase-positive, catalase-positive cocci); however, in **sexually active adults, *Neisseria gonorrhoeae* is a common cause** (gonococcal arthritis). Septic arthritis is usually **monoarticular** and tends to involve the larger joints. Gonococcal arthritis specifically usually involves the knee, and occurs after *N. gonorrhoeae* (Gram-negative, kidney bean–shaped diplococci) has been sexually transmitted to the patient.

Septic arthritis is characterized by **pus in the joint spaces** and presents as a **hot, erythematous, swollen, tender joint.** It is more common in diabetics and immunosuppressed patients, and if left untreated can lead to severe joint destruction. In this patient, septic arthritis can be ruled out by the lack of an elevated temperature, elevated WBCs, comorbid disease, or pain in the larger weight-bearing joints. One long-term sexual partner also points away from septic arthritis as a diagnosis. If the patient did have a large, swollen joint and the diagnosis was unclear, the joint must be aspirated and the fluid sent for analysis and culture.

Related Basic Science

Joint synovium

Mobile joints possess a capsule that defines the boundary between articular and periarticular tissues. This capsule is lined by a thin layer of cells called the synovium. The synovium covers all of the intracapsular structures, except for the cartilage at the end of the epiphysis. This flexible lining collapses upon itself to minimize the volume of the joint space it encloses. The synovial cells produce a proteoglycan-rich fluid that **lubricates the capsule and reduces the frictional stress placed on the articulating cartilage.** The synovium is supported by a bed of fenestrated capillaries, lymphatic vessels, and nerve fibers.

Facial nerve

The facial nerve (cranial nerve VII) exits through the stylomastoid foramen and enters the parotid gland posteriorly. Within the parotid gland it gives rise to five radiating branches: the temporal, zygomatic, buccal, mandibular, and cervical branches. The facial nerve innervates the muscles of facial expression, and damage to it causes ipsilateral facial paralysis, also known as **Bell palsy.** Bell palsy can be idiopathic or it may be a complication of **diabetes, Lyme disease,** herpes zoster, AIDS, facial tumors, trauma, or sarcoidosis.

Osteomyelitis

Osteomyelitis is an acute, pyogenic infection of bone that most often starts at the metaphysis. Although antibiotics may resolve an acute infection, chronic osteomyelitis can lead to bone necrosis **(sequestrum)** and new surrounding bone growth **(involucrum).** Skin sinuses may form, leading to drainage of pus from the infected bone. Bacteria that cause osteomyelitis include **S. aureus** (most common), *N. gonorrhoeae, Pseudomonas aeruginosa* (common in IV drug users), **Salmonella species (common in patients with sickle cell disease),** and group B streptococcus or *Escherichia coli* in newborns.

Seronegative arthritides

The seronegative arthritides are a group of arthritic diseases that are not associated with rheumatoid factor, yet are similar to rheumatoid arthritis. These diseases are much more likely to occur in patients that have HLA-B27.

Ankylosing spondylitis is characterized by **back pain** that progresses to a **rigid spine** secondary to fusion of the intervertebral disks. Radiographs reveal a "rugby jersey" spine. It is associated with **apical lung fibrosis,** aortic insufficiency, and cauda equina syndrome.

Reiter syndrome is associated with chlamydia infection and is characterized by the triad of **urethritis, conjunctivitis,** and **arthritis.**

Psoriatic arthritis is a sequela of psoriasis and occurs in approximately 10% of patients with psoriatic disease. The **distal interphalangeal** joints of the fingers and toes, the sacroiliac joints, and the spine are usually involved. The disease usually remits; however, progression to chronic, severe arthritis can occur and produce the classic radiographic finding of the **"pencil in a cup"** deformity of the distal phalanges.

Pharmacologic treatment for rheumatoid arthritis

Nonsteroidal anti-inflammatory drugs (NSAIDs)

NSAIDs, like aspirin, inhibit the enzymes cyclooxygenase (COX) I and COX II, blocking the pathway of prostaglandin production (Figure 41-2). This blockade results in anti-inflammatory, analgesic, antipyretic (prostaglandin E_2 synthesis blockade), and antiplatelet effects.

Felty syndrome is rheumatoid arthritis accompanied by splenomegaly and neutropenia.

Caplan syndrome is interstitial pneumoconiosis associated with rheumatoid arthritis.

Synovial fluid bathes the joint cartilage and provides it with its only source of nutrition.

Although *S. aureus* is still the leading cause of osteomyelitis, patients with sickle cell disease have a high incidence of salmonella osteomyelitis.

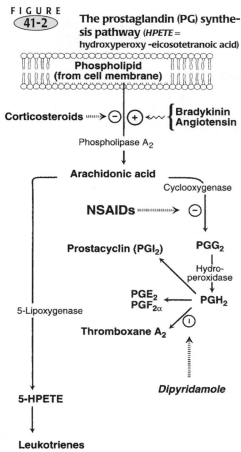

FIGURE 41-2 The prostaglandin (PG) synthesis pathway (*HPETE = hydroxyperoxy -eicosotetranoic acid*)

(Reprinted with permission from Mycek MJ, Harvey RA, Champe PC. Lippincott's Illustrated Reviews in Pharmacology, 2nd Ed. Philadelphia: Lippincott Williams & Wilkins, 2000, p 403.)

COX II inhibitors

Unlike the NSAIDs, which target COX I and II, the COX II inhibitors are more specific and target COX II only. Specific **blockade of COX II provides the analgesic effect and decreases the unwanted side effects of the NSAIDs (most notably GI bleeding),** which are supposedly associated with inhibition of COX I.

Gold salts

Gold salts are thought to suppress phagocytosis and lysosomal enzyme activity in macrophages. This slows down the destruction of articular cartilage and bone seen in arthritis. The **gold salts are slow acting** and require 4 to 6 weeks of administration before an effect is seen.

Methotrexate

Methotrexate is a **folic acid analog** that **inhibits the enzyme dihydrofolate reductase.** It is an S-phase specific antimetabolite. It is typically used in arthritis refractory to other medications. Because it is administered in smaller doses than those used for chemotherapy, it has fewer side effects.

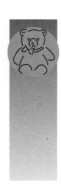

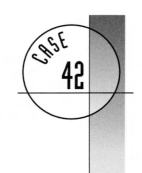

"My baby's skin turns blue when he's playing. He also seems to squat frequently."

OBJECTIVES

1. Develop a differential diagnosis and an appropriate workup for cyanosis in young children
2. Differentiate among five common congenital heart defects
3. Review fetal circulation and the embryology of the heart
4. Describe the anatomy and electrophysiology of the heart

HISTORY AND PHYSICAL EXAMINATION

A 14-month-old boy has had **recurrent bouts of cyanosis** since birth. His parents report that the child cannot keep up with other children his age. According to the parents, the child frequently turns blue and seems to breathe very heavily upon exertion. He often **squats to catch his breath.** These symptoms have been worsening. There is no family history of congenital heart defects or lung disease. Physical examination reveals a systolic ejection murmur, cyanosis, clubbing of the fingernails, and a parasternal heave.

APPROPRIATE WORKUP

Chest X-ray, EKG, echocardiogram

DIFFERENTIAL DIAGNOSIS

Tetralogy of Fallot, total anomalous pulmonary venous return, transposition of the great arteries, tricuspid atresia, and truncus arteriosus

DIAGNOSTIC LABORATORY TESTS AND STUDIES

Chest radiograph:
  Enlarged right ventricle
  "Boot-shaped" heart
EKG:
  Right ventricular hypertrophy

Echocardiogram:
  Ventricular septal defect (VSD)
  Aorta overriding interventricular septum
  Pulmonic stenosis
  Right ventricular hypertrophy

DIAGNOSIS: TETRALOGY OF FALLOT

Tetralogy of Fallot is one of the most common congenital heart defects. Its characteristics include **pulmonary stenosis, right ventricular hypertrophy, overriding aorta, and VSD** (Figure 42-1). While infections (e.g., toxoplasmosis, rubella, cytomegalovirus, herpes) can cause congenital heart defects, the etiology of Tetralogy of Fallot is often unknown. Tetralogy of Fallot results from an anterior displacement of the **infundibular septum.** Venous blood pumped from the right atrium into the right ventricle spills into the left ventricle via

FIGURE
42-1   **Anatomic abnormalities in Tetralogy of Fallot**

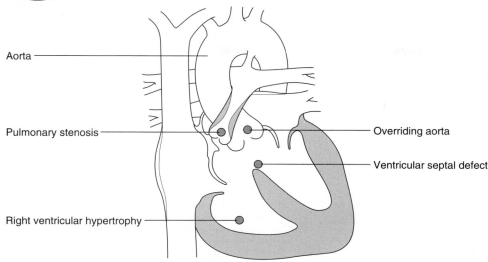

Aorta

Pulmonary stenosis — Overriding aorta

— Ventricular septal defect

Right ventricular hypertrophy

the VSD because of the pulmonic valve stenosis. As a result of this **right-to-left shunt,** babies become cyanotic. Evidence of hypoxemia is seen, with clubbing of the fingernails as well as polycythemia. Older children are known to **squat,** which increases venous return and increases systemic resistance, thereby decreasing right to left shunting. Since babies cannot "squat," they tend to fold their knees into their chest as a compensatory mechanism. Symptoms are directly proportional severity of the pulmonary stenosis. EKG typically reveals right ventricular hypertrophy. Echocardiography is the gold standard for diagnosis. Surgery is necessary for repair; however, some untreated patients survive into adulthood.

EXPLANATION OF DIFFERENTIAL

The five major congenital heart defects that lead to cyanosis in babies are Tetralogy of Fallot, total anomalous pulmonary venous return, transposition of the great arteries, tricuspid atresia, and truncus arteriosus. In all these defects, cyanosis results from **right to left shunting,** which causes hypoxemia. Many congenital heart defects do not present with cyanosis in the affected infants (Table 42-1).

Total anomalous pulmonary venous return is a condition in which no pulmonary veins directly enter the left atrium. Instead, primitive connections drain oxygenated blood to various sites. The common pulmonary vein does not develop embryologically. A patent foramen ovale or ASD allows mixing of blood. Right ventricular hypertrophy develops. Treatment is surgical.

In **transposition of the great arteries,** two separate circuits are created when the aorta arises from the right ventricle and the pulmonary artery empties the left ventricle. This defect is incompatible with life unless there is also a compensatory defects such as VSD, atrial septal defect (ASD), patent ductus arteriosus (PDA), or patent foramen ovale. Patients present with severe cyanosis hours to weeks after birth. Surgical correction is necessary emergently if there is no compensatory defect.

Tricuspid atresia involves agenesis of the tricuspid valve. Blood must cross the atrial septum to exit the right atrium. This defect is associated with transposition of the great vessels in 25% of cases. Symptoms and presentation depend on the severity of pulmonic outflow obstruction. Definitive treatment is surgical.

Truncus arteriosus is a defect in which the embryologic division of the truncus arteriosus into the aorta and pulmonary artery fails to occur. While cyanosis is not always present because of increased pulmonary blood flow with mixing, patients often experience congestive heart failure (CHF) in the first days of life. Survival is 2 to 3 months if the condition is not treated surgically.

ASDs are associated with paradoxic embolization, by which a thrombus from the systemic venous circulation passes to the arterial systemic circulation. The consequence can be cerebrovascular accident.

The conversion of a left-to-right shunt to a right-to-left shunt from progressive pulmonary hypertension is called **Eisenmenger syndrome.**

Administration of indomethacin precipitates closure of a PDA by inhibiting prostaglandin synthesis. Administration of alprostadil (PGE1) maintains a PDA. PDA is associated with congenital rubella infection.

Coarctation of the aorta is associated with the bicuspid aortic valve in 50% of cases. Incidence is four times greater in men than women, but this anomaly is common in Turner syndrome.

TABLE 42-1 Other Common Forms of Congenital Heart Defects

Defect	Clinical Presentation	Pathology
VSD (33% of defects)	• Small: asymptomatic, loud holosystolic murmur; may close spontaneously • Large: symptomatic including CHF at 4 to 6 weeks of age; soft systolic murmur • Incidence greater in males than in females	Left-to-right shunt • Membranous septum (high) 90% • Muscular
PDA (10% of defects)	• Continuous, **harsh "machinery" murmur** • Premature infants • Infants with hypoxemia	• Left-to-right shunt • Persistence of embryonic connection between pulmonary artery and aorta
ASD (5% of defects)	• Usually asymptomatic into older adulthood • Systolic murmur • Incidence greater in women than in men	Left-to-right shunt • Secundum (90%): fossa ovalis +/− septum primum, secundum, or both • Primum: low septum • Sinus venosus: high septum
Coarctation of the aorta (5% of defects)	• **Weak femoral pulses** • Holosystolic murmur • **Hypertension in arms only** • **Rib notching** on radiograph from collateral flow through intercostal vessels	Aortic narrowing of two types: • Infantile: proximal to a PDA; lower body cyanosis • Adult: opposite ligamentum arteriosum; asymptomatic
Bicuspid aortic valve (2% of general population.)	• **Asymptomatic through early life** • Angina • Syncope • Increased incidence of sudden death	• Usually caused by incomplete separation of two cusps • **Progressive calcification** leading to stenosis, regurgitation with left ventricular hypertrophy, or both • Increased risk of infective endocarditis

ASD, atrial septal defect; CHF, congestive heart failure; PDA, patent ductus arteriosus; VSD, ventricular septal defect.

Related Basic Science

Development of the heart

The primitive heart forms from the fusion of the endocardial tubes at gestational week 3. The heart begins to pump around **day 24 of fetal life** (see Figure 42-2). As the heart develops, venous return flows through the cardinal veins and the sinus venosus to the inferior portion of the heart. By fetal day 28, the heart has folded and the primitive atrium has moved superiorly. The **truncus arteriosus** gives rise to the **aorta and the pulmonic trunk.** The primary ventricle gives rise to the left ventricle, and the **bulbus cordis** gives rise to the right ventricle and the aortic outflow tract.

Fetal circulation (Figure 42-2)

The third aortic arches form the carotid arteries. The fourth aortic arches form the aorta on the left and a portion of the right subclavian artery. The sixth aortic arches form the ductus arteriosus and a portion of the pulmonary trunk. The **vitelline veins** form the adult hepatic sinusoids, portal vein, inferior vena cava, superior and inferior mesenteric veins, and ductus venosus. The **ligamentum teres** is a remnant of the umbilical vein. The anterior cardinal vein forms the superior vena cava and internal jugulars, while the posterior cardinal vein forms the common iliac veins, azygos, and renal veins.

Structure of the heart (Figure 42-3)

The heart is an organ of the middle mediastinum in the thorax. The base resides at approximately the level of the third rib. The **aorta and the pulmonary trunk** exit at the superior aspect, and their valves can be auscultated at the **right and left second intercostal spaces,** respectively. The **apex of the heart** is found at the **fifth intercostal space** in the midclavicular line. It is the site of the point of maximal impulse and **best auscultation of the mitral valve.**

QUICK HIT

Lithium use during pregnancy can result in Ebstein anomaly. The tricuspid valve is displaced downward, leading to a large right atrium and small right ventricle. Tricuspid regurgitation is a common finding.

F I G U R E
42-2   **Fetal circulation**

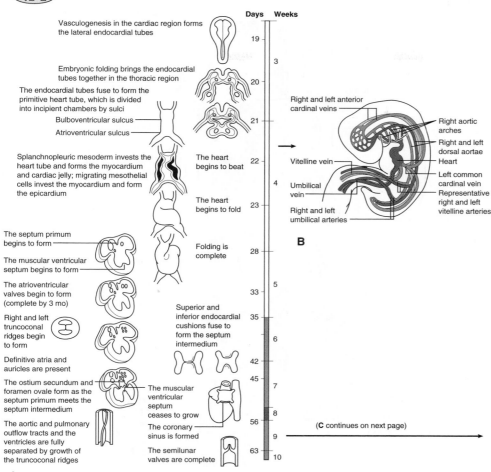

Vasculogenesis in the cardiac region forms the lateral endocardial tubes

Embryonic folding brings the endocardial tubes together in the thoracic region

The endocardial tubes fuse to form the primitive heart tube, which is divided into incipient chambers by sulci

Bulboventricular sulcus

Atrioventricular sulcus

Splanchnopleuric mesoderm invests the heart tube and forms the myocardium and cardiac jelly; migrating mesothelial cells invest the myocardium and form the epicardium

The heart begins to beat

The heart begins to fold

Folding is complete

The septum primum begins to form

The muscular ventricular septum begins to form

The atrioventricular valves begin to form (complete by 3 mo)

Right and left truncoconal ridges begin to form

Superior and inferior endocardial cushions fuse to form the septum intermedium

Definitive atria and auricles are present

The ostium secundum and foramen ovale form as the septum primum meets the septum intermedium

The muscular ventricular septum ceases to grow

The aortic and pulmonary outflow tracts and the ventricles are fully separated by growth of the truncoconal ridges

The coronary sinus is formed

The semilunar valves are complete

Days Weeks

19

3

20

21

22

4

23

28

5

33

35

6

42

45

7

56

8

9

63

10

A

Right and left anterior cardinal veins

Right aortic arches

Right and left dorsal aortae

Vitelline vein

Heart

Umbilical vein

Left common cardinal vein

Right and left umbilical arteries

Representative right and left vitelline arteries

B

(**C** continues on next page)

(Adapted from Larsen WJ. Human Embryology. New York: Churchill Livingstone, 1993, p 132; and Mehta S, Milder EA, Mirarchi AJ. Step-Up: A High-Yield, Systems-Based Review for the USMLE Step 1. Philadelphia: Lippincott Williams & Wilkins, 2000, p 40.)

F I G U R E
42-2   *(Continued)*

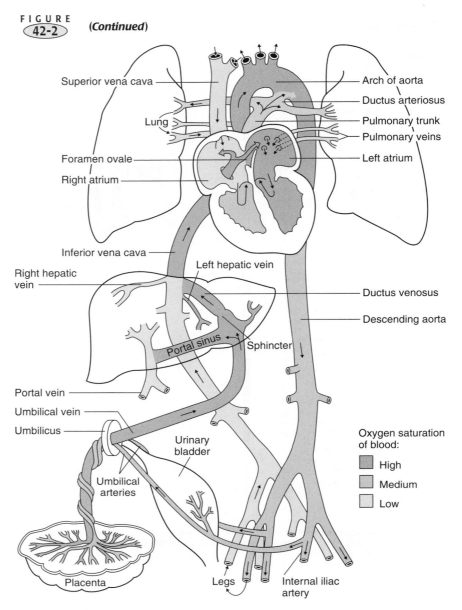

C

FIGURE
42-3

The anatomy and electrical physiology of the heart

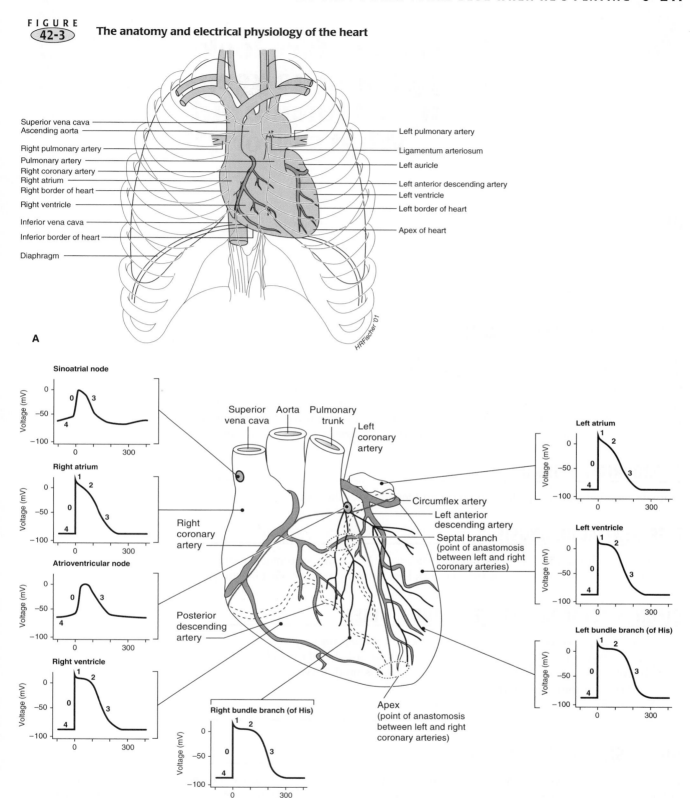

A

B

(Part B from Mehta S, Milder EA, Mirarchi AJ. Step-Up: A High-Yield, Systems-Based Review for the USMLE Step 1. Philadelphia: Lippincott Williams & Wilkins, 2000, p 43.)

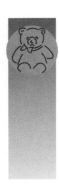

"My baby's face looks strange, and he keeps sticking his tongue out. What's wrong?"

OBJECTIVES

1. Develop a differential diagnosis for genetic disorders in infants
2. Describe the appropriate workup during pregnancy to detect genetic defects
3. Learn pathognomonic findings and karyotypes of common genetic disorders
4. Review modes of inheritance of genetic-based diseases

HISTORY AND PHYSICAL EXAMINATION

A 4-week-old male patient presents for a well baby examination. He is the product of an uncomplicated pregnancy of a **40-year-old mother.** The mother reports having **low α-fetoprotein (AFP)** levels during pregnancy. On physical examination, the patient is noted to have a flat occiput; white spots in his iris (**Brushfield spots**); a large, protruding tongue; small, low-set ears; broad, short feet and hands; a flexion crease across his palms (**simian crease**); clinodactyly (curvature) of the fifth digit; a systolic ejection **murmur**; split S2; and **hypotonia.**

APPROPRIATE WORKUP

Mother's blood chemistries, fetal karyotype, and fetal echocardiogram

DIFFERENTIAL DIAGNOSIS

Cri du chat syndrome (5p-), Down syndrome (trisomy 21), Edwards syndrome (trisomy 18), fragile X syndrome, Patau syndrome (trisomy 13), fetal alcohol syndrome, cleft lip and palate

DIAGNOSTIC LABORATORY TESTS AND STUDIES

Maternal triple screen:
   Maternal serum AFP = Decreased
   Unconjugated estriol = Decreased
   Human chorionic gonadotropin
      (hCG) = Increased

Echocardiogram:
   Endocardial cushion defect
Chromosomal karyotype:
   Trisomy 21

DIAGNOSIS: DOWN SYNDROME

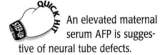

An elevated maternal serum AFP is suggestive of neural tube defects.

Down syndrome (trisomy 21) is the most common somatic chromosomal disorder and one of the most common causes of congenital mental retardation. Ninety-five percent of Down syndrome cases are due to meiotic **nondisjunction,** and the rest are due to either mosaicism or **robertsonian translocations** (Figure 43-1). While cases of maternal meiotic nondisjunction are dependent on maternal age (increased risk over 35 years of age), paternal nondisjunction, mosaicism, and robertsonian translocations are not related to age.

   Patients with Down syndrome present with typical physical findings (Figure 43-2), including those mentioned earlier. Several medical problems occur with greater frequency

FIGURE 43-1

Trisomy 21 syndrome (Down syndrome)

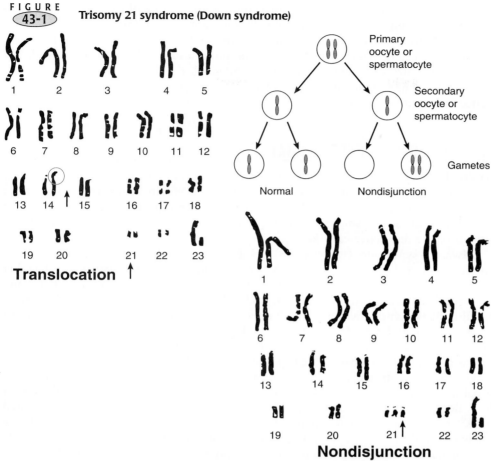

Translocation ↑

Primary oocyte or spermatocyte

Secondary oocyte or spermatocyte

Gametes

Normal   Nondisjunction

Nondisjunction

(Redrawn from Levsen WJ. Human Embryology. New York: Churchill Livingstone, 1993, pp 23–24.)

FIGURE 43-2

A. Down syndrome abnormalities. B. Down syndrome

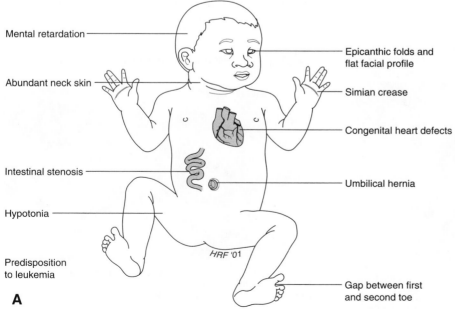

Mental retardation

Abundant neck skin

Intestinal stenosis

Hypotonia

Predisposition to leukemia

A

Epicanthic folds and flat facial profile

Simian crease

Congenital heart defects

Umbilical hernia

Gap between first and second toe

HRF '01

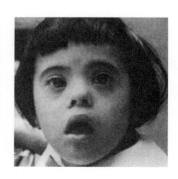

B

(Reprinted with permission from McMillan JA, DeAngelis CD, Feigin RD, et al. Oski's Pediatrics: Principles and Practice, 3rd Ed. Philadelphia: Lippincott Williams & Wilkins, p 2232.)

in these patients, such as duodenal obstruction or atresia (3% of patients), **acute lymphocytic leukemia** (risk is approximately 20 times greater than the general population), structural heart defects (about 40% of patients), conductive or neural hearing loss, hypothyroidism, and moderate to severe **mental retardation.** Males with Down syndrome are sterile, and 40% of females fail to ovulate. In middle age, changes in the brain consistent with **Alzheimer disease** appear since the gene associated with Alzheimer's is also located on chromosome 21.

EXPLANATION OF DIFFERENTIAL

Cri du chat syndrome (5p-), also known as cat's cry syndrome, is caused by deletion of the short arm of chromosome 5. The majority of cases (85%) are de novo deletions. Cri du chat syndrome is characterized by low birth weight, microcephaly, hypertelorism, low-set ears, epicanthal folds, a simian crease, hypotonia, and mental retardation (Figure 43-3). Patients have a distinctive **cat-like cry.**

Edwards syndrome (trisomy 18) results from **nondisjunction** associated with advanced maternal age in 80% of cases. Mosaicism and translocation account for the other cases. Edwards syndrome is characterized by low birth weight; a prominent occiput; **micrognathia;** malformed, low-set ears; **rocker-bottom feet;** overlapping of the second and fifth digits over the third and fourth digits; an increased incidence of congenital heart disease; and **mental retardation** (Figure 43-4). These patients are born with hypertonia, not hypotonia. There is also an association with genital anomalies, renal anomalies, and various hernias. Patients have a life expectancy of less than 1 year.

Fragile X syndrome is the most common cause of inherited mental retardation. Females are usually heterozygotes with milder disease than males. There is an expansion of the FMR1 gene on the X chromosome, where a trinucleotide repeat of 50 copies is increased to 200 or more copies. The inheritance pattern is X-linked dominant. Fragile X syndrome is characterized by macrocephaly, **large ears,** a **long face,** a prominent jaw, hypermobile joints, **macroorchidism** in postpubertal males, and mental retardation (Figure 43-5).

Patau syndrome (trisomy 13) is primarily due to nondisjunction associated with advanced maternal age in 75% of cases. The other cases result from mosaicism or translocation. Patau syndrome is characterized by **microcephaly,** microphthalmia, **polydactyly, cleft lip and palate,** congenital heart defects, and mental retardation (Figure 43-6). Other associations include omphaloceles, genital abnormalities, renal anomalies, and seizures. Like Edwards syndrome, patients have a life expectancy of less than 1 year.

> **QUICK HIT**
> Elevated AFP is also a marker of hepatocellular carcinoma and endodermal sinus (yolk sac) tumors of both the testis and ovary.

> **QUICK HIT**
> The most common cause of mental retardation in the United States is **fetal alcohol syndrome.**

> **QUICK HIT**
> Up to 50% of Down syndrome patients have heart defects. These defects include ventricular septal defect, patent ductus arteriosus, and **endocardial cushion defects.**

FIGURE 43-3 Cri du chat syndrome

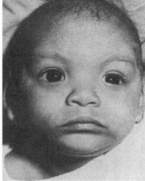

(Reprinted with permission from McMillan JA, DeAngelis CD, Feigin RD, et al. Oski's Pediatrics: Principles and Practice, 3rd Ed. Philadelphia: Lippincott Williams & Wilkins, p 2232.)

FIGURE 43-4 Trisomy 18 syndrome (Edwards syndrome)

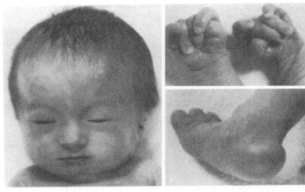

(Reprinted with permission from McMillan JA, DeAngelis CD, Feigin RD, et al. Oski's Pediatrics: Principles and Practice, 3rd Ed. Philadelphia: Lippincott Williams & Wilkins, p 2230.)

FIGURE 43-5 Fragile X syndrome

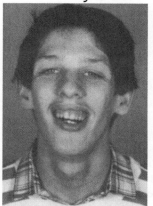

(Reprinted with permission from McMillan JA, DeAngelis CD, Feigin RD, et al. Oski's Pediatrics: Principles and Practice, 3rd Ed. Philadelphia: Lippincott Williams & Wilkins, p 2232.)

FIGURE 43-6 Trisomy 13 syndrome (Patau syndrome)

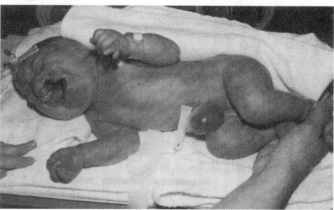

(Reprinted with permission from McMillan JA, DeAngelis CD, Feigin RD, et al. Oski's Pediatrics: Principles and Practice, 3rd Ed. Philadelphia: Lippincott Williams & Wilkins, p 2229.)

Fetal alcohol syndrome is the most common cause of mental retardation in the United States. It is present in newborns of mothers who consumed significant amounts of alcohol during pregnancy, especially between the 3rd to 8th weeks of fetal development (organogenesis). Newborns are at a high risk for pre- and postnatal developmental retardation, heart and lung fistulas, limb dislocations, and microcephaly.

Cleft lip occurs when the maxillary and median nasal processes fail to fuse during embryological development. **Cleft palate** is due to the failure of the nasal septum, lateral palatine processes, or the median palatine processes to fuse. These facial deformities are often correctable with surgery.

Related Basic Science

Maternal prenatal screening

The typical prenatal screen includes serum **AFP, unconjugated estriol**, and **hCG.** This is known as the **triple screen** and is usually performed between 16 and 18 weeks' gestation.

AFP is a protein similar to albumin and is produced by the yolk sac and fetal liver. Because AFP can diffuse across the fetal membranes into the mother's serum, it can be easily measured in the mother's blood. While pregnancies in which the fetus has a neural tube defect have **increased AFP levels,** pregnancies in which the fetus has Down syndrome have **decreased AFP levels.** In fact, this test alone can identify approximately 40% of Down syndrome pregnancies. The accuracy of Down syndrome screening is increased to approximately 70% by measuring serum levels of unconjugated estriol (decreased) and hCG (increased)

Genetics

Translocation

A translocation is the exchange of DNA between nonhomologous chromosomes. The two basic types of translocations are reciprocal and robertsonian translocations.

Reciprocal translocations are caused by two breaks on two different chromosomes with a subsequent exchange of genetic material between these chromosomes. This results in a balanced translocation; these individuals still have all of their DNA but on the wrong chromosome. Phenotypically, these individuals are completely normal. However, their offspring may have a partial trisomy or a partial monosomy with a subsequent abnormal phenotype.

Robertsonian translocations occur when the short arms of two nonhomologous chromosomes are lost and the long arms fuse at the centromere, forming a single chromosome. This is only known to occur on chromosomes 13, 15, 21, and 22. Carriers of a robertsonian translocation lose no essential material (the short arms contain nonessential genetic material) and are phenotypically normal. However, they carry only 45 chromosomes in each cell. The offspring of these individuals will end up with a full trisomy or a full monosomy and an abnormal phenotype.

Imprinting

Imprinting is the process in which DNA is expressed differently depending on if it is inherited from the mother or father. While the mechanism for this process is not entirely understood, it probably involves inactivation of specific genes by **methylation.** Prader-Willi syndrome (paternal imprinting) (Figure 43-7) and Angelman syndrome (maternal imprinting) (Figure 43-8) are examples of this process. While both diseases are caused by a deletion of the same segment of chromosome 15, they demonstrate different phenotypes. The reason for this is that the deleted "critical" region has some genes that are active only on the chromosome inherited from the father and other genes that are active only on the chromosome inherited from the mother. When the single active copy of one of these regions is lost, no gene products are produced and the disease results.

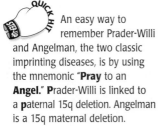

An easy way to remember Prader-Willi and Angelman, the two classic imprinting diseases, is by using the mnemonic "**Pray** to an **Angel.**" **P**rader-Willi is linked to a **p**aternal 15q deletion. Angelman is a 15q maternal deletion.

FIGURE 43-7 Prader-Willi syndrome results when there is deletion of paternal 15q11–13. It is characterized by small hands and feet, hypogonadism, marked obesity, and mild to moderate mental retardation. Behavior problems are common, such as outbursts of rage, especially when denied food.

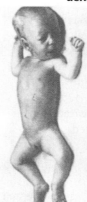 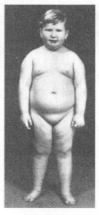

(Reprinted with permission from McMillan JA, DeAngelis CD, Feigin RD, et al. Oski's Pediatrics: Principles and Practice, 3rd Ed. Philadelphia: Lippincott Williams & Wilkins, p 2246.)

FIGURE 43-8 Angelman syndrome results when there is deletion of maternal 15q11–13. It is characterized by hypopigmentation, a large mouth with a protruding tongue, ataxia, inappropriate laughter, no speech, and mental retardation

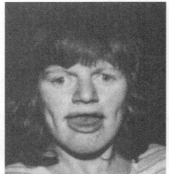 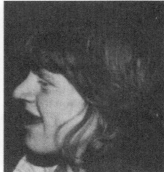

(Reprinted with permission from McMillan JA, DeAngelis CD, Feigin RD, et al. Oski's Pediatrics: Principles and Practice, 3rd Ed. Philadelphia: Lippincott Williams & Wilkins, p 2234.)

Abnormal complements of sex chromosomes (Table 43-1)

TABLE 43-1	Genetic Abnormalities Caused by Abnormal Sex Chromosomes		
Syndrome	**Genotype**	**Description**	
Turner syndrome	45, XO	• **Monosomy** of the X chromosome • Absent Barr body • Short stature • Webbed neck • Widely spaced nipples • Wide "shieldlike" chest • Wide carrying angle of arms • Lack of sexual maturity • Amenorrhea • Coarctation of the aorta	
Klinefelter syndrome	47, XXY	• Tall with long limbs • Often presents with gynecomastia • Hyalinization of seminiferous tubules • Lack of spermatogenesis leading to sterility • One Barr body	
XYY syndrome	47, XYY	• Normal-appearing male, often tall • Often associated with **aggressive behavior** • May be over-represented in the population of incarcerated males	
XXX syndrome	47, XXX	• Usually asymptomatic • Rarely associated with **menstrual irregularities** and mild mental retardation • Two Barr bodies	

Adapted with permission from Mehta S, Milder EA, Mirarchi AJ. Step-Up: A High-Yield, Systems-Based Review for the USMLE Step 1 Examination. Philadelphia: Lippincott Williams & Wilkins, 2000, p 159.

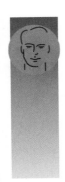

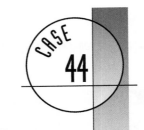

"I feel very run down and I've been losing weight."

OBJECTIVES

1. Develop a differential diagnosis and an appropriate workup for fatigue and unintentional weight loss
2. Review how retroviruses replicate
3. Understand the functions and key features of cell-mediated immunity
4. Learn the purpose and process of performing a Western Blot test
5. Discuss the serologic course of HIV and AIDS
6. Understand how homosexual activity can increase the risk for HIV transmission
7. Review key features associated with opportunistic infections of AIDS
8. Understand the pharmacoptherapy regimen for HIV and AIDS

HISTORY AND PHYSICAL EXAMINATION

A 34-year-old man reports **weight loss of 20 pounds** and **increased fatigue** over the past year. He has had recurring bouts of **diarrhea,** but denies any constipation, nausea, or vomiting. The patient works as an accountant, is married, states that he is monogamous, and has no past history of IV drug use or blood transfusion. After further questioning, however, the patient admits that he had **unprotected sexual intercourse** with a prostitute 5 years ago. Physical examination reveals a tall, frail-appearing man with **lymphadenopathy** palpable in the cervical and inguinal areas. Otherwise, physical examination is unremarkable.

APPROPRIATE WORKUP

Blood chemistries and stool culture

DIFFERENTIAL DIAGNOSIS

Colon cancer, gastroenteritis, HIV infection, infectious mononucleosis

DIAGNOSTIC LABORATORY TESTS AND STUDIES

Blood chemistry:
Carcinoembryonic antigen (CEA)
 = 0.2 ng/mL (N)
Heterophil antibody test = negative
HIV ELISA test = positive

HIV Western blot test = positive
CD4$^+$ count = 400/μL of blood (L)
Stool:
Heme = negative

DIAGNOSIS: HIV INFECTION

HIV causes a chronic infection with a variable course. In 50% of people, there is a 10-year period between infection with HIV and development of fulminant AIDS. HIV **infects CD4$^+$ (helper) T cells,** causing a decline in immune function, which results in **opportunistic infections, malignancies,** and **neurologic problems.** Most AIDS cases are caused by infection with HIV-1 retrovirus. There is an HIV-2 retrovirus that is mostly found in West Africa. The HIV-1 infection can be divided into three stages which may overlap.

The first stage is the early illness or seroconversion stage, which occurs a few weeks or a few months after infection. Although most patients are **asymptomatic,** living virus and viral antigens can be found in the blood. About 40% of patients may manifest a brief illness that usually resolves within a few weeks and is characterized by headache, fever, skin rash, and lymphadenopathy. The majority of people who are infected **develop antibody within 3 to 6 months of exposure.**

The second stage is a latent period, which occurs in almost all people infected with HIV. During this stage, there is **no clinical illness,** yet virus can be detected and is replicating. The host is able to contain the infection. However, with time the virus alters the host's immune response and causes a decline in the CD4$^+$ T-cell count. Some patients may have minor viral or bacterial infections, which tend to be more common as the duration of the infection increases.

The final stage, known as advanced symptomatic HIV infection, manifests as AIDS. AIDS is **defined clinically by the documentation of specific opportunistic infections or malignancies,** by a **CD4$^+$ count of less than 200/μL** of blood, and by **evidence of HIV in the blood.**

EXPLANATION OF DIFFERENTIAL

Colon cancer is the **most common neoplasm** in the developed world and most commonly occurs between 60 and 80 years of age. Risk factors include diet (**high in animal fat, low in fiber**), the presence of **inflammatory bowel disease,** and genetic factors. Colon cancer can present with different symptoms depending on the location of the tumor. Right-sided (ascending colon) tumors typically present with **iron deficiency anemia** due to chronic, insidious blood loss. These tumors **do not typically obstruct,** unless they are very large, because the stool is less formed on this side of the colon. Tumors of the left side (descending colon and rectosigmoid) tend to **obstruct early** because the stool is formed and hardened at this point. These tumors can present with **intermittent obstruction and diarrhea,** but do not usually cause an iron deficiency anemia. CEA is often elaborated (produced) by colonic tumors and can be used to monitor their progression. However, CEA is not specific to colon cancer and is not useful for initial diagnosis. In this patient, colon cancer could cause general malaise, weight loss, and diarrhea, but a normal CEA is not typical for this diagnosis.

Gastroenteritis commonly presents with anorexia, **nausea, vomiting, diarrhea,** and abdominal pain. This patient has diarrhea and weight loss, but gastroenteritis is less likely due to the absence of the other common symptoms. In addition, gastroenteritis would not cause lymphadenopathy or a 20-pound weight loss over 1 year because it is a self-limiting disease.

Classic signs of **infectious mononucleosis** include generalized **lymphadenopathy, splenomegaly,** and **chronic fatigue.** Infectious mononucleosis can be caused by the **Epstein-Barr virus** or the **cytomegalovirus.** Infection with the Epstein-Barr virus is diagnosed with a **Monospot test,** which demonstrates the presence of the **heterophil** antibody. However, this antibody is not present in cases of cytomegalovirus infection, so the diagnosis must be made by clinical impression. This patient's heterophil antibody test was negative, and the ELISA and Western blot tests were confirmatory for HIV infection. Note, however, that this patient could have infectious mononucleosis in addition to HIV infection.

FIGURE 44-1 Viral replication (*snRNP* = small nuclear ribonucleoprotein)

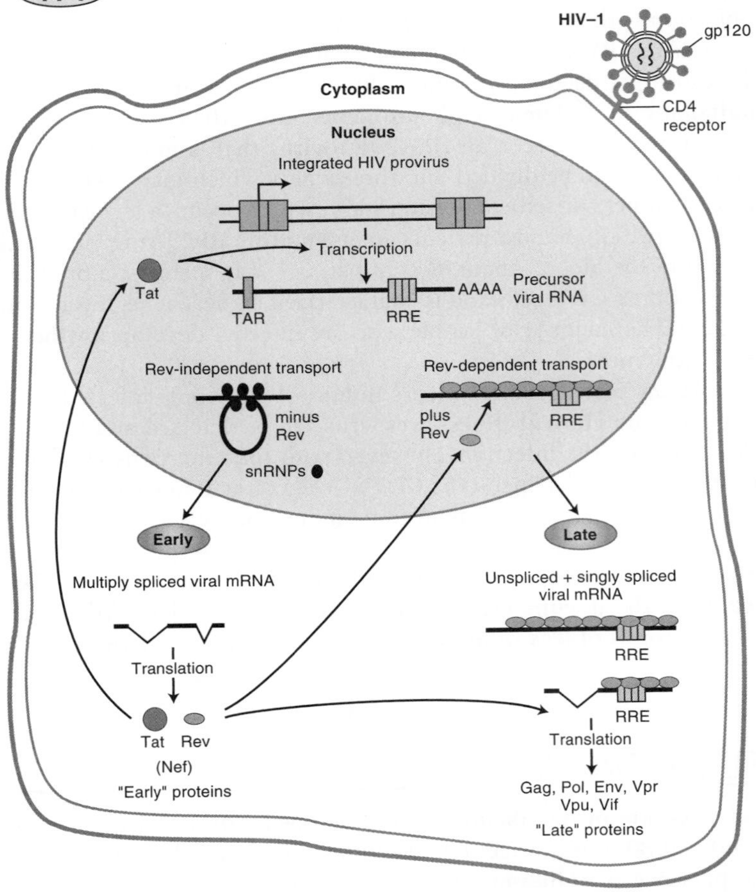

(Reprinted with permission from Mehta S, Milder EA, Mirarchi AJ. Step-Up: A High-Yield, Systems-Based Review for the USMLE Step 1 Examination. Philadelphia: Lippincott Williams & Wilkins, 2000, p 173.)

Related Basic Science

Retroviral replication (Figure 44-1)

Retroviruses are single-stranded RNA viruses characterized by the presence of **reverse transcriptase,** which is an enzyme that uses retroviral RNA to serve as a template for the synthesis of DNA. The DNA that is synthesized, called cDNA, can be inserted into the genome of the host cell and expressed. Because it is made from mRNA, which forms after the splicing process, **cDNA does not contain introns.**

Immune response

The immune response is made up of **cell-mediated and humoral (antibody-mediated) immunity. Cell-mediated immunity** (Figure 44-2) **consists mainly of T lymphocytes** and inhibits organisms such as fungi, parasites, and certain intracellular bacteria and kills virus- and tumor-infected cells. There are two components of cell-mediated immunity. The **T helper cells (CD4⁺) and macrophages** defend against the **intracellular bacteria and fungi,** while the **cytotoxic T cells (CD8⁺)** defend against viruses by **destroying virus-infected cells.** Cell-mediated immunity has four major functions: **host defense against infection, allergic reactions, graft and tumor rejection,** and **regulation of the antibody response.** Three major features, including **diversity, memory,** and **specificity,** character-ize the cell-mediated response itself. Cell-mediated immunity is specific for an invading

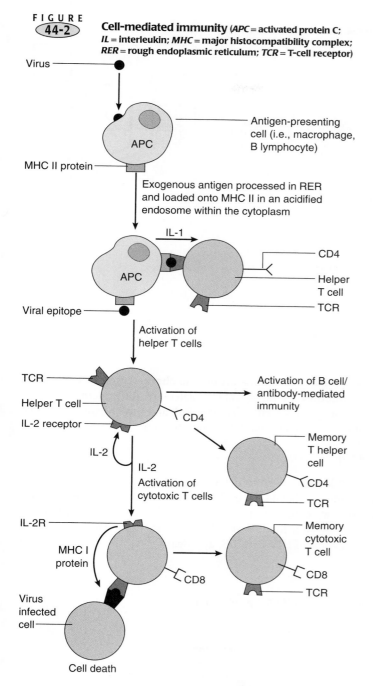

FIGURE 44-2

Cell-mediated immunity (*APC* = activated protein C; *IL* = interleukin; *MHC* = major histocompatibility complex; *RER* = rough endoplasmic reticulum; *TCR* = T-cell receptor)

Virus

Antigen-presenting cell (i.e., macrophage, B lymphocyte)

APC

MHC II protein

Exogenous antigen processed in RER and loaded onto MHC II in an acidified endosome within the cytoplasm

IL-1

APC

CD4

Helper T cell

Viral epitope

TCR

Activation of helper T cells

TCR

Helper T cell

IL-2 receptor

Activation of B cell/ antibody-mediated immunity

CD4

IL-2

IL-2

Activation of cytotoxic T cells

Memory T helper cell

CD4

TCR

IL-2R

MHC I protein

Memory cytotoxic T cell

CD8

TCR

CD8

TCR

Virus infected cell

Cell death

organism and acts by recognizing a foreign organism and activating immune cells to produce a response (through the action of cytokines and interleukins) to target that organism. Upon exposure, memory T cells are produced that last for many years and will cause a more rapid response on next exposure to the same organism.

Western blot test

The Western blot test is used to confirm a positive ELISA for diagnosis of HIV infection to decrease the rate of false-positive results. The test looks for antibodies to viral proteins. A protein sample is separated via electrophoresis on a gel and then transferred to a filter that has many invisible bands of proteins. The protein to be studied is visualized by labeled

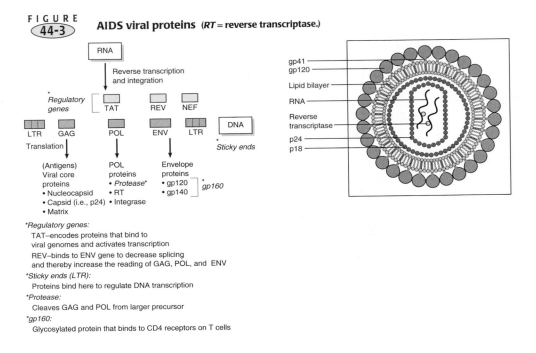

FIGURE 44-3 **AIDS viral proteins** (*RT* = reverse transcriptase.)

*Regulatory genes:
    TAT—encodes proteins that bind to
    viral genomes and activates transcription
    REV—binds to ENV gene to decrease splicing
    and thereby increase the reading of GAG, POL, and ENV
*Sticky ends (LTR):
    Proteins bind here to regulate DNA transcription
*Protease:
    Cleaves GAG and POL from larger precursor
*gp160:
    Glycosylated protein that binds to CD4 receptors on T cells

antibody probes specific to that protein. Western blot is used to **characterize the expression of a protein or to assay for antibodies.** In the case of HIV detection, the protein to be studied is antibody to the **HIV viral antigens, specifically Gag, Pol,** and **Env** (Figure 44-3). The Western blot test is positive if it has bands to two HIV gene products.

Course of HIV and AIDS (Figure 44-4)

Both CD4$^+$ counts and the viral load are used to determine the severity of HIV infection, the risk of opportunistic infections (Table 44-1), and the prognosis and response to therapy. The plasma HIV RNA can now be measured by a polymerase chain reaction. Evidence shows that the higher the ratio of viral load to HIV RNA levels, the greater the risk of opportunistic infections, progression of HIV to AIDS, and death.

QUICK HIT
The Southern blot test uses a technique similar to the Western blot test, only the sample to be studied is DNA. A radioactive DNA probe is hybridized with the sample to detect specific segments of the DNA. The Northern blot test is also similar to the Western blot test, except it involves an RNA sample that is hybridized with a radioactive DNA probe.

FIGURE 44-4 **Serologic profile of HIV infection** (*gp* = glycoprotein)

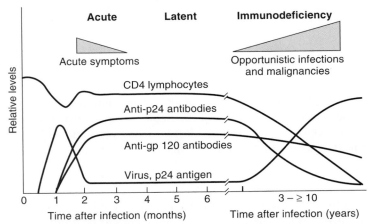

Serologic profile of HIV infection

(Reprinted with permission from Mehta S, Milder EA, Mirarchi AJ. Step-Up: A High-Yield, Systems-Based Review for the USMLE Step 1 Examination. Philadelphia: Lippincott Williams & Wilkins, 2000, p 173.)

TABLE 44-1 Opportunistic Infections of AIDS

Kaposi sarcoma	• This is a **malignant vascular tumor** that most often occurs in AIDS patients. • It is characterized by **red-purple plaques** or nodules that arise on the skin on all parts of the body. • It is likely of viral origin, specifically **human herpesvirus 8.**
Pneumocystis carinii pneumonia (PCP)	• PCP is the **most common opportunistic infection of AIDS.** • Signs and symptoms are cough and hypoxia, and the chest x-ray may be normal or show interstitial infiltrates. • Prophylaxis should be considered at a CD4$^+$ count <400/μL of blood. • At least 80% of AIDS patients will be infected with PCP once in their lifetime if no prophylaxis is given. • Trimethoprim/sulfamethoxazole or pentamidine are used for prophylaxis.
Cryptococcus neoformans	• *C. neoformans* is a fungal infection that may cause **meningitis** in approximately 10% of AIDS patients. • It manifests with fever, nausea, and vomiting. • Fever may be the only sign of meningitis in AIDS patients. • A lumbar puncture should always be considered in these patients and will show increased pressure, increased lymphocytes, increased protein, and decreased glucose. • *C. neoformans* has a **large capsule** that is visible on microscopic analysis with **India ink.**
Candida albicans	• *C. albicans* is a fungal infection that is very common in AIDS patients. • It causes oral thrush (white plaques in the mouth that leave a red, bleeding base when scraped with a tongue depressor). • It also causes esophagitis.
Mycobacterium avium-intracellulare (MAI) (also known as *Mycobacterium avium* complex)	• MAI is one of the major systemic bacterial infections of AIDS patients, usually occurring late in the course of disease. • It presents with fever, night sweats, diarrhea, and elevated liver function tests. • Bacteria disseminate throughout the body, causing a chronic wasting.
Cytomegalovirus (CMV)	• CMV is in the herpes simplex virus family. • It causes severe lung disease in patients with T-cell deficiencies. • CMV can also cause chorioretinitis and blindness.

Homosexuality

Male homosexual activity was the number one mode of transmission of HIV in the United States and Europe through the 1980s. Currently, heterosexual activity is the most common form of transmission of the virus in Africa. Receptive anal intercourse appears to increase the risk of transmission due to mucosal trauma of the thin rectal wall. The DSM-IV considers homosexuality to be a normal variant of sexual expression, not a dysfunction.

Pharmacotherapy for HIV and AIDS

Currently, there are two primary classes of drugs used to treat HIV infection: **reverse transcriptase inhibitors** and **protease inhibitors.** Reverse transcriptase inhibitors can be either nucleoside analogs or non-nucleoside analogs. The nucleoside reverse transcriptase inhibitors include zidovudine (AZT), didanosine (ddI), zalcitabine (ddC), stavudine (d4T), lamivudine (3TC), and abacavir. The non-nucleoside reverse transcriptase inhibitors include nevirapine and others. The protease inhibitors include saquinavir, ritonavir, nelfinavir, and indinavir. At this time, the best treatment method is the use of **triple therapy** to prevent resistance.

In general, the goal of HIV therapy is to **reduce the viral load** as much as possible to delay or reverse the deterioration of the immune system. AZT is the first-line medication because it has been shown to reduce mortality and opportunistic infections in symptomatic HIV-infected patients, delay the progression to AIDS, and decrease maternal-to-infant transmission of HIV. The other reverse transcriptase inhibitors also reduce the viral RNA load, increase CD4 counts, and slow the progression to AIDS. These agents are usually added to AZT to provide more effective therapy and to prevent the emergence of AZT resistance. As for the protease inhibitors, ritonavir can be used alone in patients with CD4 counts less than 500/μL of blood to increase the CD4 counts and decrease the plasma

QUICK HIT In AIDS patients with blindness, one also must think about brain masses caused by toxoplasmosis and lymphoma.

QUICK HIT Paraphilias involve the use of unusual objects of sexual desire or unusual sexual activities and are not considered a normal variant. Paraphilias usually occur in men.

viremia. When added to the two reverse transcriptase inhibitors, ritonavir has been shown to cause a greater increase in CD4 counts and a greater reduction in viral levels than using the two reverse transcriptase inhibitors alone.

The nucleoside analogs must first be **converted to their nucleotide form** to exert their antiretroviral effect. These activated nucleotides are then **incorporated into the growing chain of viral DNA by reverse transcriptase.** They then **cause termination of DNA synthesis** because they lack a key component; therefore, viral replication cannot take place. Protease inhibitors **inhibit the protease enzyme** that is necessary to **cleave the precursor polyprotein into viral proteins** necessary for the assembly and release of the virus. Although none of these drugs is curative, they interfere with the multiplication of the virus and significantly slow the progression of the disease.

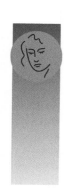
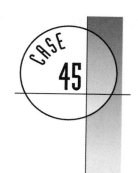
"I have extremely painful periods, and I can't get pregnant."

OBJECTIVES

1. Develop a differential diagnosis and an appropriate workup for dysmenorrhea, menorrhagia, and infertility
2. Compare and contrast the synthesis and roles of estrogen and progesterone during the menstrual cycle, pregnancy, breast development, and lactation
3. Discuss the treatment options for endometriosis

HISTORY AND PHYSICAL EXAMINATION

A 29-year-old woman presents with **chronic pelvic pain**. She describes her menstrual cycle with a **heavy flow** lasting 5 days or more with **excruciating pain**. She is currently taking ibuprofen to relieve menstrual cramps. She also complains of significant pain during sexual intercourse. She has never been pregnant with no history of prior surgeries. However, she has been **trying to conceive for the past year.** She recalls her mother having a surgery which "stopped her periods" when she was 50 years old.

A pelvic exam reveals **adnexal tenderness**. Indurations in the pouch of Douglas with **several small nodules** are palpable through the posterior fornix. Her temperature is 98.6°F.

APPROPRIATE WORKUP

Cervical culture, Serum β-hCG test, pelvic ultrasound (US), pelvic laparoscopy

DIFFERENTIAL DIAGNOSIS

Endometriosis, pelvic inflammatory disease, adenomyosis, leiomyomata, and benign ovarian tumor

DIAGNOSTIC LABORATORY TESTS AND STUDIES

Culture of cervix:
Negative for *Neisseria gonorrhoeae*
Negative for *Chlamydia trachomatis*
Serum β-hCG test:
(β-hCG): Negative

US, pelvic:
Cystic enlargement of ovaries
Laparoscopy, pelvis:
"Chocolate cysts" on both ovaries; thickening of uterosacral ligaments (Figure 45-1)

DIAGNOSIS: ENDOMETRIOSIS

Endometriosis is caused by **retrograde menstruation** through the fallopian tubes resulting in the presence of **normal endometrial tissue in extrauterine locations**, most commonly in the dependent portions of the female pelvis (i.e., posterior and anterior cul-de-sac,

FIGURE
45-1   **Chocolate cysts**

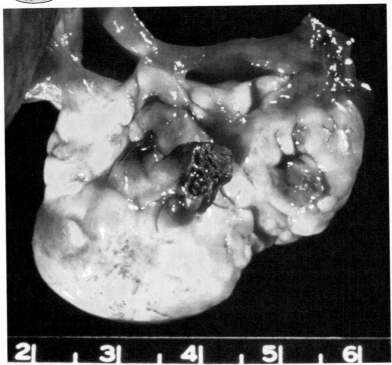

(From Rubin E, Farber JL. Pathology, 3rd Ed. Philadelphia: Lippincott Williams & Wilkins, 1999.)

Chlamydia trachomatis is the most common STD and is also the leading cause of blindness in the world. Because fetuses delivered via an infected birth canal can develop inclusion conjunctivitis, infants are routinely given prophylactic erythromycin drops.

N. gonorrhoeae is a Gram-negative, intracellular diplococcus that is a common cause of PID and septic arthritis (usually of only one joint).

Lactobacillus acidophilus maintains the normal vaginal pH at < 4.5.

Key diagnostic clues: Malodorous discharge with fishy odor on KOH: bacterial vaginosis/*Gardnerella vaginalis* White, cheesy discharge with hyphae on microscopy: vaginal candidiasis/*Candida albicans*

uterosacral ligaments, and ovaries). This ectopic endometrial tissue **possesses the same steroid receptors** as normal endometrium with the same cycle of proliferation, secretory activity, and cyclic sloughing of endometrium (both normal and ectopic) in response to progesterone and estrogen. During menstruation, this sloughing results in **inflammation, infertility,** and **chronic pelvic pain,** which most often brings females to physicians for evaluation. The **chocolate cysts** found on laparoscopic examination are ovarian cysts filled with blood that develop when endometrial tissue implants and grows on ovaries. Recurrent hemorrhages can result in scarring and fibrous adhesions in the pelvis causing distortion of the ovaries and fallopian tubes, and hence infertility.

Family history for endometriosis is common with as much as a sevenfold increase in risk of endometriosis in first-degree relatives. The negative pregnancy test eliminates the suspicion for an intrauterine pregnancy or ectopic pregnancy.

EXPLANATION OF DIFFERENTIAL

Pelvic inflammatory disease (PID) is an infection of the upper genital tract with *Neisseria gonorrhoeae* or *Chlamydia trachomatis*. Clinically, symptoms of PID are similar to endometriosis with **bilateral adnexal tenderness** and **dyspareunia**. This patient has no fever, which often suggests an infection. A **positive chandelier sign** is often diagnostic. The sign is provoked by moving tender and inflamed fallopian tubes and pelvic structures. Moreover, there is often a **purulent cervical discharge** with a cervical smear for chlamydia or gonorrhea.

Long-term complications of PID include **infertility or ectopic pregnancy** as tubal strictures develop from the inflammatory process. Treatment includes **doxycycline** for *C. trachomatis*, an obligate intracellular parasite, and a broad-spectrum antibiotic, such as **ceftriaxone**, if cervical culture reveals a polymicrobial infection.

Adenomyosis can also cause **dysmenorrhea** with an ingrowth of endometrial glands and stroma into the **myometrium** resulting in **symmetric uterine enlargement**. Patients can also complain of heavy menstrual bleeding (menorrhagia). Adenomyosis is associated with significant cyclic changes in size, consistency, and tenderness of the uterine fundus. During the **follicular phase**, it is **small and firm**. Prior to **menses**, the **glands are enlarged, tender, and softer**.

Leiomyomata (singular: leiomyoma) are benign local proliferations of **smooth muscle cells** in the uterus. They are **estrogen sensitive**. Therefore, the **endogenous estrogens of oral contraceptives** can promote the growth of leiomyomata. In addition, increased estrogen levels during pregnancy can enhance growth. Often after menopause, uterine fibroids shrink in size and become asymptomatic. Clinical presentation includes menorrhagia, chronic pelvic pain, and dyspareunia. Pelvic exam would yield an **enlarged, irregular uterus**.

Benign ovarian tumors may be solid, cystic, or mixed and are **often clinically silent** until well developed. They can cause mild pelvic, lower back pain, and/or dyspareunia. Menstruation can be abnormal with changes in menstrual flow, length of periods, and intervals between periods. On physical exam, there may be **lower quadrant tenderness**, adnexal masses, and a sensitive pelvic exam.

Related Basic Sciences

Progesterone versus estrogen (Table 45-1)

QUICK HIT Endometritis is general inflammation of the uterus that does not extend to the myometrium and does not increase the uterine size.

QUICK HIT Leiomyosarcomas are malignant tumors derived from the smooth muscle cells of the uterus. Benign fibroids are not believed to be a risk factor for developing leiomyosarcoma.

QUICK HIT Meigs syndrome consists of a triad of ascites, hydrothorax, and ovarian fibromas.

QUICK HIT After birth, estrogen and progesterone levels decrease and lactation occurs. It is maintained by suckling, which stimulates both prolactin and oxytocin secretion.

QUICK HIT During lactation, ovulation is suppressed because hypothalamic GnRH is inhibited and consequently LH and FSH secretion is inhibited.

TABLE 45-1 Estrogen and Progesterone

	Estrogen	Progesterone
Synthesis	Theca cells produce testosterone; **aromatase** in nearby granulosa cells convert **testosterone to 17β-estradiol (positive feedback by FSH)**	LH in theca cells converts **cholesterol to pregnenolone,** which is converted to progesterone
Menstrual cycle	• Follicular phase: estrogen levels increase and cause **proliferation of the uterus**; suppress LH and FSH by negative feedback on the anterior pituitary • Ovulation: **estrogen burst** has positive feedback on LH and FSH (**LH surge**) • Luteal phase: estrogen produced by the corpus luteum	Luteal phase: progesterone has **negative feedback** effects on LH and FSH via the hypothalamus; **increases basal body temperature** by acting on the **hypothalamic thermoregulatory center**
Pregnancy	Synthesis: • **1st trimester:** produced by **corpus luteum** which is stimulated by placental hCG • **2nd trimester: fetal adrenal gland** synthesizes intermediate (**DHEA-S**) which is transferred to placenta and aromatized to estrogen • Function: increases throughout pregnancy to maintain the endometrium for the fetus, inhibits FSH and LH, suppressing ovarian follicular development; **sensitizes uterus to contractile stimuli** with an increased estrogen/progesterone ratio	Synthesis: • 1st trimester: same as estrogen • 2nd trimester: produced by placenta • Function: increases throughout pregnancy to maintain the endometrium for the fetus, inhibits FSH and LH, suppressing ovarian follicular development; increases the threshold for uterine contraction during parturition
Breast development	Stimulates **growth and development**	Stimulates **growth and development**
Lactation	• **Stimulates prolactin secretion** from **anterior pituitary** • Blocks the action of prolactin on the breast during pregnancy	• Blocks the action of prolactin on the breast during pregnancy

Treatment of Endometriosis

The anterior pituitary releases FSH and LH in response to a ***pulsatile* secretion of GnRH** from the hypothalamus. **Leuprolide** is a GnRH analog with a ***prolonged* secretion** that inhibits the pituitary release of gonadotropins. Suppression of FSH and LH secretion places the woman in an artificial state of menopause with no estrogen or progesterone production. Without estrogenic stimulation, the endometrial tissue cannot proliferate and progesterone cannot stimulate the maturation and eventual sloughing of the endometrium and ectopic endometrial tissue. Side effects are similar to those that occur with menopause: **risk of osteoporosis**, **hot flashes**, **vaginal dryness**, and **headaches. NSAIDs** are used for symptomatic relief of dysmenorrhea with **anti-inflammatory**, **antipyretic**, and **analgesic** properties. They inhibit prostaglandin synthesis by **inhibition of the cyclooxygenase (COX) enzyme**, both COX-1 and COX-2 isoforms. COX-1 is responsible for the production of protective prostaglandins in the gastric mucosa. These prostaglandins function to protect gastric mucosa by increasing mucus and bicarbonate secretion. They also **stimulate local vasodilation**, maintaining a steady energy supply to the gastric mucosa and preventing ischemia.

Danazol is a derivative of testosterone that decreases pituitary FSH and LH secretion. This promotes the regression of endometrial implants with significant pain relieved. Common side effects include hirsutism, voice deepening, and reversible adverse effects on serum lipids (decreased HDLs and increased LDLs).

Conservative laparoscopic surgery is aimed at destroying endometrial foci and ablating any adhesions. It is considered the first-line option to increase fertility and treat pain that may be unresponsive to the above pharmacologic therapies. There is always the risk of recurrence of disease that may require further medical or surgical treatment. A more invasive but permanent surgery is a **total abdominal hysterectomy with bilateral salpingo-oophorectomy** with removal of the uterus, fallopian tubes, and ovaries. It is important to remove ovaries even if they are not the site of ectopic endometrial tissue since the estrogens produced by the ovaries can stimulate the menstrual cycle. The risk of recurrence is significantly reduced with irreversible loss of fertility. With this procedure, it is important to ensure and discuss with the patient the permanence of the procedure and the resulting **loss of fertility.**

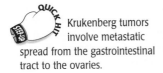

NSAIDs, specifically indomethacin, can be used to close PDAs. Prostaglandin is used to keep PDAs open in conditions such as transposition of the great vessels. **In**domethacin **in**hibits PDAs while **pro**staglandins **prop** open PDAs.

Postmenopausal vaginal bleeding is a "red flag" for endometrial carcinoma. The risk for endometrial hyperplasias and carcinomas due to hyperestrinism can be increased with obesity, exogenous estrogen (i.e., oral contraceptives) diabetes, and nulliparity.

Krukenberg tumors involve metastatic spread from the gastrointestinal tract to the ovaries.

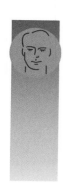

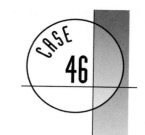

"I've started coughing up blood!"

OBJECTIVES

1. Develop a differential diagnosis and an appropriate workup for cough with hemoptysis
2. Review the location, histology, and clinical features of lung neoplasms
3. Differentiate among paraneoplastic syndromes
4. Describe common interstitial and environmental lung diseases
5. Review the characteristics of substance abuse and the difference between psychologic and physical dependence

HISTORY AND PHYSICAL EXAMINATION

A 73-year-old African American man complains of **coughing up bright-red blood.** He states that he has had a "chest cold" with a **productive cough** for the past few months, but it was just yesterday that he noticed blood in his sputum. The patient also complains of **dyspnea and weakness,** and states that over the past few weeks his "cough seemed different." He admits to an **86 pack-year history of smoking,** and was diagnosed with **chronic bronchitis** 10 years ago. He states that he has drunk "at least one six-pack of beer" every night for the past 20 years. All other past medical and surgical history is unremarkable; however, the patient notes that he has not been eating much lately and has **lost 10 pounds over the past few weeks.** In general, the patient appears frail and suffers from poor nutrition. Pertinent findings on physical examination include **tachypnea, positive end-expiratory wheezing,** and **clubbing of the digits.** Lung auscultation reveals decreased breath sounds on the right side.

APPROPRIATE WORKUP

Blood chemistries, chest X-ray, sputum culture, urinalysis, and lung biopsy

DIFFERENTIAL DIAGNOSIS

Bronchiectasis, Goodpasture syndrome, pneumonia, pulmonary neoplasm (squamous cell carcinoma, large cell carcinoma, small cell carcinoma), tuberculosis

DIAGNOSTIC LABORATORY TESTS AND STUDIES

Blood chemistry:
  WBCs = 8,500/μL(N)
  Hct = 31% (L)
  Mean corpuscular volume
    = 99 μm^3 (H)
  Calcium = 12.8 mg/dL (H)
Chest radiograph:
  Large hilar mass on the right
  Enlarged lymph nodes on the right,
    especially the lower lobe

Sputum culture:
  Normal respiratory flora
  No acid-fast bacilli
Urinalysis:
  Ketones = none
  Leukocyte esterase = none
  Bacteria = none
Lung biopsy:
  Keratin-producing cells
  Intracellular bridging

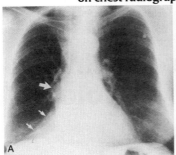
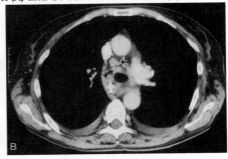

FIGURE 46-1 A mass can be seen affecting the right lower lobe of the lung on chest radiograph (A) and CT scan of the thorax (B)

(Reprinted with permission from Brant WE, Helms CA. Fundamentals of Diagnostic Radiology, 2nd Ed. Philadelphia: Lippincott Williams & Wilkins, 1999, p 392.)

DIAGNOSIS: SQUAMOUS CELL CARCINOMA OF THE LUNG (FIGURE 46-1)

Squamous cell carcinoma is most commonly found in men with a **smoking history.** As with most neoplasms of the lung, squamous cell carcinoma presents as a **cough with a recent change in character, hemoptysis, airway obstruction,** and **weight loss.** It typically **spreads locally** and metastasizes later than other lung cancers. On a chest radiograph, it appears as a **large hilar mass** with evidence of **cavitation** and **enlarged hilar lymph nodes.** Histologically, **keratin production** and **intracellular bridging** can be seen in the well-differentiated forms. This type of lung cancer can produce a parathyroid hormone–related peptide, leading to **hypercalcemia.**

EXPLANATION OF DIFFERENTIAL

Bronchiectasis, a form of emphysema (see Figure 46-2), is an abnormal and permanent dilation of the bronchi caused by **inflammatory destruction,** which is typically due to *Pseudomonas, Haemophilus influenzae,* or bronchial obstruction from a **tumor.** Smoking

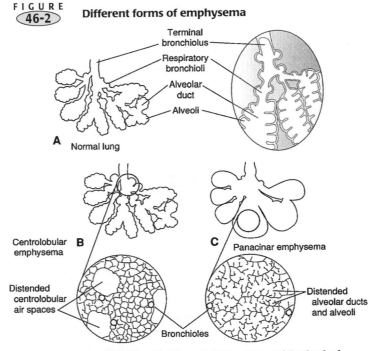

FIGURE 46-2 Different forms of emphysema

(Reprinted with permission from Damjanov I. A Color Atlas and Textbook of Histopathology. Baltimore: Williams & Wilkins, 1996, p 146.)

has been implicated as a contributing factor. Bronchiectasis presents with recurrent **cough, purulent sputum,** and **hemoptysis.** On lung examination, **crackles, rhonchi,** and **wheezing** may all be heard. A chest radiograph may reveal **diffuse parenchymal changes** consisting of prominent **cystic spaces.**

Goodpasture syndrome is a disease affecting both the **lungs and the kidneys.** Its pathogenic factor is an **anti–basement membrane antibody,** but its cause is unknown. A biopsy of the kidney with immunofluorescence demonstrating smooth **deposition of immunoglobulin G along the glomerular basement membrane** is diagnostic. Goodpasture syndrome presents with severe hemoptysis (pneumonitis), dyspnea, and hematuria (glomerulonephritis).

Pneumonia is commonly caused by aspiration; other portals of entry include respiratory droplets, contiguous spread, and traumatic inoculation. The most common causes of pneumonia include **respiratory syncytial virus in infants,** *Mycoplasma pneumoniae* **in young adults,** and *Streptococcus pneumoniae* **in the elderly.** Pneumonia typically presents acutely with **fever, purulent sputum, pleuritic chest pain,** and **lobar lung infiltrate on chest radiograph.** Persistent pneumonia can be the presenting symptom of lung cancer.

Mycobacterium tuberculosis is an **acid-fast bacillus** that is an **obligate aerobe.** Active tuberculosis is usually due to **reactivation of a primary infection** secondary to an immunocompromised state, which is often associated with advanced age, immunosuppressive drugs, or AIDS. Tuberculosis often presents with **hemoptysis** associated with weakness, **cough, night sweats,** and **weight loss.** Chest radiograph reveals localized consolidation, possibly with cavitation. Old calcified lesions of tuberculosis may also be present. This patient's clinical presentation is characteristic of tuberculosis. He is immunocompromised due to excessive alcohol intake and poor nutrition, but tuberculosis is less likely due to the absence of lung lesions on the chest radiograph and acid-fast bacilli in the sputum.

Related Basic Science

Lung neoplasms (Figure 46-3 and Table 46-1)

While lung cancer is the **second most common cancer,** it is the **leading cause of cancer death for both men and women** in the United States. Symptoms include cough, hemoptysis, airway obstruction, weight loss, and paraneoplastic syndromes. Smoking is the most important risk factor for most types of lung cancer.

Paraneoplastic syndromes

A paraneoplastic syndrome (Table 46-2) is a clinical syndrome caused by abnormal elaboration of a hormone from a neoplasm.

Interstitial lung diseases

Interstitial lung diseases (Table 46-3) are a group of noninfectious, nonmalignant conditions characterized by inflammation and pathologic changes of the alveolar wall. Differentiation and diagnosis often require histologic evaluation of the lung.

QUICK HIT STEP-UP Metastatic cancer is more common than primary cancer in the lung. On radiograph, metastatic cancer to the lung presents as multiple "cannonball lesions."

QUICK HIT STEP-UP Horner syndrome is characterized by ptosis, miosis, and anhydrosis. This syndrome occurs with any lesion that disrupts the cervical sympathetic chain. Pancoast tumor, which involves the apex of the lung, is a common cause.

QUICK HIT STEP-UP Syndrome of inappropriate antidiuretic hormone is similar in clinical findings to psychogenic polydipsia, a compulsion to drink excess water. Both conditions result in hyponatremia. Diabetes insipidus, a deficit in antidiuretic hormone that causes excessive water loss, has the opposite effect of syndrome of inappropriate antidiuretic hormone and, therefore, results in hypernatremia.

QUICK HIT STEP-UP Transudative pulmonary edema is a noninflammatory edema resulting from altered hydrostatic (heart failure) or osmotic (nephrotic syndrome) pressure. Exudative pulmonary edema is an inflammatory edema due to increased vascular permeability from sepsis or lung disease.

QUICK HIT STEP-UP Birbeck granules are cytoplasmic inclusions resembling tennis rackets.

FIGURE 46-3 **Lung cancer** (*ACTH* = adrenocorticotropic hormone; *ADH* = antidiuretic hormone; *PTH* = parathyroid hormone)

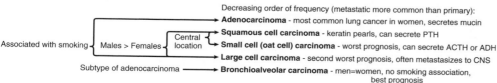

Decreasing order of frequency (metastatic more common than primary):

Associated with smoking — Males > Females — Central location

Adenocarcinoma - most common lung cancer in women, secretes mucin

Squamous cell carcinoma - keratin pearls, can secrete PTH

Small cell (oat cell) carcinoma - worst prognosis, can secrete ACTH or ADH

Large cell carcinoma - second worst prognosis, often metastasizes to CNS

Subtype of adenocarcinoma — **Bronchioalveolar carcinoma** - men=women, no smoking association, best prognosis

TABLE 46-1 Lung Neoplasms

Tumor	Location and Histology	Clinical Features
Adenocarcinoma	**Peripheral;** subpleural; usually on pre-existing **scars;** glandular	**Most common type;** may be related to smoking; CEA positive; K-ras oncogenes
Bronchioalveolar	**Peripheral;** subtype of adenocarcinoma; tumor cells line alveolar walls	**Less strongly associated with smoking;** autoantibodies to surfactant may exist
Carcinoid	Major bronchi; spread by direct extension	Increased secretion of **5-HT;** flushing; wheezing; heart disease; low malignancy
Large cell	**Peripheral;** undifferentiated; giant cells with pleomorphism	Poor prognosis; metastasis to the brain; smoking
Metastasis	**Cannonball** lesions	**Higher incidence than primary lung cancer**
Small cell (oat cell)	**Central;** undifferentiated; **most aggressive;** small dark-blue cells	Poor prognosis; increased in smokers; ectopic ACTH and ADH secretion
Squamous cell	**Central;** mass from bronchus; keratin pearls; cavitation	Increased in smokers; secretion of **PTH-like peptide**

ACTH, adrenocorticotropic hormone; ADH, antidiuretic hormone; CEA, carcinoembryonic antigen; 5-HT, serotonin metabolite; PTH, parathyroid hormone.
Reprinted with permission from Mehta S, Milder EA, Mirarchi AJ. Step-Up: A High-Yield, Systems-Based Review for the USMLE Step 1 Examination. Philadelphia: Lippincott Williams & Wilkins, 2000, p 80.

Environmental lung diseases

Environmental lung diseases (Table 46-4) are often caused by workplace exposure to various organic and chemical irritants. A careful history and pulmonary function testing are often important for diagnosis.

Substance abuse

> **QUICK HIT**
> Ferruginous bodies are yellowish-brown, rod-shaped bodies with clubbed ends that stain with Prussian blue stain.

Substance abuse is a significant cause of morbidity and mortality in the United States. **Alcohol** is the **most widely abused** drug; however, marijuana, cocaine, and heroin are also commonly abused. Addiction is defined as habitual psychologic and physiological dependence on a substance or practice that is **beyond voluntary control.** It is mediated by **dopamine,** the neurotransmitter linked to the pleasure and reward center of the brain. The most common **predisposing factor** to addiction is **low self-esteem.**

Psychologic dependence on addictive substances involves **impairment of social, physical, or occupational functioning.** It is considered a compulsive disorder and has a

TABLE 46-2 Common Paraneoplastic Syndromes

Syndrome	Hormone	Common Cause
Hypercalcemia	PTH-related peptide	Squamous cell lung carcinoma
SIADH	ADH	Small cell lung carcinoma
Cushing syndrome	ACTH	Small cell lung carcinoma
Acromegaly	GHRH	Bronchial carcinoid tumors
Gynecomastia	hCG	Testicular cancer
Hypoglycemia	IGF-II	Sarcomas

ACTH, adrenocorticotropic hormone; ADH, antidiuretic hormone; GHRH, growth hormone–releasing hormone; hCG, human chorionic gonadotropin; IGF, insulin-like growth factor; PTH, parathyroid hormone; SIADH, syndrome of inappropriate antidiuretic hormone.

TABLE 46-3 Interstitial Lung Disease

Disease	Pathophysiology	Population Most at Risk	Clinical Features
Eosinophilic granuloma	Presence of Langerhans-like cells and **Birbeck granules;** subset of histiocytosis X	Former **smokers**	Lesions in lung or ribs; pneumothorax
Goodpasture syndrome	Pulmonary hemorrhage; anemia; glomerulonephritis; **anti-basement membrane antibodies**	Males; middle-aged people	**Hemoptysis;** hematuria
Idiopathic pulmonary fibrosis	Chronic **inflammation of alveolar wall;** fibrosis; cystic spaces	Sixth generation of life	**Honeycomb lung;** fatal within years
Sarcoidosis	Interstitial fibrosis; diagnosis based on biopsy showing **noncaseating granulomatous lesions;** uveitis; polyarthritis	**Young African American females**	Dyspnea on exertion, dry cough, fever, fatigue and bilateral hilar lymphadenopathy
Hypersensitivity pneumonitis (farmer's lung)	Prolonged exposure to organic antigens in atopic individuals; interstitial inflammation; alveolar damage leads to chronic, fibrotic lung	People with an occupational history of farming or bird-keeping	**Dry cough, chest tightness** general malaise and fever

Reprinted with permission from Mehta S, Milder EA, Mirarchi AJ. Step-Up: A High-Yield, Systems-Based Review for the USMLE Step 1 Examination. Philadelphia: Lippincott Williams & Wilkins, 2000, p 74.

high rate of relapse after rehabilitation. In a psychologically dependent state, the majority of a person's time is spent thinking about, doing, and getting the money to buy the substance they are dependent on.

Physical dependence is a state in which the body has adapted to the **chronic presence of a substance.** A person can be physically dependent on a drug and not be addicted; physical dependence is not an absolute criterion in the development of addiction. Withdrawal occurs after a substance is lowered in dosage or is terminated. Its symptoms are opposite of the drug's primary effects. The severity of withdrawal depends on the amount of drug used per day, length of time the drug has been used, and length of time allowed for withdrawal.

QUICK HIT

Naloxone is given to counter the effects of opioids and can precipitate an acute withdrawal effect if too much is given too quickly.

TABLE 46-4 Environmental Lung Diseases (Pneumoconiosis)

Disease	Pathophysiology	Clinical Features
Anthracosis	Carbon dust ingested by alveolar macrophages; visible **black deposits**	Usually asymptomatic
Asbestosis	Asbestos fibers ingested by alveolar macrophages; fibroblast proliferation; interstitial fibrosis (lower lobes); **asbestos bodies and ferruginous bodies;** pleural plaques and effusions	Increased risk of bronchogenic carcinoma and **malignant mesothelioma;** synergistic effect of asbestos and tobacco
Coal worker's pneumoconiosis	Carbon dust ingested by alveolar macrophages forms bronchiolar **macules;** may progress to fibrosis	Plaques as asymptomatic; often benign, may progress to fibrosis; may be fatal due to pulmonary hypertension and **cor pulmonale**
Silicosis	Silica dust ingested by alveolar macrophages causing release of harmful enzymes; **silicotic nodules**	Nodules may obstruct air or blood flow; concurrent tuberculosis common (**silicotuberculosis**)
Berylliosis	Induction of cell-mediated immunity leads to noncaseating granulomas; several organ systems affected; histologically identical to sarcoidosis	Increased lung cancer

Reprinted with permission from Mehta S, Milder EA, Mirarchi AJ. Step-Up: A High-Yield, Systems-Based Review for the USMLE Step 1 Examination. Philadelphia: Lippincott Williams & Wilkins, 2000, p 75.

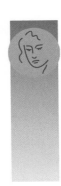

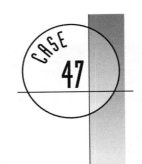
"I've had terrible throbbing headaches, and now I can't see out of my right eye."

OBJECTIVES

1. Develop a differential diagnosis and an appropriate workup for throbbing headaches and unilateral loss of vision
2. Review the pathology, anatomy, and clinical manifestations of peripheral vascular diseases
3. Understand the regulation of blood pressure
4. Describe the three major types of headaches and associated treatment

HISTORY AND PHYSICAL EXAMINATION

A 68-year-old Caucasian woman presents with a **severe headache** on the right side. The patient states that she has had headaches, **fevers,** general malaise, and stiffness of her neck, shoulders, and hips over the past few months. She states that she has had periods of intermittent **blindness in her right eye** today. She does not report photophobia. On examination, she has a fever, with **tenderness along the right side of her face** and a nodular, **pulseless** cord over her right temple. Pulses in the patient's extremities are normal.

APPROPRIATE WORKUP

Blood chemistries

DIFFERENTIAL DIAGNOSIS

Amaurosis fugax, migraine, multiple sclerosis (MS), retinal detachment, Takayasu arteritis, temporal arteritis

DIAGNOSTIC LABORATORY TESTS AND STUDIES

> **Blood chemistry:**
> **ESR = 150 mm/h (H)**
> Hgb = 9 g/dL (L)
> Mean corpuscular volume (MCV) = 90 um^3 (N)
> Mean corpuscular Hgb concentration = 32 g/dL (N)
> Alkaline phosphatase = 435 (H)

DIAGNOSIS: TEMPORAL ARTERITIS

Temporal arteritis, also known as giant cell arteritis, is the **most common vasculitis** in the United States. It is a nodular inflammation of the large arteries, most commonly the branches of the carotid. It also tends to affect the **temporal artery. Granulomatous inflammation** involves mononuclear cells, which may form giant cells. Temporal arteritis is most common in caucasian women older than 60 years of age. Familial clusters and an association with **HLA-DR4** suggest a genetic predisposition.

Temporal arteritis is often associated with **polymyalgia rheumatica,** a group of symptoms that consists of **myalgias, periarticular pain,** and **morning stiffness.** Common presentation of temporal arteritis usually is a severe unilateral headache with a palpable pulseless nodule on the affected side. Double vision, blurry vision, and even **blindness** are other possible symptoms. Accompanying jaw pain may result from **claudication** in the muscles of mastication. The history may include fatigue, fevers, malaise, and weight loss. Laboratory findings will reveal a markedly elevated **ESR,** a normocytic, normochromic anemia, and an elevated alkaline phosphatase level. The gold standard for diagnosis is **biopsy** of the temporal artery. Treatment is high-dose **steroids** and should be implemented quickly to prevent permanent loss of vision.

EXPLANATION OF DIFFERENTIAL

Amaurosis fugax is loss of vision resulting from transient interruption of blood flow to the retina. Patients describe a sensation like a curtain falling over the eye. The most common cause is an **embolus,** and the most common source is carotid atherosclerosis. If the embolus breaks up, no permanent damage occurs. Otherwise, the retina infarcts, and funduscopic examination reveals a **cherry red fovea** on a white retina. Patients who experience amaurosis fugax are at risk for **cerebrovascular accident (CVA)** and require evaluation of their carotid arteries.

A **migraine** is a headache that lasts between 4 and 72 hours. Described as a **pulsating or throbbing** pain, a migraine is normally unilateral and tends to worsen with stress or exertion. Migraines are more common in women. Associated symptoms are nausea, vomiting, light sensitivity (**photophobia**), and sound sensitivity (**phonophobia**). In a classic migraine, an **aura** precedes the headache. An aura may be visual or olfactory. The visual symptoms (**scotomata**) are usually flashing lights, zigzag patterns, or both. There may be loss of central vision, which can expand outward. Olfactory symptoms include sweet or noxious odors.

MS is the most common **demyelinating** disease. Areas of demyelination, called plaques, are scattered through the brain and spinal cord. **Paraventricular plaques** are commonly seen on CT or MRI. The cause is unclear. Increased immunoglobulins in the cerebrospinal fluid (CSF) (**oligoclonal bands** on electrophoresis) suggest viral or immune causes. Increased incidence in **Northern Europeans** and association with HLA-B7, DR2, and DW2 suggest genetic factors. Patients can present with a wide variety of symptoms. Visual changes or loss, lower extremity weakness, and urinary incontinence are some common early symptoms. Over the course of the disease, there are acute exacerbations with remissions, or periods of stability. Eventually, the patient's condition deteriorates physically and mentally. There is no cure, but steroids are a mainstay in therapy (see Case 29).

Retinal detachment manifests as flashing lights and "floaters." These vision changes are in the **periphery** where the detachment has occurred. The detachment usually begins with a tear in the retina, which allows vitreous humor to flow into the subretinal space. Prior trauma and myopic vision are risk factors. Surgical repair is usually possible.

Takayasu arteritis is an inflammatory disease of medium and large arteries. Its common presentation is inflammation of the aortic arch and its branches, which can lead to **stenosis.** This disease is most common in **young Asian women.** Like temporal arteritis, Takayasu arteritis is associated with **HLA-DR4.** Symptoms of general malaise, fever, and weight loss may precede the vascular pathology by months. Clinical manifestations include weak or absent ulnar and radial pulses and **visual** problems if the carotids are involved. ESR and immunoglobulin levels are elevated, and the patient is usually anemic. Death can occur from CVA or congestive heart failure (CHF). Some cases spontaneously remit. Treatment involves steroids and surgery.

Related Basic Science

The vascular system

Blood vessels vary greatly in composition. Most vessels are composed of three basic layers (Figure 47-1). The **tunica intima** starts with the endothelium, which is in contact with the flowing blood. These cells are supported by a basal lamina that separates them from

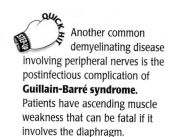

QUICK HIT Another common demyelinating disease involving peripheral nerves is the postinfectious complication of **Guillain-Barré syndrome.** Patients have ascending muscle weakness that can be fatal if it involves the diaphragm.

QUICK HIT The combination of nystagmus, intention tremor, and scanning speech is referred to as **Charcot triad,** and is classically seen in MS.

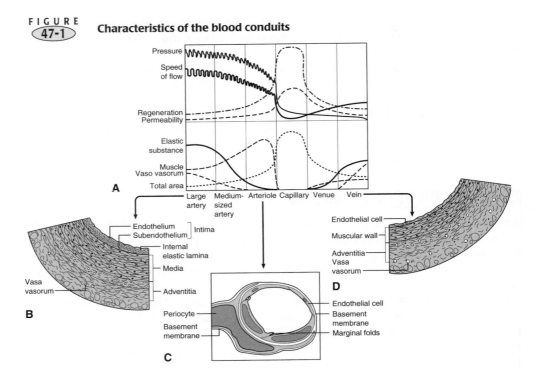

FIGURE 47-1 Characteristics of the blood conduits

the subendothelial layer. The tunica intima is composed of longitudinally arranged connective tissue and sometimes smooth muscle. The **tunica media** is composed of smooth muscle. In capillaries **pericytes** replace the smooth muscle. Pericytes have contractile function but also use their pluripotency to serve a primary role in capillary generation and repair. The final layer is the **tunica adventitia.** Here, longitudinally arranged collagen and elastin blend with the surrounding connective tissue of the organ or muscle the vessel is supplying. In large vessels, unable to rely on diffusion, the tunica adventitia and media are supplied blood through the **vaso vasorum.**

Peripheral vascular diseases

Peripheral vascular diseases (PVDs) come in many forms and often have systemic manifestations. See Table 47-1.

Blood pressure

Arterial pressure is closely regulated to maintain perfusion. The baroreceptor mechanism mediates acute response. **Baroreceptors** are stretch receptors found in the **carotid sinus** (Figure 47-2) and along the aortic arch. Increased arterial pressure activates the baroreceptor, increasing firing along **cranial nerve X.** The signal reaches the **vasomotor center** in the brainstem, and a parasympathetic response ensues. Consequently, heart rate, contractility of the myocardium, and tonic vasomotor tone decrease (lowering total peripheral resistance [TPR]).

The renin–angiotensin–aldosterone system accomplishes long-term regulation of blood pressure. Instead of being neuronal, this response is hormonal. Changes are made to blood volume. With decreased blood pressure, there is decreased perfusion of the kidneys (Figure 47-3). The juxtaglomerular apparatus releases renin, which catalyzes the conversion of angiotensinogen to angiotensin I in the blood. In the lung angiotensin-converting enzyme (ACE) converts angiotensin I to angiotensin II. Angiotensin II causes release of adrenal aldosterone and directly increases TPR by causing arteriolar vasoconstriction. Aldosterone acts on the distal tubule of the kidney to increase salt resorption. Water follows, and blood volume increases.

QUICK HIT
The pathophysiology of the vasculitides is thought to be mediated by immunopathology.

QUICK HIT
Serum sickness, a generalized deposition of immune complexes, is now rare because of decreased administration of animal serum.

TABLE 47-1 Peripheral Vascular Diseases

Disease	Pathology	Vessels Affected	Clinical Manifestations	Notes
Churg-Strauss	Eosinophilic, **granulomatous** inflammation	Small and medium vessels	**Asthma; elevated plasma eosinophils;** heart disease	May be associated with antineutrophil antibodies (p-ANCA)
Henoch-Schönlein purpura	**IgA** immune complex–mediated acute inflammation; renal deposits in mesangium	Arterioles; capillaries; venules	Hemorrhagic urticaria; palpable purpura; fever; RBC casts in urine; **atopic** patient	Often associated with **URI children**
Kaposi sarcoma	Viral origin; component of **AIDS**	Cutaneous and visceral vasculature	Malignant vascular tumor, especially in **homosexual** men	May be related to HHV-8 infection
Kawasaki disease	Acute necrotizing inflammation	Large, medium, and small vessels	Fever; conjunctival lesions; lymphadenitis; coronary artery aneurysms	Affects **young children**
Rendu-Osler-Weber syndrome	**Autosomal dominant** hereditary hemorrhagic telangiectasia	Dilatation of venules and capillaries	Epistaxis; GI bleeding	Increased frequency in **Mormon** population
Polyarteritis nodosa (PAN)	**p-ANCA** lead to necrotizing degeneration of media; aneurysms	Small and medium arteries	Fever; weight loss; abdominal pain (GI); hypertension (renal)	Associated with **hepatitis B infection**
Thromboangiitis obliterans (Buergerdisease)	Acute, full-thickness inflammation of vessels; may extend to nerves; occlusive lesions in extremities	Small and medium arteries	Cold, pale limb; pain; **Raynaud phenomenon;** gangrene	Typical patient is a young **Jewish** man who **smokes heavily**
von Hippel-Lindau disease	**Autosomal dominant;** localized to chromosome 3	Visceral vasculature	**Hemangioblastomas** of the cerebellum, brain stem, and retina; hepatic, renal, and pancreatic cysts	Increased incidence of **renal cell carcinoma**
Wegener granulomatosis	Anti-neutrophil antibodies (**c-ANCA**) cause necrotizing, **granulomatous lesions** in **kidney** and **lung**	Small arteries; small veins	Cough; ulcers of sinuses and **nasal septum;** RBC casts in urine	More common in males

HHV-8, human herpesvirus 8.
From Mehta S, Milder E, Mirarchi A. *Step-Up: A High-Yield, Systems-Based Review for the USMLE Step 1.* Philadelphia: Lippincott Williams & Wilkins, 2000, pp 58–59.

Raynaud disease

Raynaud disease is a recurrent **vasospasm** in small arteries. This spasm leaves the affected areas (usually fingers or toes) pale or cyanotic. Raynaud disease is common in young women, and it leaves no serious damage. **Raynaud phenomenon** is similar to Raynaud disease, but it is secondary to a systemic illness such as **systemic lupus erythematosus (SLE)** or **scleroderma.**

Headache and migraine pharmacotherapy

Several different types of headache have various clinical presentations. Treatment often includes nonsteroidal anti-inflammatory drugs (NSAIDs); however, migraines are more difficult to control, and pharmacotherapy varies for them. See Table 47-2 and Figure 47-4 for more information.

Chemicals producing vasoconstriction include **TXA-2,** LTC-4, LTD-4, and LTE-4. Mediators of vasodilation include PGI-2, PGD-2, **PGE-2,** PGF-2α, and bradykinin.

The posterior pituitary releases **antidiuretic hormone** (ADH, vasopressin) when cells in the atria sense an acute drop in blood pressure, causing vasoconstriction (V1 receptors) and increased resorption of water in the distal tubule (V2 receptors). Blood pressure increases.

The atria release **atrial natriuretic peptide** (ANP) when blood pressure increases. ANP inhibits vasoconstriction (decreasing TPR) and release of renin. It also promotes salt and water wasting by the kidney. Blood pressure drops.

Cluster headaches are associated with cigarette smoking and ethanol consumption.

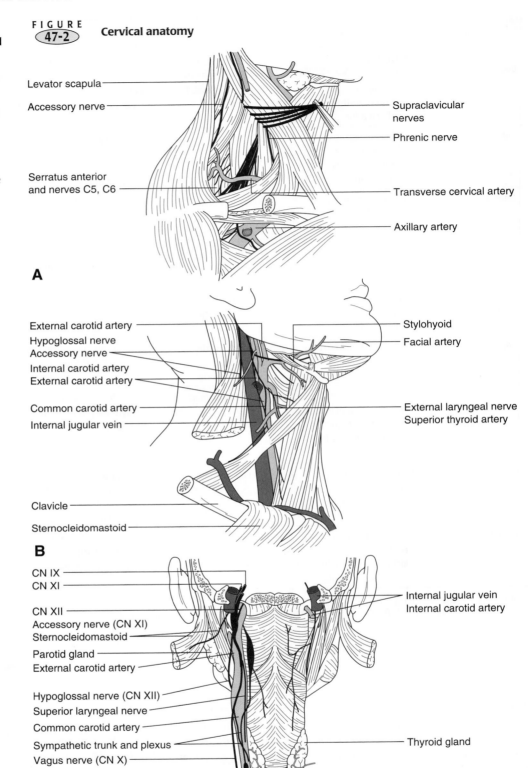

F I G U R E
47-2 **Cervical anatomy**

A

Levator scapula
Accessory nerve
Serratus anterior and nerves C5, C6

Supraclavicular nerves
Phrenic nerve
Transverse cervical artery
Axillary artery

B

External carotid artery
Hypoglossal nerve
Accessory nerve
Internal carotid artery
External carotid artery
Common carotid artery
Internal jugular vein
Clavicle
Sternocleidomastoid

Stylohyoid
Facial artery
External laryngeal nerve
Superior thyroid artery

C

CN IX
CN XI
CN XII
Accessory nerve (CN XI)
Sternocleidomastoid
Parotid gland
External carotid artery
Hypoglossal nerve (CN XII)
Superior laryngeal nerve
Common carotid artery
Sympathetic trunk and plexus
Vagus nerve (CN X)
Left recurrent laryngeal nerve

Internal jugular vein
Internal carotid artery
Thyroid gland
Esophagus
Right recurrent laryngeal nerve

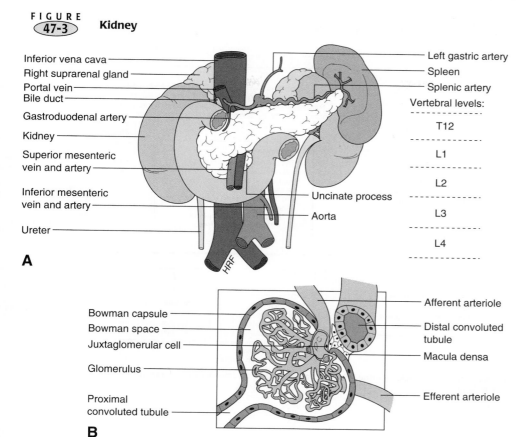

FIGURE 47-3   Kidney

A

- Inferior vena cava
- Right suprarenal gland
- Portal vein
- Bile duct
- Gastroduodenal artery
- Kidney
- Superior mesenteric vein and artery
- Inferior mesenteric vein and artery
- Ureter

- Left gastric artery
- Spleen
- Splenic artery
- Vertebral levels:
  - T12
  - L1
  - L2
  - L3
  - L4
- Uncinate process
- Aorta

HRF

B

- Bowman capsule
- Bowman space
- Juxtaglomerular cell
- Glomerulus
- Proximal convoluted tubule

- Afferent arteriole
- Distal convoluted tubule
- Macula densa
- Efferent arteriole

TABLE 47-2   Characteristics of Migraine, Cluster, and Tension-Type Headaches

	Migraine	Cluster	Tension Type
Family history	Yes	No	Yes
Sex	Women more often than men	Men more often than women	Women more than men
Onset	Variable	During sleep	Under stress
Location	Usually unilateral	Behind or around one eye	Bilateral in band around head
Character, severity	Pulsating, throbbing	Excruciating, sharp, steady	Dull, persistent, tightening/pressing
Duration	2 to 72 hr per episode	15 to 90 min per attack	30 min to 7 days per episode
Associated symptoms	Visual auras, sensitivity to light and sound, pale facial appearance, nausea and vomiting	Unilateral or bilateral, sweating facial flushing, nasal congestion, ptosis, lacrimation, pupillary changes	Mild intolerance to light and noise, anorexia

From Harrey RA, Champe PC. *Pharmacology, 2nd Ed.* Philadelphia: Lippincott Williams & Wilkins, 2000, p 425.

FIGURE
47-4   **Migraine pharmacotherapy**

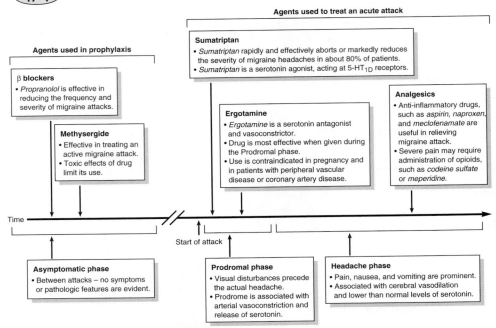

Agents used to treat an acute attack

Sumatriptan
- *Sumatriptan* rapidly and effectively aborts or markedly reduces the severity of migraine headaches in about 80% of patients.
- *Sumatriptan* is a serotonin agonist, acting at 5-HT$_{1D}$ receptors.

Agents used in prophylaxis

β blockers
- *Propranolol* is effective in reducing the frequency and severity of migraine attacks.

Methysergide
- Effective in treating an active migraine attack.
- Toxic effects of drug limit its use.

Ergotamine
- *Ergotamine* is a serotonin antagonist and vasoconstrictor.
- Drug is most effective when given during the Prodromal phase.
- Use is contraindicated in pregnancy and in patients with peripheral vascular disease or coronary artery disease.

Analgesics
- Anti-inflammatory drugs, such as *aspirin, naproxen,* and *meclofenamate* are useful in relieving migraine attack.
- Severe pain may require administration of opioids, such as *codeine sulfate* or *meperidine.*

Time

Start of attack

Asymptomatic phase
- Between attacks – no symptoms or pathologic features are evident.

Prodromal phase
- Visual disturbances precede the actual headache.
- Prodrome is associated with arterial vasoconstriction and release of serotonin.

Headache phase
- Pain, nausea, and vomiting are prominent.
- Associated with cerebral vasodilation and lower than normal levels of serotonin.

(Redrawn from Harvey RA, Champe PC. Pharmacology, 2nd Ed. Philadelphia: Lippincott Williams & Wilkins, 2000, p. 427.)

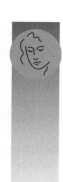

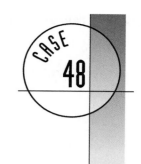

"I'm very tired and feverish. My knees are swollen, I can't concentrate, and I've had this rash on my face all summer."

OBJECTIVES

1. Develop a differential diagnosis and an appropriate workup for fatigue, swollen joints, and a malar rash
2. Learn the etiology and clinical presentation for common nephrotic glomerular diseases
3. Review the distribution of total body water and the kidney's function in maintaining fluid balance
4. Review skeletal muscle anatomy and physiology of contraction
5. Describe the actions of hormones on the nephron
6. Differentiate between the classic and alternative pathways of the complement cascade

HISTORY AND PHYSICAL EXAMINATION

A 20-year-old African American woman complains of **general malaise, joint pain, and a rash.** She has been feeling so poorly that she cannot continue her job as a lifeguard. She reports that the rash usually appears after she has been at work and especially bothers her because it is on her face. She indicates that the joint pain waxes and wanes, mostly in her hands and knees. The patient states that she has not been outside in grassy fields or woods recently and denies a history of prescription drug use. Physical examination reveals swelling in the proximal interphalangeal joints and knees. A **rash is noted on sun-exposed areas,** especially the **malar "butterfly" region of her face.** Lymphadenopathy is also present.

APPROPRIATE WORKUP

Blood chemistries, urinalysis, and serology

DIFFERENTIAL DIAGNOSIS

Dermatomyositis, drug-induced lupus, Lyme disease, rheumatoid arthritis (RA), systemic lupus erythematosus (SLE)

DIAGNOSTIC LABORATORY TESTS AND STUDIES

Blood chemistry:
  HgB = 10.0 g/dL (L)
  WBC = 3,000/dL (L)
  Platelets = 65,000/dL (L)
Urinalysis:
  Protein = 3+ (H)
  Cellular casts = positive
Serology:
  Antinuclear antibody = positive
  Anti-ds DNA = positive

Anti-Smith antibody = positive
C3 and C4 complement levels
  = decreased
Antihistone antibody = negative
Rheumatoid factor (IgM anti-IgG
  antibodies) = negative
Serum CK = 45 ng/dL (N)
ELISA for *Borrelia burgdorferi*
  = negative

DIAGNOSIS: SYSTEMIC LUPUS ERYTHEMATOSUS (SLE)

SLE, commonly called "lupus," is an autoimmune disorder with multiple manifestations and complications, ranging from arthritis to kidney failure. The disease usually presents in **women** 14 to 45 years of age, is **more common in African Americans,** and has a strong familial correlation.

SLE is a **systemic inflammatory process** involving IgG, IgM, IgA, and complement deposition. Antigen-specific B cells and T cells are also implicated. An **anemia of chronic inflammation** is also present which can be normochromic and normocytic or hypochromic and macrocytic. Diagnosis is made when the patient has four of the criteria listed in Figure 48-1 at one time.

The autoantibodies in SLE attack virtually all areas of the body, especially the connective tissues. The most characteristic lesion is the **"butterfly" rash** that appears over the **malar** region of the face. Skin manifestations result from inflammatory cells that attack the

Patients with lupus may have a false-positive result when given a VDRL test for syphilis.

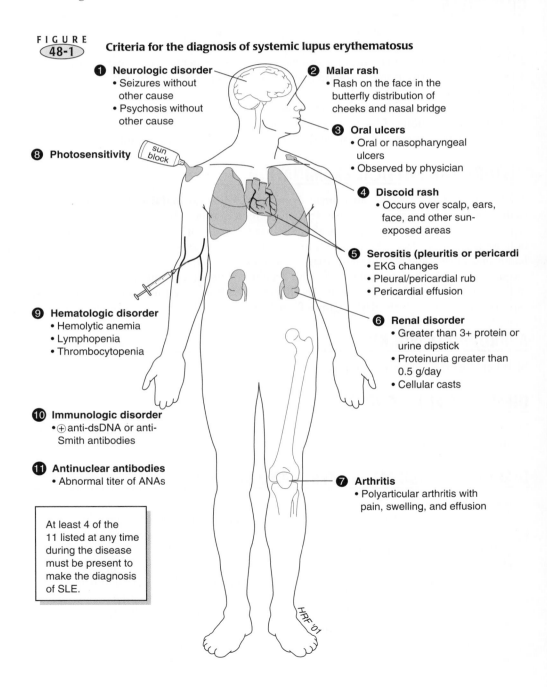

FIGURE 48-1 Criteria for the diagnosis of systemic lupus erythematosus

1 Neurologic disorder
• Seizures without other cause
• Psychosis without other cause

2 Malar rash
• Rash on the face in the butterfly distribution of cheeks and nasal bridge

3 Oral ulcers
• Oral or nasopharyngeal ulcers
• Observed by physician

8 Photosensitivity

sun block

4 Discoid rash
• Occurs over scalp, ears, face, and other sun-exposed areas

5 Serositis (pleuritis or pericardi
• EKG changes
• Pleural/pericardial rub
• Pericardial effusion

9 Hematologic disorder
• Hemolytic anemia
• Lymphopenia
• Thrombocytopenia

6 Renal disorder
• Greater than 3+ protein or urine dipstick
• Proteinuria greater than 0.5 g/day
• Cellular casts

10 Immunologic disorder
• ⊕ anti-dsDNA or anti-Smith antibodies

11 Antinuclear antibodies
• Abnormal titer of ANAs

7 Arthritis
• Polyarticular arthritis with pain, swelling, and effusion

At least 4 of the 11 listed at any time during the disease must be present to make the diagnosis of SLE.

HRF '01

dermal-epidermal junction, causing bullae formation and macular/papular lesions that resemble psoriasis. Other manifestations of SLE include **symmetrical and bilateral arthralgias** and arthritidis with effusions. The joints degenerate and can appear similar to RA, with deviations and subluxations. The most clinically important manifestation is the autoantibody effect on the kidneys, as **renal failure** is the major cause of death in patients with SLE. **Subendothelial immune complexes** deposit in the glomeruli, causing thickening of the basement membrane and formation of the characteristic **wire-loop appearance.** The resultant nephropathy results in a **nephrotic syndrome** characterized by hypoalbuminemia, massive edema, hyperlipidemia, and proteinuria greater than 4 g/day (Table 48-1).

SLE also affects the lungs, leading to interstitial fibrosis, diffuse alveolitis, and even pulmonary hypertension and embolism. Cardiac manifestations include **pericarditis, Libman-Sacks endocarditis** (verrucous lesions usually found on the mitral valve), pericardial effusions, and tamponade.

TABLE 48-1 **Nephrotic Glomerular Diseases**

Glomerular Disease	Etiology	Clinical Features	Notes
Minimal change disease (lipoid nephrosis)	Fusion of foot processes on the basement membrane leads to loss of negative charge and changes the protein selectivity; altered appearance of villi on epithelial cells	Electron microscopy shows **fusion of podocyte foot processes,** and lipid-laden renal cortices	**Common in young children** (usually under 5 years of age); responds well to steroids; albumin usually selectively secreted
Membranous glomerulonephritis	Idiopathic; secondarily caused by SLE, hepatitis B, syphilis, gold, penicillamine, malignancy	Basement membrane thickening; **"spike and dome"** with **subepithelial IgG and C3 deposits**	Common in young adults
Diabetic nephropathy	Microangiopathy leading to thickening of basement membrane	Basement membrane thickening	Two types: diffuse and nodular glomerulosclerosis; nodular has **Kimmelstiel-Wilson nodules;** usually leads to renal failure
Renal amyloidosis	Subendothelial/mesangial amyloid deposits; associated with multiple myeloma	Stains: periodic acid-Schiff (PAS) (−); **Congo Red (+)**	Increasing severity leads to renal failure
Lupus nephropathy	**Anti ds-DNA**	WHO Classifications: • WHO I: normal • WHO II: mesangial proliferation; little clinical relevance • WHO III (focal proliferative): <1/2 of glomeruli affected • **WHO IV (diffuse proliferative):** worst prognosis; **wire-loop lesions;** (subendothelial immune complex deposition of IgM and IgG + C3) • WHO V: membranous glomerulonephritis	Degree of kidney involvement correlates to SLE prognosis; may have nephritic qualities
Focal and segmental glomerulosclerosis	Has four possible etiologies: idiopathic; superimposed on pre-existing pathology; associated with loss of renal mass; secondary to other disorders (e.g., heroine abuse or HIV)	Sclerosis of some glomeruli; only capillary tuft is involved in affected glomeruli	Clinically similar to minimal change disease, but affects older population

C_3, third component of complement; SLE, systemic lupus erythematosus; ds-DNA, double-stranded deoxyribonucleic acid; *WHO,* World Health Organization.
Mehta S, Milder E, Mirarchi A. Step-Up: A High-Yield, Systems-Based Review for the USMLE Step 1. Philadelphia: Lippincott Williams & Wilkins, 2000, p 116–117, Tbl 5-5.

SLE is usually treated with glucocorticoids prophylactically and high-dose corticosteroids for acute debilitating exacerbations. Other immunosuppressants such as azathioprine can be used to control active disease.

EXPLANATION OF DIFFERENTIAL

Dermatomyositis results in muscle damage and skin rash caused by lymphocytic infiltration. It is assumed to be **autoimmune** in nature and is often associated with other connective tissue disorders such as **SLE and RA.** Characteristically, the disease causes profound **proximal muscle weakness** (Figure 48-2), dysphagia, EKG changes, and myocardial necrosis. The classic **lilac-colored (heliotropic) rash** is found on the face, chest, knees, and knuckles. Diagnosis is made by an **increased serum CK level,** electromyography, and muscle biopsy. In this patient, no specific evidence of muscle weakness was noted, and the serum CK level was within normal limits.

Drug-induced lupus is an adverse drug reaction that presents similarly to SLE. It can occur with the administration of many drugs, but the most notable offenders are **hydralazine and procainamide.** The most common complaints in this form of lupus include generalized malaise and arthralgias, with occasional pleuropericarditis. **Renal and CNS manifestations are rare.** This disease can be differentiated from SLE by antibody testing. Both diseases cause antinuclear antibodies (ANAs), but only **drug-induced lupus causes antihistone antibodies.** Also anti-dsDNA antibodies and low levels of complement do not usually occur in drug-induced lupus.

Lyme disease is caused by the **spirochete *B. burgdorferi*** and is **spread by tick bites.** Incidence is greatest between May and August. Lyme disease is most prevalent in the wooded and grassy areas of the Northeast, upper Midwest, and northern California. After an incubation period of 7 to 10 days, the classic **erythema migrans** shin rash and general malaise develop. The disease can progress in weeks or months and cause chronic neurologic and cardiac symptoms as well as asymmetric oligoarthritis. The presence of a lymphoplasmacytic infiltrate with endothelial proliferation is characteristic of Lyme arthritis. Erythema migrans may persist as the disease progresses. Diagnosis is based on a **positive ELISA** test result, but must be confirmed with a **Western blot.** Antibiotic treatment is curative. In this patient, a diagnosis of Lyme disease can be ruled out based on the negative history of exposure to wooded areas or grassy fields, no erythema migrans rash, and more specifically by the negative ELISA result. Lyme disease, however, should always be considered in a previously young healthy person who presents with a rash, generalized weakness, and malaise.

RA is an autoimmune inflammatory disease that affects the joints and tendons. It usually presents with **morning stiffness** that **improves with use.** RA is associated with **rheumatoid factor** on serologic testing. RA causes **pannus formation** (hypergranulation tissue over articular cartilage) as well as subcutaneous nodules. **Swan-neck and boutonnière deformities of the fingers** are also characteristic. Distal interphalangeal (DIP) joints are not affected. RA is seen more commonly in women and is associated with **HLA-DR4.** In this patient, findings on physical examination and serologic testing exclude the diagnosis of RA. This patient's examination reveals swelling but no deformity in the finger joints, and no evidence of pannus formation or subcutaneous nodules. Serologic testing results in this case are negative for rheumatoid factor.

Skeletal Muscle Anatomy and Contraction

Please refer to Figure 48-2.

Related Basic Science

Body water and renal function

Total body water is 60% of total body weight for men and 50% for women. Total body water is 66% intracellular fluid (ICF) and 33% extracellular fluid (ECF). ECF is made up of 25% plasma and 75% interstitial fluid.

FIGURE
48-2   **Skeletal muscle anatomy and contraction** (*T* = troponin)

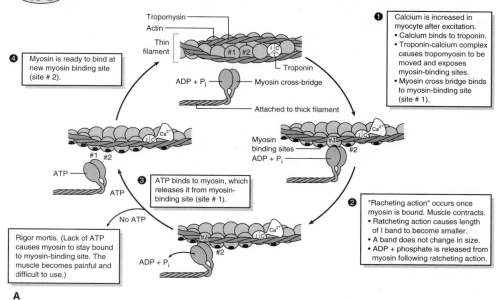

❹ Myosin is ready to bind at new myosin binding site (site # 2).

❶ Calcium is increased in myocyte after excitation.
• Calcium binds to troponin.
• Troponin-calcium complex causes tropomyosin to be moved and exposes myosin-binding sites.
• Myosin cross bridge binds to myosin-binding site (site # 1).

❸ ATP binds to myosin, which releases it from myosin-binding site (site # 1).

❷ "Racheting action" occurs once myosin is bound. Muscle contracts.
• Ratcheting action causes length of I band to become smaller.
• A band does not change in size.
• ADP + phosphate is released from myosin following ratcheting action.

Rigor mortis. (Lack of ATP causes myosin to stay bound to myosin-binding site. The muscle becomes painful and difficult to use.)

A

B. Gross, histologic, microscopic anatomy of skeletal muscle

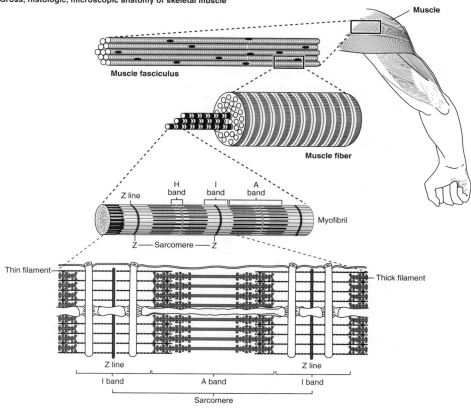

(Modified from Mehta S, Milder E, Mirarchi A. Step-Up: A High-Yield, Systems-Based Review for the USMLE Step 1. Philadelphia: Lippincott Williams & Wilkins, 2000, pp 193–194.)

The function of the kidneys in fluid balance is to primarily control the volume of the ECF. This regulation then helps to maintain ICF balance. A complicated process involving several different hormones maintains the balance of fluid.

The renin–angiotensin–aldosterone axis is a key player in the control of ECF balance. The juxtaglomerular apparatus (JGA) secretes renin in response to a decreased plasma volume, which is measured by the baroreceptors of the macula densa. Renin cleaves angiotensinogen to angiotensin I, which is then cleaved to form angiotensin II. Angiotensin II acts on the zona glomerulosa of the adrenal gland to make aldosterone and stimulates release of antidiuretic hormone (ADH) and adrenocorticotropic hormone (ACTH). It also stimulates thirst and causes vasoconstriction. Angiotensin II acts directly on the nephron to promote Na^+ –H exchange and HCO_3^- absorption. Through aldosterone and ADH, angiotensin II causes increased Na^+ resorption and increased H_2O resorption, thereby increasing ECF.

Hormone action on the nephron

Please refer to Figure 48-3.

Complement function (Figure 48-4)

Complement functions to defend against Gram-negative bacteria by causing direct lysis of bacterial cells. The complement system has two pathways. IgG and IgM antibodies that are bound to bacterial antigen activate the **classic pathway.** This **antigen–antibody** complex stimulates the activation of C1, which starts the complement cascade. The **alternative pathway** is initiated by the surface of bacteria, aggregated IgA, endotoxin, and other factors. The alternative pathway begins with the **activation of C3.** Both the classic and alternative

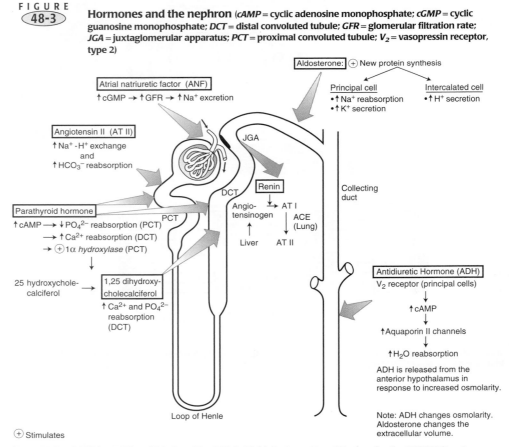

FIGURE
48-3

Hormones and the nephron (*cAMP* = cyclic adenosine monophosphate; *cGMP* = cyclic guanosine monophosphate; *DCT* = distal convoluted tubule; *GFR* = glomerular filtration rate; *JGA* = juxtaglomerular apparatus; *PCT* = proximal convoluted tubule; *V₂* = vasopressin receptor, type 2)

(From Mehta S, Milder E, Mirarchi A. Step-Up: A High-Yield, Systems-Based Review for the USMLE Step 1. Philadelphia: Lippincott Williams & Wilkins, 2000, p 112.)

FIGURE
48-4   **Complement cascade**

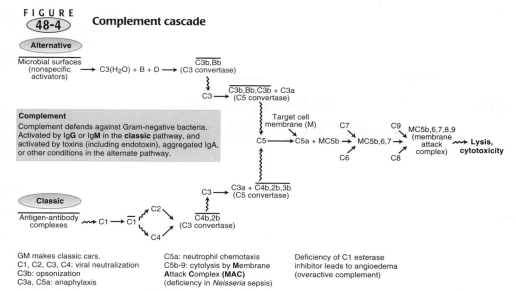

Alternative

Microbial surfaces
(nonspecific ⟶ C3(H₂O) + B + D ⟶ $\overline{\text{C3b,Bb}}$ (C3 convertase)
activators)

$\overline{\text{C3b,Bb,C3b}}$ + C3a
C3 ⟶ (C5 convertase)

Complement
Complement defends against Gram-negative bacteria.
Activated by Ig**G** or Ig**M** in the **classic** pathway, and
activated by toxins (including endotoxin), aggregated IgA,
or other conditions in the alternate pathway.

Target cell
membrane (M)   C7   C9   MC5b,6,7,8,9
                                (membrane
C5 ⟶ C5a + MC5b ⟶ MC5b,6,7 ⟶ attack ⤳ **Lysis,**
                C6   C8   complex) **cytotoxicity**

C3a + $\overline{\text{C4b,2b,3b}}$
C3 ⟶ (C5 convertase)

Classic

Antigen-antibody ⤳ C1 ⟶ $\overline{\text{C1}}$ C2
complexes $\overline{\text{C4b,2b}}$
                          C4   (C3 convertase)

GM makes classic cars.   C5a: neutrophil chemotaxis   Deficiency of C1 esterase
C1, C2, C3, C4: viral neutralization   C5b-9: cytolysis by **M**embrane   inhibitor leads to angioedema
C3b: opsonization   **A**ttack **C**omplex **(MAC)**   (overactive complement)
C3a, C5a: anaphylaxis   (deficiency in *Neisseria* sepsis)

**(From Mehta S, Milder E, Mirarchi A. Step-Up: A High-Yield, Systems-Based Review for the USMLE Step 1.
Philadelphia: Lippincott Williams & Wilkins, 2000, p 210.)**

pathways result in the formation of the **membrane attack complex (MAC)** (C5b-6–7–8–9)
that causes bacterial cell lysis.

The various factors of complement, in addition to promoting the formation of the
MAC, are also biologically active. C1 through C4 are active in viral neutralization. **C3b** is
involved with **opsonization.** C5a produces anaphylatoxin II and functions in neutrophil
and macrophage chemotaxis.

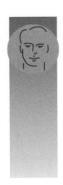
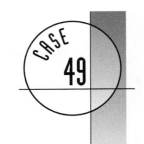

"My stomach hurts so much; I can't stand it!"

OBJECTIVES

1. Develop a differential diagnosis and an appropriate workup for acute abdominal pain with characteristic pain radiation patterns
2. Review the development of the pancreas
3. Describe pancreatic histology and key features
4. Discuss the causes, clinical presentation, and diagnosis of chronic pancreatitis and pancreatic adenocarcinoma

HISTORY AND PHYSICAL EXAMINATION

A 35-year-old man presents in the ED with **abdominal pain.** The pain began when the patient woke up and has progressively worsened over the past few hours. He describes the pain as extremely intense, localized to the **epigastrium,** and **radiating to the back.** He recalls no previous episodes of such pain. Extreme **nausea** and pain have kept the patient from eating anything this morning. He has had only two glasses of water today. The patient did vomit once; the vomitus was clear. His history is positive for excessive alcohol use (about six beers per day for 10 years); the patient admits to drinking about 20 beers the night before. He denies any drug use. Vital signs are as follows: pulse 110 bpm (H); respirations 30 bpm (H); blood pressure 95/50 mm Hg (L); temperature 101.2°F (H). Physical examination reveals marked epigastric tenderness, mild **abdominal distention,** and **diminished bowel sounds.**

APPROPRIATE WORKUP

Blood chemistries, urinalysis, and abdominal radiograph, CT, and US

DIFFERENTIAL DIAGNOSIS

Abdominal aortic aneurysm, acute cholecystitis, acute pancreatitis, intestinal obstruction, perforated peptic ulcer, urolithiasis

DIAGNOSTIC LABORATORY TESTS AND STUDIES

Blood chemistry:
Hgb = 14.5 g/dL (N)
Hct = 45% (N)
Leukocyte count
    = 16,000 (N)
Glucose = 135 mg/dL (H)
Amylase = 225 U/L (H)

Lipase = 40 U/dL (H)
Ca = 7.5 mg/dL (L)
Urinalysis:
Protein = trace (N)
Leukocytes = 0/hpf (N)
Red cells = 1/hpf (N)

Abdominal radiograph:	Abdominal CT:
Dilated loop suggestive of a partial ileus	Edematous pancreas No pseudocysts
No air under the diaphragm or any other evidence of GI perforation	**Abdominal US:**
No evidence of nephrolithiasis	Gallbladder not distended No evidence of stones

DIAGNOSIS: ACUTE PANCREATITIS

Acute pancreatitis is characterized by inflammation, edema, and necrosis of pancreatic tissue. In the United States, the two most common causes are chronic alcohol use and **cholelithiasis.** With activation of the digestive pancreatic enzymes, the pancreatic parenchyma and surrounding tissues are destroyed. Amylase and lipase leak into the systemic circulation, causing markedly elevated levels of these enzymes. Calcium is consumed in reactions with fatty acid soaps (saponification), resulting in hypocalcemia. Death can result from shock, acute renal failure, or respiratory distress. Most cases resolve in 3 to 6 days.

EXPLANATION OF DIFFERENTIAL

Rarely, problems of the aorta can cause abdominal pain. Abdominal **aortic aneurysms** most often are secondary to atherosclerosis. The rate of expansion increases as the aneurysm grows. These aneurysms can remain asymptomatic until a sharp, tearing pain signals aortic rupture. Aortic rupture carries greater than a 50% mortality.

Acute cholecystitis can occur secondary to cholelithiasis or infection. Certain conditions such as high cholesterol level or chronic hemolysis predispose to gallstone formation. Sharp, localized **pain in the right upper quadrant (RUQ),** fever, nausea, and vomiting are all part of the typical clinical presentation. This patient had no predisposing factors for cholecystitis and no pain in the RUQ. Furthermore, his gallbladder appeared normal on US.

Intestinal obstruction presents with abdominal pain, nausea, vomiting, abdominal distention, and diminished bowel sounds. Some common causes are **hernias, adhesions,** volvulus, **tumors,** postoperative ileus, and, in children, **intussusception.** Obstruction has a characteristic appearance on abdominal radiograph, including diffuse air-fluid levels. Obstruction was not seen on this patient's radiograph.

Perforation is a serious complication of **peptic ulcer disease (PUD).** Affected patients typically present with a history of gnawing or burning epigastric pain. GI perforation is often diagnosed by a history of hematemesis and visualization of air under the diaphragm on an upright abdominal radiograph. This patient did not have a long-term history of epigastric pain or hematemesis, and air did not appear under the diaphragm on abdominal radiograph.

Urolithiasis, or renal stones, can cause abdominal pain or renal colic. Stone formation is more common in men than women and is most frequently associated with hypercalcemia. The location and constant nature of this patient's pain is more suggestive of pancreatitis. Also, the patient had normal results on urinalysis, including no red cells, which are common in urolithiasis.

Related Basic Science

Development of the pancreas

The pancreas develops from the distal **foregut** initially as **dorsal and ventral pancreatic buds.** These buds originate from the endoderm and grow between the layers of the mesentery. As the duodenum grows and rotates, the ventral bud comes to lie posteriorly. Eventually the two buds fuse as do their ducts. The main pancreatic duct is normally the original ventral pancreatic duct. The dorsal pancreatic duct occasionally persists as an accessory duct. The dorsal bud forms the tail, body, and most of the head of the adult pancreas. The ventral bud forms part of the head and the uncinate process.

QUICK HIT
A severe, tearing abdominal pain that radiates to the back also occurs with **aortic dissection.** This condition occurs when weakness in the aortic vessel wall allows blood to gain access to the intramural space. **Chronic hypertension** and **Marfan syndrome** predispose to this event.

QUICK HIT
Gallstones can block the ampulla of Vater and simultaneously cause cholecystitis and pancreatitis.

QUICK HIT
The vascular components and surrounding connective tissue of the pancreas are derived from mesoderm. All other parts of the pancreas, including acinar and islet cells, are of **endodermal** origin.

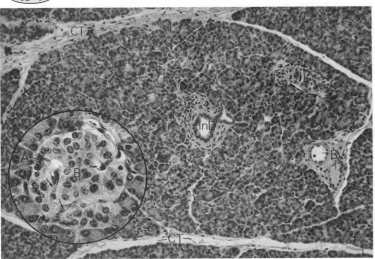

F I G U R E
49-1   (See also Color Plate 49-1.) Pancreatic histology

From Ross MH, Romrell LJ, Kaye GI. Histology: A Text and Atlas, 3rd Ed. Philadelphia: Lippincott Williams & Wilkins, 1995, p 529.)

Maternal diabetes exposes the fetus to elevated glucose levels and causes accelerated development of the pancreatic islet cells. These babies, which are often large for gestational age, are born with elevated insulin levels and are at risk for developing hypoglycemia.

Developmental anomalies of the pancreas are rare. Of these, the **annular pancreas** is probably the best known. It occurs when the pancreatic buds fuse both posteriorly and anteriorly. As a result, the pancreas forms as a ring around the duodenum. This condition, which is more common in **men,** can cause duodenal **obstruction** in the neonate or adult.

Pancreatic histology (Figure 49-1)

The pancreas has both exocrine and endocrine functions. The functional unit of the exocrine pancreas is the **acinus,** which produces digestive enzymes. The functional unit of the endocrine pancreas is the **islet of Langerhans,** which produces insulin, glucagon, and somatostatin. It is the pancreatic duct system under the influence of secretin that produces bicarbonate to neutralize stomach acid in the duodenal lumen.

Chronic pancreatitis

While chronic alcohol use or gallstones often cause acute pancreatitis, chronic pancreatitis almost always occurs secondary to **alcoholism.** Chronic pancreatitis often follows a relapsing course with intermittent attacks. With each attack, there is progressive **parenchymal fibrosis** and **loss of function** of the exocrine pancreas. Calcifications and pseudocysts can form and be visualized by radiograph and CT. Didanosine (ddI), a nucleoside reverse transcriptase inhibitor used to treat HIV, can cause fatal pancreatitis.

Pancreatic adenocarcinoma

Dysfunction of the exocrine pancreas leads to malabsorption, especially of fats. Deficiencies of fat-soluble vitamins (A, D, E, K) can ensue, with night-blindness being one of the earliest symptoms.

Pancreatic cancer develops most often from the ductal epithelium of the exocrine pancreas. The most common location is the head of the pancreas, where the growing tumor can cause **obstructive jaundice.** Other symptoms of pancreatic cancer are **weight loss** and **abdominal pain.** Patients with pancreatic cancer are also at increased risk for migratory thrombophlebitis (Trousseau sign) and **depression** (occurring before the diagnosis of pancreatic cancer). The one-year survival rate for this deadly cancer is less than 20%.

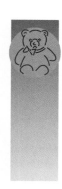
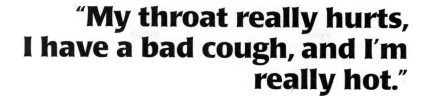

"My throat really hurts, I have a bad cough, and I'm really hot."

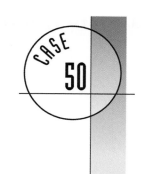
OBJECTIVES

1. Develop a differential diagnosis and an appropriate workup for the presenting symptoms of cough, fever, and a sore throat
2. Review the cough reflex
3. Understand viral genetics and appropriate chemotherapeutic agents
4. Describe the mechanism of action and side effects of acetaminophen
5. Differentiate between measles and mumps

HISTORY AND PHYSICAL EXAMINATION

A man brings his 9-year-old son to the office in **early December**. According to the father, the boy has had a very bad cough, sore throat, and fever over the past 4 days. The cough is nonproductive. The patient also has had chills, headache, and a runny nose. The child's immunizations are all current, but he has not received an influenza (flu) shot this year. The boy says that many of his friends at school have gotten the flu over the past 2 weeks. He denies drinking from anyone's cup or sharing food. On physical examination, he has a **fever** (102.3°F), facial flushing, erythematous conjunctiva, and a **swollen throat** that is painful on swallowing.

APPROPRIATE WORKUP

Blood chemistries, throat culture, and laryngoscopy

DIFFERENTIAL DIAGNOSIS

Adenovirus infection, croup, epiglottitis, influenza virus infection, rhinovirus infection

DIAGNOSTIC LABORATORY TESTS AND STUDIES

Blood chemistry:
WBC = 3000/mm³ (L)
Throat culture:
Flu virus Type A

Laryngoscopy of the epiglottis:
No swelling or erythema

DIAGNOSIS: INFLUENZA

Flu is an **orthomyxovirus** that travels in **respiratory secretions**. There are three antigenic types: A, B, and C. These three types are based on their complement-fixing antibodies to nuclear and matrix proteins. Additionally, flu has two **surface glycoprotein** antigens, hemagglutinin (HA) and neuraminidase (NA), that permit virus entry and infection.

Flu viruses are characterized by their antigenic strain, and new strains can be created by mutations in HA and NA (**antigenic drift**). Antigenic drift produces flu epidemics, which occur most commonly in the fall and winter. **Antigenic shift**, which occurs when entire strains of genomes recombine (e.g., human and avian Type A strains), causes flu pandemics.

Flu symptoms include fever, runny nose, nonproductive cough, headache, chills, myalgias, arthralgias, malaise, and inflamed mucous membranes. Fever and other constitutional symptoms (e.g., headache, myalgias, arthralgias) distinguish the flu from the common cold. Initial presentation of the flu is mild upper respiratory symptoms, such as cough and runny nose; later, lower respiratory symptoms may result. The face may become erythematous and flushed, and the oropharynx can also become erythematous. Often, the conjunctiva will be inflamed. **Leukopenia** is common, and the virus may be isolated from respiratory secretions and cultured in cells.

During the second week of infection, complement-fixing and hemagglutination-inhibiting antibodies are created. Prophylactically, the flu virus vaccine can be administered, which gives partial immunity for a few months (up to 1 year). The vaccine is created each year with the antigens that were prevalent in strains of the previous year. The trivalent (types A, B, C) flu vaccine is recommended for the elderly; children and adolescents on chronic aspirin therapy; patients with diabetes; those with chronic lung, heart, or renal disease; and healthcare workers. Chemoprophylaxis with **amantadine** or rimantadine significantly reduces the infection rate and symptoms if taken within 10 days after exposure. Treatment is supportive with analgesics and cough medicine.

EXPLANATION OF DIFFERENTIAL

Adenovirus and **rhinovirus** can produce URIs with such symptoms as conjunctivitis, rhinitis, sore throat, fever, and cough. Adenovirus and rhinovirus are among the most common URIs in children. They typically lack the headaches, myalgias, and arthralgias of flu. The cough of adenovirus infection is sometimes mistaken for pertussis; adenovirus also is responsible for **pink eye.**

Croup is a parainfluenza infection that causes upper respiratory symptoms in children. The fusion protein (F-protein) is the virulence factor responsible for spreading croup, which produces swelling of the pharynx and larynx and narrowing of the airway. Barking cough and stridor are characteristic presentations in croup. Presentation is similar to epiglottitis, but epiglottitis lacks the barking cough. Laryngoscopy reveals a normal-sized epiglottis that may be erythematous.

Haemophilus influenza type B bacteria most commonly cause **epiglottitis.** Epiglottitis presents acutely with a sore throat, high fever, dysphagia, hoarseness, drooling, and respiratory distress. Laryngoscopy, in a controlled setting, can be used to visualize the stiffened and erythematous epiglottis but should not be relied on for diagnosis, which is based on clinical signs. Because the inflamed epiglottis obstructs the airway, suspected epiglottitis must be treated emergently.

Related Basic Science

Pharynx (Figure 50-1)

The pharynx functions in both the GI and respiratory systems and is located between the nasal and oral cavities posterior to the larynx. It is bounded superiorly by the base of the skull and inferiorly by the cricoid cartilage anteriorly and C6 posteriorly. Pharyngeal walls are comprised mainly of three constrictor muscles and internal longitudinal muscles. These muscles cooperate to elevate the larynx and pharynx in deglutition and phonation. Branches of cranial nerves (CN) IX and X innervate the pharynx.

Cough reflex

The cough reflex is a protective mechanism of the respiratory system that forces air out rapidly to keep the respiratory system clear of harmful material. When an irritant comes

Reye syndrome causes **hepatic encephalopathy** and results from the administration of aspirin after a viral infection (e.g., flu) in children.

Bordalella pertussis is a Gram-negative rod that causes pertussis (whooping cough) by infecting the bronchial epithelium via an "A" subunit (that increases cyclic adenosine monophosphate [cAMP]) and a "B" subunit (that causes attachment). An acellular pertussis vaccine is given at 2, 4, and 6 months of age.

Respiratory syncytial virus (RSV) is the most common cause of pneumonia in infants younger than 6 months of age.

FIGURE 50-1 **The pharynx** (*CN* = cranial nerve)

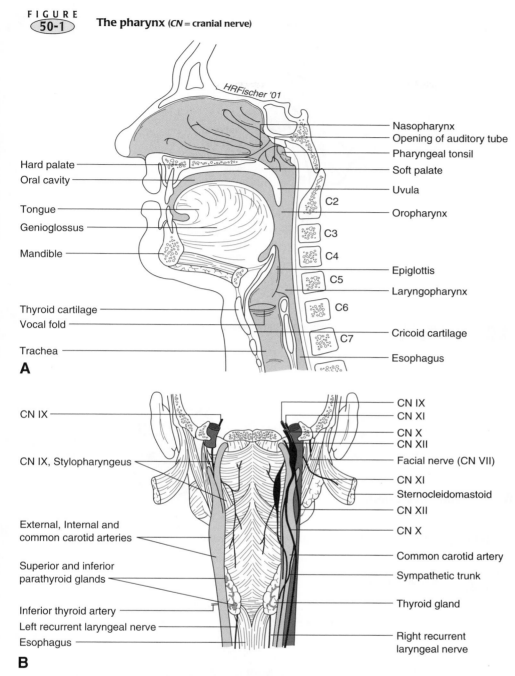

HRFischer '01

A

Nasopharynx
Opening of auditory tube
Pharyngeal tonsil
Hard palate
Oral cavity
Soft palate
Uvula
C2
Tongue
Genioglossus
Oropharynx
C3
Mandible
C4
Epiglottis
C5
Laryngopharynx
Thyroid cartilage
C6
Vocal fold
Cricoid cartilage
C7
Trachea
Esophagus

B

CN IX
CN IX
CN XI
CN X
CN XII
CN IX, Stylopharyngeus
Facial nerve (CN VII)
CN XI
Sternocleidomastoid
CN XII
External, Internal and
common carotid arteries
CN X
Common carotid artery
Superior and inferior
parathyroid glands
Sympathetic trunk
Thyroid gland
Inferior thyroid artery
Left recurrent laryngeal nerve
Esophagus
Right recurrent
laryngeal nerve

(Adapted from Moore K, Agur A. Essential Clinical Anatomy. Baltimore: Williams & Wilkins, 1995, pp 440–441.)

in contact with the glottis, trachea, or bronchi, sensory signals are relayed to the medulla, which helps generate a motor response. While the glottis is closed, respiratory muscles forcefully contract to create pressure in the lungs. When the glottis is opened, the pressurized air blows out the irritant. The cough reflex is mediated by the glossopharyngeal nerve (CN IX) (Figure 50-2).

Viral genetics and relevant chemotherapeutics

Viruses (Figure 50-3) are obligate intracellular parasites that use host machinery to replicate. Most chemotherapeutic agents prevent viral replication by destroying both the virus and host machinery (Figure 50-4).

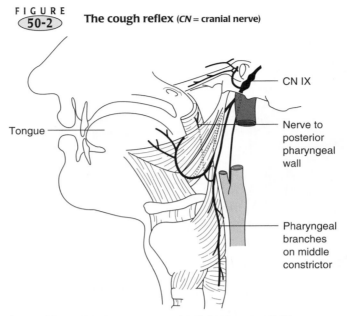

The cough reflex (*CN* = cranial nerve)

CN IX

Nerve to posterior pharyngeal wall

Tongue

Pharyngeal branches on middle constrictor

(Adapted from Moore K, Agur A. Essential Clinical Anatomy. Baltimore: Williams & Wilkins, 1995, p 458.)

F I G U R E
50-3 **Viruses**

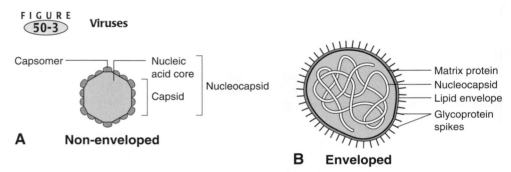

Capsomer

Nucleic acid core

Capsid

Nucleocapsid

A   **Non-enveloped**

Matrix protein
Nucleocapsid
Lipid envelope
Glycoprotein spikes

B   **Enveloped**

(Adapted from Bhushan V, Le T. First Aid for the USMLE Step 1. Stamford: Appleton & Lange, 1999, p 195.)

F I G U R E
50-4 **Antiviral chemotherapy**

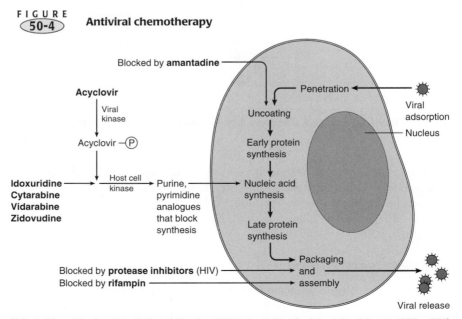

Blocked by **amantadine**

Penetration

Viral adsorption

Acyclovir

Viral kinase

Uncoating

Nucleus

Acyclovir —Ⓟ

Early protein synthesis

Idoxuridine
Cytarabine
Vidarabine
Zidovudine

Host cell kinase

Purine, pyrimidine analogues that block synthesis

Nucleic acid synthesis

Late protein synthesis

Packaging and assembly

Blocked by **protease inhibitors** (HIV)
Blocked by **rifampin**

Viral release

(Adapted from Bhushan V, Le T. First Aid for the USMLE Step 1. Stamford: Appleton & Lange, 1999, p. 271.)

Acetaminophen (Figure 50-5)

Acetaminophen is an analgesic and antipyretic that inhibits CNS prostaglandin synthesis but has **no effect on platelet function or inflammation.** Acetaminophen is less effective than other drugs (e.g., nonsteroidal anti-inflammatory drugs [NSAIDs]) as an anti-inflammatory agent because it does not **inhibit cyclooxygenase** (COX) in the periphery. Acetaminophen is the agent of choice for **analgesia** and **antipyrexia** in children, as it does not cause **Reye syndrome** unlike aspirin. Acetaminophen is metabolized in the liver by the **cytochrome p-450** system and rarely has side effects if used appropriately. With large doses, the toxic metabolite N-acetylbenzoquineimine reacts with sulfhydryl groups of proteins in the liver and can produce liver necrosis. **N-acetyl-cysteine** is the antidote given for acetaminophen overdose because it has sulfhydryl groups that react with the acetaminophen.

NSAIDs are effective in the periphery as anti-inflammatory drugs, as they inhibit COX-1 and COX-2 (enzymes that mediate the inflammatory process). The newer COX-2 inhibitors (celecoxib and rofecoxib) are more specific for inflammation and produce fewer GI side effects, as they do not affect the COX-1 pathway.

Mumps and measles

Mumps and measles are viral disorders often affecting children; however, a live-attenuated vaccine is given to children for both diseases. Mumps results in painful parotid gland swelling, painful testicular inflammation, and possible meningitis and encephalitis. A patient with the measles will have a prodrome causing high fever, hacking cough, conjunctivitis, photophobia, and malaise. This prodrome is followed by development of Koplik spots (small, red-based blue-white lesions in the mouth) and a rash that spreads from head to toe.

> **QUICK HIT**
> There is a 20% risk of fetal death if a pregnant woman acquires measles early in her pregnancy.

> **QUICK HIT**
> Subacute sclerosing panencephalitis is a slow form of encephalitis that can occur many years after infection with measles.

FIGURE 50-5   **Acetaminophen metabolism**

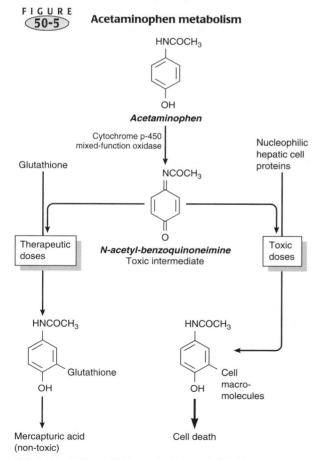

(Adapted from Mycek M, Harvey R, Champe P. LIR Pharmacology, 2nd Ed. Philadelphia: Lippincott Williams & Wilkins, 1997, p 413.)

Questions

1. A 22-year-old student presents to student health with coryza, headache, cough with minimal sputum production, and fever. Prior to these symptoms, he had a sore throat with a nonproductive cough. Gram stain of the sputum was negative along with blood and sputum cultures. The leukocyte count was within normal limits. The cold agglutinin titer was elevated. What is the most common organism responsible for this patient's symptoms and the most appropriate treatment?

   A. *Streptococcus pneumoniae;* penicillin.

   B. *Mycoplasma pneumoniae;* erythromycin.

   C. *Staphylococcus aureus;* methicillin.

   D. *Pneumocystis carinii;* TMP-SMX.

2. Three days after a 42-year-old woman returns from a trip to Mexico, she experiences severe diarrhea. Stool analysis reveals mucus and blood with nonmotile cysts that have four nuclei. The diarrhea subsides in a few weeks. However, several weeks later, she becomes febrile with pain in her right upper quadrant. An abdominal ultrasound reveals a cyst in the right hepatic lobe. What is a common side effect of the medication used to treat this infection?

   A. Cough.

   B. Lupus-like syndrome.

   C. Disulfiram-like reaction with alcohol.

   D. Agranulocytosis.

3. A 55-year-old man presents with severe pain in his left big toe which seemed to worsen the morning after a wine and cheese party. On physical exam, his MTP joint is red, warm, and sensitive to touch. An aspirate of the joint will most likely reveal:

   A. Calcium pyrophosphate crystals.

   B. Antibodies to double-stranded DNA.

   C. Monosodium urate crystals.

   D. Anti-IgG antibodies.

4. A 40-year-old patient presents with complaints of excessive vomiting and diarrhea that is black in color. She appears pale and feels more fatigued than normal. She also complains of hot flashes. A CBC reveals anemia with an unusually high reticulocyte count. You suspect a possible carcinoid tumor. Which of the following would be the most likely location of the tumor and which element might be abnormal in a urinalysis?

   A. Small intestine; norepinephrine.

   B. Appendix; serotonin.

   C. Liver; VIP.

   D. Large intestine; epinephrine.

5. A pediatrician is unable to decipher the gender of a newborn. A lab exam reveals low serum cortisol, low sodium, high potassium, and high testosterone levels. An abdominal CT reveals enlarged adrenal glands. Which enzyme is mostly likely deficient in this patient?

A. 17α-hydroxylase.

B. 11β-hydroxylase.

C. Insulin.

D. 21α-hydroxylase.

6. A 24-year-old patient presents to the ER with pelvic pain, acute onset of left knee pain, and a fever of 100.8°C. Pelvic exam is significant for a positive chandelier sign, bilateral adnexal tenderness, and cervical discharge that on culture reveals Gram-negative diplococci. The patient denies any recent trauma but admits to multiple sexual partners with minimal, if any, contraception. What is the most likely cause of this patient's findings?

A. *Chlamydia trachomatis.*

B. *Staphylococcus saprophyticus.*

C. *Lactobacillus acidophilus.*

D. *Neisseria gonorrhea.*

7. A 25-year-old female presented to the ER 2 years ago with acute pancreatitis with elevated calcium levels cited as the cause. She reports a history of ulcers for which she takes sucralfate. Increased serum parathyroid hormone levels prompted excision of two of her parathyroid glands with a postoperative return to normal calcium levels. One year later, she presents with decreased visual acuity and milk discharge from her breasts. What is the most likely diagnosis?

A. MEN II/IIa.

B. Overdose on antipsychotic medications.

C. Chronic renal disease.

D. MEN I.

8. A 22-year-old female who lives in an apartment with her roommates suspects they are spying on her by tapping her phone lines for the past year. For this reason, she has decided to live alone. She dresses strangely, is not well groomed, and seems preoccupied with what she claims are voices from the FBI. Neuropsychological evaluation of this patient will most likely reveal which of the following:

A. Mental retardation.

B. Frontal lobe dysfunction.

C. Memory loss.

D. Lack of orientation to person and place.

9. A 30-year-old patient with chronic asthma presents for a yearly physical. He is currently on no medications and significant family history includes his father's passing at age 50 from an acute myocardial infarction. He reports allergies to a trimethoprim sulfamethoxazole (TMP-SMX) medication he took several years ago to treat a *Salmonella* infection. On physical exam, there are no remarkable findings except a blood pressure of 155/102. Given this patient's history, which is the best medication to prescribe?

A. Propranolol.

B. Clonidine.

C. Atenolol.

D. Furosemide.

10. A 24-year-old male presents with a resting tremor which has become progressively worse over the past year. A slit lamp examination indicates yellowish brown deposits at the limbus of the cornea. Lab studies reveal elevated AST and ALT. What is the correct trend of plasma ceruloplasmin, total serum copper, and free copper, respectively?

    A. Decreased, decreased, increased.

    B. Increased, decreased, decreased.

    C. Decreased, increased, increased.

    D. Decreased, decreased, decreased.

11. A 55-year-old male presents with diarrhea and abdominal cramps. Stool specimens reveal blood and mucus but no parasites or ova. Within 2 weeks, the patient's condition improves. However, his history indicates that intermittent episodes of pain and diarrhea have occurred during the past 15 years. Colonoscopy revealed superficial, uninterrupted mucosal inflammation extending from the rectum to the transverse colon. This patient is at highest risk for developing which complication?

    A. Fistula.

    B. Pseudomembranous colitis.

    C. Fat malabsorption.

    D. Adenocarcinoma of the colon.

12. The most common pathological finding in Alzheimer disease is:

    A. Neuronal loss in the caudate nucleus and putamen.

    B. Neuronal loss in the zona compacta of the substantia nigra, the locus ceruleus, and the dorsal nucleus of the vagus nerve.

    C. Neurofibrillary tangles and senile plaques.

    D. Negri bodies.

    E. Copper deposits in the brain, liver, cornea, and kidney.

13. A 65-year-old male complains of postprandial epigastric pain for the past 6 months. Endoscopy reveals an erythematous patch on the lower esophageal mucosa with a biopsy of the lesion showing basal squamous epithelial hyperplasia. Based on these findings, what is the patient most likely at risk for developing?

    A. Esophageal varices.

    B. Scleroderma.

    C. Esophageal adenocarcinoma.

    D. Iron deficiency.

14. At autopsy, the heart of an 84-year-old female showed marked right ventricular and right atrial dilation and hypertrophy. Minimal atherosclerosis was present in the aorta and the pulmonary trunk showed moderate atherosclerosis. Which of the following conditions is the most likely predisposing factor?

    A. Chronic obstructive pulmonary disease.

    B. Pulmonary embolism.

    C. Tetralogy of Fallot.

    D. Hypertrophic cardiomyopathy.

15. A 45-year-old male presents with flank pain and complaints of blood in urine which was confirmed by a urinalysis. An abdominal ultrasound reveals bilaterally enlarged kidneys replaced with cysts. Which of the following would be a likely finding in this patient?

   A. Hemoptysis.

   B. White cell casts in urine.

   C. Hypertension.

   D. Proteinuria.

16. An 8-year-old female presents to the ER with excessive coughing and wheezing. Her parents relay that she has a history of such attacks with difficulty breathing. A sputum sample examined microscopically revealed increased numbers of eosinophils and lab testing indicated elevated serum IgE levels. Which of the following is the most likely histologic finding?

   A. Hypertrophy and inflammation of the bronchial wall muscle and thickening of the pulmonary epithelial basement membrane.

   B. Dilation and inflammatory destruction of bronchi walls.

   C. Hyaline membrane lining of alveoli with interstitial and alveolar edema.

   D. Patchy areas of consolidation around bronchioles with neutrophils in the alveoli.

17. A woman recently gave birth to a baby girl. Physiologically, what is the hormonal stimulus for lactation?

   A. Decreased estrogen and progesterone levels.

   B. Dopamine.

   C. Increased estrogen and progesterone levels.

   D. Bromocriptine.

18. A 4-month-old female is brought to her pediatrician with recurrent infections ranging from *E. coli*, *Candida albicans*, rotavirus, and cytomegalovirus. The patient died 2 months later despite aggressive treatment. What was the cause of this patient's death?

   A. DiGeorge syndrome.

   B. Wiskott-Aldrich syndrome.

   C. Severe combined immunodeficiency.

   D. Selective IgA deficiency.

19. A 3-year-old child presents for an annual physical and a harsh, machinery-like murmur is auscultated in the upper chest. Echocardiography reveals no abnormalities in valves. However, angiography shows moderate pulmonary hypertension. Which is the best way to correct this defect?

   A. Indomethacin.

   B. Steroids.

   C. Prostaglandin E.

   D. N-acetylcysteine.

20. A 13-year-old mentally retarded female presents for a regular check-up. On physical exam, she had palpebral fissures with epicanthal folds. Her palms both have transverse creases. On auscultation of the chest, a grade II/VI systolic murmur is heard. Which of the following diseases is she predisposed to developing at an unusually early age?

A. Heart failure.

B. Subarachnoid hemorrhage.

C. Hipercholesterolemia.

D. Alzheimer disease.

21. A 59-year-old male who has smoked two packs of cigarettes for the past 43 years develops a cough with hemoptysis that has persisted for 2 months. He has also noticed a 7-pound weight loss over a 6-month time period. Serum calcium concentration is elevated with low phosphorous levels. Albumin levels are on the upper end of normal. What is the most common histologic finding in this patient?

A. Deposition of IgG along the glomerular basement membrane.

B. Small, dark blue cells.

C. Tennis racket–shaped cytoplasmic inclusions.

D. Keratin pearls.

22. An 80-year-old female presents to her family physician with headaches for the past several months. On physical exam, she has a pulsating left temporal artery that is painful to touch. A biopsy of the thickened temporal artery reveals focal granulomatous inflammation. What is the best therapy to treat this condition and the associated complication if left untreated?

A. Lovastatin; malignant hypertension.

B. Corticosteroids; blindness.

C. Penicillin; aortic aneurysm.

D. Smoking cessation; gangrene.

23. A 55-year-old female presents to the ER with a ruptured abdominal aortic aneurysm and is rushed to the OR. In order to correct the aneurysm, the surgeon had to clamp the abdominal aorta above the bifurcation of the renal arteries for approximately 90 minutes. On postoperative evaluation, the patient's BUN was 80mg/dL and creatinine was 4.1 mg/dL. Her GFR declined to 8 ml/minute with diminished urine output. What would be a likely finding in this patient's urinalysis?

A. White cell casts.

B. Epithelial cell casts.

C. Protein.

D. Glucose.

24. A mother brings her 6-year-old son to the ER. For the past 3 hours, he has failed to respond to any external stimuli. The mother reports that her son suffered a sore throat, fever, and cough for almost 5 days. Lab testing reveals a total bilirubin level of 6.5 mg/dL, direct bilirubin of 4.5 mg/dL, alkaline phosphatase of 98 U/L, AST of 541 U/L, and ALT of 698 U/L in serum. Blood ammonia concentration was 104 μmol/L. What is the most likely cause of this patient's emergent condition?

A. Chloramphenicol.

B. Trimethoprim-sulfamethoxazole (TMP-SMX).

C. Aspirin.

D. Ciprofloxacin.

25. A 43-year-old alcoholic presents to the ER with acute epigastric abdominal pain. He also complains of nausea and vomiting. Physical exam reveals a fever, blood pressure of 95/70 mm Hg, tachycardia, and a tender epigastric region. Lab tests indicate elevated lipase and amylase, leukocytosis, and hypocalcemia. Which of the following is a common cause of this condition?

A. Alcohol abuse.

B. Hypercalcemia.

C. Hypertriglyceridemia.

D. Cystic fibrosis.

26. A 32-year-old African American female presents with feelings of fatigue for the past several months. She has noticed a rash on her cheeks that worsens with sun exposure. Blood work reveals positive antinuclear antibodies and a hypochromic, microcytic anemia. Urinalysis shows mild proteinuria. Which medication might this patient be taking that predisposed her to these symptoms?

A. Spironolactone.

B. Lithium.

C. Quinidine.

D. Amiodarone.

27. A 70-year-old male, long-time smoker is hospitalized for over 3 weeks due to complications from a hip replacement. He suddenly experienced severe dyspnea and died within 1 hour despite resuscitative measures. What is the most likely cause of death in this patient?

A. Acute right heart failure.

B. Emphysema.

C. Asthma.

D. Bronchoconstriction.

28. A 4-year-old boy is unable to play with his classmates because he becomes increasingly tired and is unable to keep up. His mother describes his gait as "clumsy" and noticed that he is having difficulty climbing stairs. His serum creatine kinase level is significantly elevated. Which of the following lab findings would confirm this patient's diagnosis?

A. Blood eosinophil count.

B. Acetylcholinesterase antibody titer.

C. Oligoclonal immunoglobulin bands in cerebrospinal fluid.

D. Immunohistochemical staining for dystrophin.

29. A 25-year-old sexually active female complains of vaginal pruritus and a yellowish vaginal discharge. On pelvic exam, the cervical os is red with no remarkable mass lesions or erosions. A Pap smear reveals numerous neutrophils but no dysplastic cells. Addition of KOH to the discharge resulted in a negative "Whiff" test. The most common cause of this patient's presentation is:

A. *Trichomonas vaginalis*.

B. *Candida albicans*.

C. *Gardnerella vaginalis*.

D. Herpes simplex virus (HSV).

30. A 40-year-old male with an unremarkable past medical history presents with complaints of chronic leg pain that began approximately 5 months ago. An X-ray of the leg reveals a 3-cm cystic lesion in the left tibial diaphysis with no erosion of the cortex or soft tissue. On biopsy, osteoclasts are increased in number with fibroblast proliferation. The most likely diagnosis is:

   A. Giant cell tumor of the bone.
   B. Parathyroid adenoma.
   C. Osteomyelitis.
   D. Secondary parathyroidism.

31. A 55-year-old female presents with pain in her left knee, right distal interphalangeal joints of her fourth and fifth fingers, low back pain, and neck pain. She has noticed more stiffness and pain in the morning that gets better as the day progresses. On the musculoskeletal exam, joint crepitus is audible on knee movement. Lab results are unremarkable with normal phosphorous, alkaline phosphatase, uric acid, and calcium levels. Given these findings, what is the most likely diagnosis?

   A. Gout.
   B. Multiple myeloma.
   C. Rheumatoid arthritis.
   D. Osteoarthritis.

32. A 25-year-old medical student uses insulin injections to control her diabetes mellitus for the past 12 years. One morning, she is unable to be awakened by her roommate and is brought to the ER unconscious. Lab findings include a high plasma level of insulin with no detectable C-peptide. Urinalysis reveals a 4+ ketone level with no blood, protein, or glucose. What is the most likely diagnosis?

   A. Excessive exogenous insulin.
   B. Nodular glomerulosclerosis.
   C. Type 2 diabetes.
   D. Zollinger-Ellison syndrome.

33. Two weeks after a normal delivery, a 29-year-old female who is nursing her infant notices fissures in the skin around her right nipple. She describes it as extremely tender and "red." There is also a purulent exudate that drains from the fissure. What is the most likely diagnosis?

   A. Intraductal papilloma.
   B. Acute mastitis.
   C. Fat necrosis.
   D. Fibroadenoma.

34. A 23-year-old female presents for her monthly prenatal checkup. She was under the impression that she would begin lactating during pregnancy and not after. What is the physiology associated with why lactation begins after parturition?

   A. Elevated FSH and LH levels.
   B. Elevated estrogen and progesterone blood levels.
   C. Depressed prolactin blood levels.
   D. Elevated hypothalamic GnRH levels.

35. A 15-year-old high school football player presents with pain and weakness in his right shoulder. He is unable to abduct his arm past 30°. He has also noticed a general sensory loss around his shoulder and upper arm areas. His shoulder appears to be anteriorly dislocated and the patient reports a hard tackle during a recent game. What is the most likely nerve involved?

A. Radial nerve.

B. Long thoracic nerve.

C. Axillary nerve.

D. Ulnar nerve.

36. A 35-year-old female presents with the skin lesion below on her lower, outer left arm.

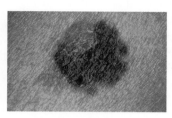

(Reprinted by the permission of the American Cancer Society.)

She has noticed it increase in size from a "small mole" to this lesion over a few weeks. When asked about her occupation, which do you think is her most likely response?

A. Radiation oncologist.

B. Corporate executive.

C. Beach lifeguard.

D. Teacher.

37. A 20-year-old male college student presents to student health with a sore throat, slight fever, and bilateral submaxillary and cervical lymphadenopathy. He complains of a dry cough and general fatigue for the past week. Physical exam reveals slight hepatosplenomegaly with enlarged posterior auricular lymphadenopathy as well. Labs reveal anemia, thrombocytopenia, elevated ALT, AST, and bilirubin, and a positive heterophil antibody test. What is the most likely cause of this patient's diagnosis?

A. *Staphylococcus aureus*.

B. Epstein-Barr virus.

C. *Chlamydia trachomatis*.

D. *Streptococcus pneumoniae*.

38. A 10-year-old child presents with a 5-month history of profuse bleeding from minor cuts and injuries. He has also suffered a severe hemorrhage into his knee joint which required multiple transfusions. His father and paternal uncle also suffer with the same condition. His PTT is prolonged and the PT is normal. Given this patient's history, what is most likely lacking?

A. Factor VIII.

B. β-globin chain.

C. α-globin chain.

D. Glucose-6-phosphate dehydrogenase.

39. A 65-year-old female presents to her gynecologist with complaints of vaginal bleeding. She has never been married or had children and has been postmenopausal for 14 years now. Her BMI is 34. On pelvic exam, her uterus does not seem enlarged and her cervix appears normal. What is the most likely risk factor that led to this patient's disease?

   A. Adenomyosis.
   B. HPV infection.
   C. Nulliparity.
   D. Smoking.

40. A 28-year-old female presents with decreased vision in her right eye. She complains of episodes of increased weakness several weeks ago which she felt attributed to being in medical school. A neurologic exam revealed left, lower weakness. A CSF analysis reveals increased IgG levels with prominent oligoclonal bands. The MRI of the brain below revealed small, 0.5-cm areas of demyelination located in periventricular white matter. With what condition is her diagnosis often associated?

   A. Berry aneurysms.
   B. Bronchogenic cancer.
   C. Horner syndrome.
   D. Medial longitudinal fasciculus (MLF) syndrome.

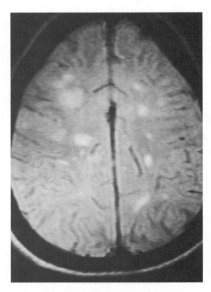

(From Tasman W, Jaeger E. The Wills Eye Hospital Atlas of Clinical Ophthalmology, 2nd Ed. Lippincott Williams & Wilkins, 2001.)

41. The gross appearance of a heart depicted in Figure7-5 at autopsy was seen in a 30-year-old patient after a short illness of less than a week. Which of the following laboratory findings was obtained during his hospital course prior to his death?

   A. Positive antineutrophil cytoplasmic autoantibody.
   B. Increased creatine kinase MB fraction.
   C. Blood culture with *Staphylococcus aureus*.
   D. Elevated anti-streptolysin O titer.

42. A 60-year-old shipyard employee experienced dyspnea for the past 2 years and eventually dies of respiratory complications. A biopsy of his lung revealed the following. (See below.) Which neoplasm is this condition most commonly associated with?

A. Bronchogenic carcinoma.

B. Esophageal adenocarcinoma.

C. Hepatocellular carcinoma.

D. Colonic adenocarcinoma.

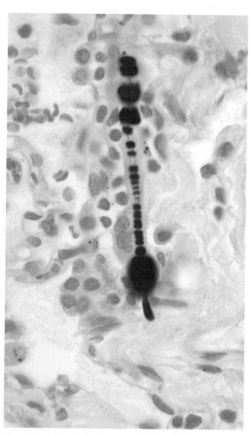

(From Cagle PT. Color Atlas and Text of Pulmonary Pathology. Philadelphia: Lippincott Williams & Wilkins, 2005.)

43. A 55-year-old man presents with a 3-year history of dyspnea on exertion and overall weakness. A radiograph of the chest reveals diffuse interstitial markings. Pulmonary function tests reveal a normal FEV_1/FVC ratio but a diminished FVC. Which of the following is the most likely pathologic finding?

A. Uniform dilation of air spaces.

B. Edematous, congested lungs and prominent hyaline membranes.

C. Inflammation of the bronchial walls with eosinophilia.

D. Honeycombed lung with alveolar septal fibrosis.

44. A 66-year-old woman presents to the emergency room with complaints of dyspnea and diaphoresis but no real chest pain or back pain. She has been nauseous and vomiting intermittently for the past 8 hours. Her daughter describes her vomit as bilious without any indication of bright-red blood or coffee-ground material. Physical exam reveals a distressed woman with a blood pressure of 115/75 mm Hg, pulse 70, and respiratory rate of 16. Jugular venous distension is 8.5 cm. Lungs are clear to auscultation with an audible S4, normal S1 and S2 without murmurs. Abdominal exam was unremarkable. Pulses are equal bilaterally. Chest X-ray revealed a "boot-shaped" heart. An ECG shows ST elevations in the inferior leads (II, III, and AVf) and reciprocal ST depressions in the anterior leads (V1, V2). Given these findings, what is the patient's most likely diagnosis?

A. Aortic dissection.

B. Right heart failure.

C. Pericardial tamponade.

D. Anterior myocardial infarction.

45. A 32-year-old complains of intermittent abdominal cramping with diarrhea that was positive for occult blood. Colonoscopy reveals many areas of mucosal edema and ulceration scattered among areas that appear normal. There are also crypt abscesses with noncaseating granulomas present in a biopsy of the small intestine. Which of the following additional findings is likely given this patient's history?

A. Inflammation limited to the mucosa.

B. Continuous lesions.

C. Hypertrophy of Brunner glands.

D. Fistulas.

46. A 40-year-old male presents with several months of worsening fatigue with headache and abdominal pain. He works in an antique shop where he cleans, polishes, and welds metals. The shop is in the basement of a high-rise building and poorly ventilated. He has noticed that he is unable to grasp his tools as well as he used to. A complete blood count reveals microcytic anemia and the peripheral smear below.

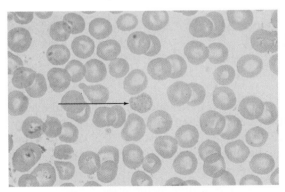

(From Anderson SC. Anderson's Atlas of Hematology. Lippincott Williams & Wilkins, 2003.)

Which of the following additional lab tests will support your diagnosis?

A. Elevated blood creatine kinase.

B. Elevated ALT and AST levels.

C. Hypocalcemia.

D. Elevated blood levels of zinc protoporphyrin.

47. A patient who was recently diagnosed with HIV presents with severe abdominal pain that began 2 days ago. He also complains of back pain and nausea. Physical exam reveals rigidity in the abdominal musculature. Labs reveal elevated amylase and lipase levels. What is the most likely cause of this patient's findings?

   A. Didanosine (ddI).

   B. Fluconazole.

   C. Isoniazid.

   D. Rifampin.

48. A 22-year-old female presents with complaints of tremor at rest which has become worse over the past 3 months. Her friends also believe she is acting strangely in social settings. A slit-lamp exam reveals corneal deposits in a ring-like pattern. Lab findings include decreased total serum protein concentration, normal albumin levels, increased total and direct bilirubin, and an elevated AST and ALT. Alkaline phosphatase was within normal limits. Which of the following lab findings would also be likely in this case?

   A. Increased serum ferritin.

   B. Decreased serum ceruloplasmin.

   C. Positive antimitochondrial antibody.

   D. Decreased α_1-antitrypsin.

49. A 25-year-old female presents with complaints of weak extraocular muscle movement and eyes that she feels are "bulging out." She has also noticed the skin on her lower legs turning unusually thick. Physical exam reveals exophthalamos with diffuse, nonpitting edema and thickening of the skin on the anterior aspect of her lower legs. What is the most likely lab finding given this patient's condition?

   A. Decreased serum TSH levels.

   B. Decreased calcium levels.

   C. Increased urinary homovanillic acid (HVA) levels.

   D. Increased urinary 5-HIAA levels.

50. A 49-year-old construction worker complains of polydipsia and polyuria. His past medical history is unremarkable except for a recent fall from a ladder while on the job in which he hit his head. Lab findings include hypernatremia, increased serum osmolality, and decreased urine specific gravity. These findings are most likely associated with a deficiency in:

   A. ADH.

   B. Prolactin.

   C. TSH.

   D. Melatonin.

Answers

1.	B	26.	C
2.	C	27.	A
3.	C	28.	D
4.	B	29.	A
5.	D	30.	B
6.	D	31.	D
7.	D	32.	A
8.	B	33.	B
9.	C	34.	B
10.	A	35.	C
11.	D	36.	C
12.	C	37.	B
13.	C	38.	A
14.	A	39.	C
15.	C	40.	D
16.	A	41.	C
17.	A	42.	A
18.	C	43.	D
19.	A	44.	B
20.	D	45.	D
21.	D	46.	D
22.	B	47.	A
23.	B	48.	B
24.	C	49.	A
25.	A	50.	A

1. **Answer: B (Case 5).** This patient exhibits signs and symptoms of atypical pneumonia. Key findings include cough with minimal sputum production, normal leukocyte count, increased cold agglutinins, and a negative Gram stain, sputum, and blood cultures. In over 50% of cases, cold agglutinin titer is increased. Because *Mycoplasma pneumoniae* lacks a cell wall, penicillins and cephalosporins are ineffective. Erythromycin is the drug of choice as it directly inhibits protein synthesis when blocking translocation when binding to the 50S ribosomal subunit. All other choices are correctly paired with their most appropriate treatment. However, since the cultures and stains for bacteria were negative, we can immediately rule out Options A and C. *Streptococcus pneumoniae* (Option A) is a common cause of bacterial pneumonia in adults older than 20 years old. However, on Gram stain, Gram-positive cocci would be visible and on blood culture, α-hemolytic, catalase-negative organisms would be observed. *Staphylococcus aureus* (Option C) is not a cause of pneumonia (Table 5-1). *Pneumocystis carinii* (Option D) is best treated with the TMP-SMX combination. However, it is a common cause of pneumonia in the immunocompromised such as AIDS patients.

2. **Answer: C (Case 12).** Severe diarrhea with mucus and blood in the stools suggests an enteroinvasive microorganism, such as *Entamoeba histolytica* or *Shigella dysenteriae*. In gastroenteritis, the diarrhea is self-limited. In this case, a liver abscess along with the description of the cyst in the stool sample (as nonmotile and with four nuclei) suggests *E. histolytica*. Mucosal and submucosal invasion by *E. histolytica* allows for access to submucosal veins that drain into the portal system and eventually the liver. The best treatment is metronidazole which also treats *Giardia lamblia* and *Trichomonas vaginalis*. Several key side effects associated with metronidazole include GI upset and a disulfiram-like reaction if taken with alcohol.

   Cough (Option A) is a common side effect of ACE inhibitors used to treat hypertension, CHF, and diabetic renal disease. Losartan is an angiotensin II receptor antagonist with the same therapeutic effect but does not cause cough. Phenytoin, procainamide, hydralazine, and isoniazid have been associated with causing a lupus-like syndrome (Option B). Agranulocytosis (Option D) is a common side effect of clozapine, carbamazepine, and colchicine. Drugs suggested in Options A, B, and D are not used to treat this patient's condition.

3. **Answer: C (Case 14).** This patient most likely has gout which was exacerbated by alcohol. The "wine and cheese" buzzword is often used on Boards to suggest a hypertensive crisis that results when tyramine in foods such as wine and cheese is ingested by patients taking monoamine oxidase inhibitors such as phenelzine and tranylcypromine. On joint aspirate, monosodium urate crystals (Option C) would be the most likely finding with crystals that are needle-shaped and negatively birefringent. Calcium pyrophosphate crystals (Option A) suggest pseudogout with rhomboid-shaped, positively birefringent crystals. The knee is often a classic location. Antibodies to double-stranded DNA (Option B) is specific for systemic lupus erythematosus (SLE) and indicates a poor prognosis. Over 90% of patients with SLE are female and additional findings such as a malar rash, photosensitivity, and arthritis would be mentioned in the clinical presentation. Anti-IgG antibodies (Option D) is specific to rheumatoid arthritis which presents with symmetric joint involvement and morning stiffness that improves with use.

4. **Answer: B (Case 18).** This patient's presentation suggests a carcinoid tumor which most often arises from the appendix (Option B), from which it usually never metastasizes. The neurotransmitter that would be elevated on a urinalysis would be serotonin because these tumors produce serotonin (5-HT), which is then broken down in the liver to 5-HIAA. Carcinoid tumors rarely affect the small intestine (Option A) and would not secrete norepinephrine. Pheochromocytomas, tumors of the chromaffin cells of the adrenal gland, secrete epinephrine (Option D) and norepinephrine. VIPomas are tumors of the pancreas that secrete vasoactive intestinal peptide (VIP). This peptide has three major functions: 1) relaxation of the GI smooth muscle, including the lower esophageal sphincter, 2) stimulation of pancreatic HCO_3^- secretion, and 3) inhibition of gastric H^+ secretion.

5. **Answer: D (Case 20).** This patient presents with 21α-hydroxylase deficiency which results in a female (XX) fetus born with ambiguous genitalia, decreased aldosterone (hence, hyponatremia, metabolic acidosis, and hyperkalemia), decreased cortisol, and increased ACTH. The latter is the cause of hyperplasia of the adrenal cortex. Precursors of

cortisol can accumulate and be shunted toward the androgen synthesis pathway, leading to virilization of the female fetus. 17α-hydroxylase (Option A) presents in teenage females who never enter puberty. Lab findings reveal increased ACTH due to decreased adrenal androgens and glucocorticoids and increased mineralocorticoids. Increased aldosterone causes hypernatremia, hypokalemia, and metabolic alkalosis with lack of pubic and axillary hair due to decreased adrenal androgens. 11β-hydroxylase (Option B) would also present with ambiguous genitalia and increased deoxycortisone which acts as a mineralocorticoid increasing sodium and decreasing potassium. Like 21α-hydroxylase deficiency, ACTH levels are increased while cortisol and aldosterone levels are decreased. Insulin (Option C) would not affect sodium, ACTH, and cortisol levels. It would cause hyperkalemia because insulin promotes potassium uptake. It would also cause metabolic acidosis with an over-production of ketoacids (β-hydroxybutyrate and acetoacetate).

6. **Answer: D (Case 22).** This patient presents with the classic symptoms of pelvic inflammatory disease (PID). Given this patient's acute onset of knee pain and the culture description, *Neisseria gonorrhea* (Option D) would be the most likely causative agent. *Chlamydia trachomatis* (Option A) is often cited as a cause of PID. However, it does not cause septic arthritis, and endocervical culture would not reveal Gram-negative diplococci. Instead, infected cells are examined for the presence of iodine-staining glycogen inclusion bodies which are unique to *C. trachomatis*. *Staphylococcus saprophyticus* (Option B) is a common cause of urinary tract infections and on culture would appear as Gram-positive cocci that are catalase positive, coagulase negative. *Lactobacillus acidophilus* (Option C) is part of the normal vaginal flora that is responsible for maintaining the vaginal pH at <4.5.

7. **Answer: D (Case 27).** Taking this patient's entire history into account, the best diagnosis would be MEN I (Wermer syndrome) which is associated with neoplasms or hyperplasia of the parathyroids, pancreas, and pituitary (Option D). Two years ago, her parathyroid gland was overactive causing hypercalcemia and acute pancreatitis. This patient also has a history of Zollinger-Ellison syndrome caused by a gastrin-secreting tumor in the pancreas resulting in recurrent ulcers. Her recent complaint of visual loss and galactorrhea suggests a pituitary adenoma.
MEN II/IIa (Option A) would be correct if there were some mention of adrenal medulla hyperplasia or neoplasm (pheochromocytoma) or medullary thyroid carcinoma. MEN II/IIa is a constellation of medullary thyroid carcinoma, pheochromocytoma, and a parathyroid tumor or adenoma. Overdose on antipsychotic medications (Option B) would explain her recent galactorrhea but does not take into account her history of pancreatic and parathyroid-related conditions. Chronic renal disease (Option C) is a secondary cause of hyperparathyroidism. Again, it does not explain the patient's 3-year history of pancreatic, parathyroid, and pituitary complications.

8. **Answer: B (Case 28).** The key findings in this case are the patient's dress, poor grooming habits, and auditory hallucinations for a period longer than 6 months which indicates this patient has schizophrenia. Neuropsychological evaluation of a patient with schizophrenia will most likely reveal frontal lobe dysfunction (Option B) with decreased glucose utilization in these lobes. Other findings include enlargement of lateral and third ventricles and decreased size of limbic structures (i.e., hippocampus and amygdala). Patients with schizophrenia usually have intact memory, orientation to person, place, and time, and are of normal intelligence. Memory loss (Option C) suggests Alzheimer disease, which is commonly associated with geriatric patients with common presentation including gradual memory loss and intellectual abilities. Neurophysiologically, acetylcholine activity decreases with reduced choline acetyltransferase (the enzyme involved in the synthesis of ACh). Brain ventricles enlarge and pathologically, senile (amyloid) plaques and neurofibrillary tangles are evident.

9. **Answer: C (Case 30).** This patient is suffering from essential hypertension given his young age, high blood pressure, and family history. There are several clues in the case that should suggest atenolol as the best treatment for this patient. He is a chronic asthmatic with sulfa allergies. Therefore, furosemide (Option D) would not be the best choice because furosemide is a sulfa drug and allergy to one sulfa drug usually eliminates treatment with other sulfas to avoid a hypersensitivity reaction. The bronchioles have β$_2$ receptors, which dilate bronchiolar smooth muscle when sympathetically stimulated. Propranolol (Option A) is a β$_1$ and β$_2$

antagonist. The β_1 antagonist effect is therapeutic for this patient's malignant hypertension, decreasing heart rate, contractility, and AV node conduction. However, the β_2 antagonist effect will constrict bronchiolar smooth muscle, further exacerbating his asthma. Atenolol (Option C) and metoprolol are only β_1 antagonists and would be the best treatment option in this patient. Clonidine (Option B) is an α_2 agonist that is mainly used to treat mild to moderate hypertension that has failed to respond to treatment with diuretics alone.

10. **Answer: A (Case 33).** This patient presents with classic Wilson disease with Kayser-Fleischer rings due to deposition of copper in the corneal limbus and a Parkinson-like syndrome. The latter is due to degeneration of the putamen and globus pallidus, manifesting as resting tremors, spasticity, and dysarthria. The primary defect in Wilson disease is a decrease in ceruloplasmin, which normally functions to bind plasma copper, leading to low total plasma copper but elevated free plasma copper. This elevation in free plasma copper is the main cause of the pathology associated with Wilson disease. The elevated plasma copper deposits in the cornea, liver, and lenticular nuclei. The treatment of this disease involves lifelong copper chelation therapy with D-penicillamine.

11. **Answer: D (Case 34).** This patient presents with clinical and histologic features that suggest ulcerative colitis. Patients with this disease have an increased risk of developing adenocarcinoma of the colon (Option D). Because inflammation is limited to the mucosa, ulcerative colitis does not predispose to fistula formation. On the other hand, Crohn disease involves full thickness inflammation and therefore, can cause fistulas (Option A) to form between the large intestine and bladder, for instance. Pseudomembranous colitis (Option B), caused by overgrowth of *C. difficile,* occurs when the normal gut flora is altered by antibiotic treatment, specifically clindamycin and ampicillin. Fat malabsorption (Option C) does not occur in ulcerative colitis because the ileum is not involved.

12. **Answer: C (Case 35).** Neuronal loss in the caudate nucleus and putamen (Option A) is characteristic of Huntington disease. Patients with this autosomal dominant disease have an expanded CAG triplet repeat (>40) associated with clinical features of progressive choreo-athetosis, early personality changes with progressive dementia, and eventual psychosis. Neuronal loss in the zona compacta of the substantia nigra, the locus ceruleus, and the dorsal nucleus of the vagus nerve (Option B) describes Parkinson disease with a decrease in dopaminergic neurons that is characterized by four cardinal signs: resting ("pill rolling" tremor), rigidity, bradykinesia, and gait disturbances/ postural instability. Neurofibrillary tangles and senile plaques (Option C) are classic for Alzheimer disease. The senile plaques are composed of a central amyloid core while the neurofibrillary tangles are phosphorylated tau proteins that form helical filaments. Negri bodies (Option D) are characteristic of Rabies disease. It should be noted that both Negri bodies and Lewey bodies (found in Parkinson disease) are intra*cytoplasmic* inclusions. Viruses, on the other hand, tend to have intra*nuclear* inclusions. Copper deposits in the brain, liver, cornea, and kidney (Option E) are characteristic of Wilson disease, which is an autosomal recessive disease. Key clinical findings include liver failure, Kayser-Fleischer rings, and elevated copper in the urine due to its effect on the kidney. There is a wide variety of movement problems (i.e., wing-beating, tremor, parkinsonism, dystonia, and chorea) that reflects the deposition of copper in the brain.

13. **Answer: C (Case 23).** The pathological changes suggest Barrett esophagus associated with reflux of acidic gastric contents into the lower esophagus (gastroesophageal reflux disease [GERD]). Patients often present with a history of "heartburn" after meals. In Barrett esophagus, which is a complication of long-standing GERD, there is columnar metaplasia of the squamous epithelium that normally lines the esophagus. Eventually, Barrett esophagus can predispose to esophageal cancer (Option C). Esophageal varices (Option A) can be associated with inflammation and mucosal ulceration overlying the varices but there is no association with epigastric pain postprandially. Esophageal varices are more often associated with alcohol abuse. Scleroderma (Option B) is associated with progressive fibrosis with stenosis and can be part of a larger constellation of findings (the CREST syndrome). Iron deficiency (Option D) can lead to the appearance of upper esophageal webs and can be part of the Plummer-Vinson syndrome with atrophic glossitis and anemia.

14. **Answer: A (Case 36).** This patient exhibits evidence of pulmonary hypertension (Option A) with moderate atherosclerosis and right-sided heart failure. Because this is secondary to lung disease, it is often called cor pulmonale or right heart failure due to an obstructive (emphysema, COPD) or restrictive lung disease (fetal/adult respiratory distress syndrome). Pulmonary embolism (Option B) can also result in cor pulmonale but with right heart dilation, *not* hypertrophy. Tetralogy of Fallot (Option C) is further discussed in Case 42. Briefly, the Tetralogy of Fallot is characterized by pulmonary stenosis, right ventricular hypertrophy, an overriding aorta, and a ventricular septal defect. This commonly will present at a much earlier age with cyanosis and characteristic EKG (right ventricular hypertrophy) and echocardiogram findings. Hypertrophic cardiomyopathy (Option D) is due to asymmetric hypertrophy involving the intraventricular septum. Over 50% of the cases are familial and autosomal dominant in inheritance. Hypertrophic cardiomyopathy is a common cause of sudden death in young athletes. In this case, the changes in this patient's autopsy were primarily on the right.

15. **Answer: C (Case 37).** This patient has an autosomal dominant form of polycystic kidney disease (APKD). Hypertension (Option C) and infection are the most common complications of this disorder. The kidney damage that occurs with APKD causes hypertension via the same mechanism as renal artery stenosis with activation of the renin–angiotensin–aldosterone system. Hemoptysis (Option A) would be an associated finding in Goodpasture disease which affects both the lungs and kidneys with symptoms of hemoptysis and hematuria, respectively. White cell casts in urine (Option B) is pathognomonic for acute pyelonephritis which would present with a different profile of clinical symptoms, including dysuria, frequent urination, fever, and CVA tenderness. Proteinuria (Option D) suggests a nephrotic syndrome such as membranous glomerulonephritis. The case would have some mention of periorbital and peripheral edema and lab tests would reveal hypoalbuminemia and hyperlipidemia.

16. **Answer: A (Case 38).** This patient is suffering from a Type I hypersensitivity reaction precipitated by presensitized IgE-coated mast cells in the mucosal and submucosal surfaces of airways. Exacerbating factors include cold weather, smoking, and exercise. These lead to degranulation of mast cells; release of mediators such as leukotrienes, prostaglandins, and histamine; attraction of eosinophils; and bronchoconstriction. Hypertrophy and inflammation of the bronchial wall muscle and thickening of the pulmonary epithelial basement membrane (Option A) is the best description of the histologic changes that follow inflammation during an "asthma attack." Dilation and inflammatory destruction of bronchi walls (Option B) refers to bronchiectasis. Hyaline membrane lining of alveoli with interstitial and alveolar edema (Option C) refers to acute alveolar damage. Bacterial pneumonia results in neutrophilic exudates and consolidation (Option D).

17. **Answer: A (Case 45).** To review prolactin secretion, the hypothalamus releases thyrotropin-releasing hormone (TRH) which acts on the anterior pituitary to stimulate prolactin secretion. Prolactin acts on the mammary glands to stimulate milk production and the development of breasts while inhibiting ovulation/spermatogenesis by decreasing gonadotropin-releasing hormone (GnRH). Dopamine (Option B), also released from the hypothalamus, acts to inhibit the anterior pituitary from releasing prolactin and hence inhibits lactation.

During pregnancy, a woman's estrogen and progesterone levels are high (Option C), blocking the action of prolactin on the breast. After parturition, estrogen and progesterone levels decrease (Option A), releasing their negative inhibition of prolactin and causing lactation. Milk production is maintained by suckling, which stimulates both oxytocin and prolactin secretion. Prolactin stimulates milk production in the mammary glands, while oxytocin causes ejection of milk from the breast. Bromocriptine (Option D) is a dopamine agonist so it would also decrease prolactin secretion.

18. **Answer: C (Case 40).** Children with susceptibility to bacterial, viral, and fungal infections most likely suffer from severe combined immunodeficiency (Option C). Lymph nodes are extremely underdeveloped with few lymphocytes and no germinal centers. The thymus, tonsils, and Peyer patches are often hypoplastic. These patients are sometimes referred to as "bubble kids" because of their increased sensitivity to infection and careful exposure to the environment. This patient would have benefited from an allogenic bone marrow transplantation with stem

cells that could give rise to normal T and B cells. DiGeorge syndrome (Option A) manifests in infancy as well with failure of cell-mediated immunity owing to T-cell deficiency. The third and fourth pharyngeal pouches fail to develop, leading to an absence of the thymus and parathyroid glands. This presents as tetany from the hypocalcemia (no PTH) and recurrent bacterial, viral, and fungal infections. Wiskott-Aldrich syndrome (Option B) refers to an inability to mount an IgM response to capsular polysaccharides of bacteria. Therefore, patients with Wiskott-Aldrich syndrome present with recurrent pyogenic infections, thrombocytopenia, and eczema. Selective IgA deficiency (Option D) often results from deficient terminal differentiation of B cells into IgA-secreting plasma cells. Lack of IgA in mucosal secretions increases susceptibility to respiratory and gastrointestinal infections.

19. **Answer: A (Case 42).** This patient most likely has a patent ductus arteriosus (PDA). Major clues include the classic description of a PDA murmur that results in pulmonary hypertension. In the fetal period, a shunt from the high pressured right side of the heart to the lower pressured left side of the heart is present. In the neonatal period, the lung resistance decreases, lowering the pressure on the right side of the heart and reversing the shunt to left to right. Patency of the duct is necessary to sustain life in transposition of the great vessels. This is maintained with prostaglandin E (Option C). However, indomethacin (Option A) is the treatment of choice to close PDAs. Steroids (Option B) are not used to correct PDAs. Instead, they are common treatments for conditions such as Takayasu and temporal arteritis, Crohn disease, multiple sclerosis, and minimal change disease. N-acetylcysteine (Option D) is the drug of choice to loosen mucous plugs in patients with cystic fibrosis and is used as an antidote to treat acetaminophen overdose.

20. **Answer: D (Case 43).** Based on the physical exam, it is clear this patient has Down syndrome. Patients with this genetic disorder are at increased risk of developing Alzheimer disease at an early age. This is believed to be due to the fact that the genetic defects for both Alzheimer disease and Down syndrome are located on chromosome 21. Patients with Marfan syndrome are at increased risk of heart failure (Option A) due to aortic dilation which causes regurgitation and aortic rupture and dissection. Subarachnoid hemorrhage (Option B) has been linked to patients with the autonomic dominant condition called polycystic kidney disease. Patients would present with a chief complaint similar to the "worst headache of their life." Finally, hypercholesterolemia (Option C) is a genetic disorder caused by defective LDL receptor in peripheral tissues, specifically the liver, which plays a key role in the clearance of cholesterol from the blood. Heterozygotes present with cholesterol levels between 300 and 500 mg/dl, whereas homozygotes can suffer from their first heart attack before age 20 with total cholesterol levels ranging from 500 to 1,000 mg/dl.

21. **Answer: D (Case 46).** This patient most likely suffers from squamous cell carcinoma with the characteristic histologic finding of keratin pearls (Option D). This neoplasm can secrete a parathyroid hormone-related peptide which explains this patient's high calcium and low phosphorous levels. Deposition of IgG along the glomerular basement membrane (Option A) is classic for Goodpasture syndrome which affects *both* the lungs and kidneys with associated hemoptysis and hematuria. Small, dark blue cells (Option B) imply small cell carcinoma, which is associated with ectopic ACTH and ADH secretion causing a Cushing-like syndrome and hyperosmotic urine, respectively. Tennis racket–shaped cytoplasmic inclusions (Option C) describes Birbeck granules which are characteristic of eosinophilic granuloma. Although common in former smokers, clinical features of eosinophilic granulomas include lesions in lungs or ribs with potential for pneumothorax.

22. **Answer: B (Case 47).** This patient presents with a classic case of temporal arteritis, which responds well to steroids. If left untreated, the patient can experience impaired vision and even blindness (Option B) with occlusion of the ophthalmic artery. Lovastatin; malignant hypertension (Option A) would relate best to a patient with familial hypercholesterolemia that should be treated with a lipid lowering drug. Without treatment, the patient is at increased risk for several cardiovascular diseases, one of them being malignant hypertension. Penicillin; aortic aneurysm (Option C) relates best to syphilis which, if left untreated by penicillin can progress to tertiary syphilis. This stage results in disruption of the vasa vasorum of the aorta,

dilation of the aorta and valve ring, and increased risk of aortic aneurysm. Smoking cessation; gangrene (Option D) relates to Buerger disease, which is seen in heavy smokers. This disease can cause thrombosing vasculitis of small and intermediate peripheral arteries and veins. The only real treatment is smoking cessation. Otherwise, complications such as gangrene can develop.

23. **Answer: B (Case 25).** This patient probably developed acute tubular necrosis (ATN) secondary to renal ischemia during her surgery. Other causes of ATN include rhabdomyolysis and drugs such as amphotericin B and aminoglycosides. In ATN, renal tubular epithelial cells (Option B) are damaged and are sloughed, blocking renal tubule lumens and impeding urine flow. This explains this patient's decreased GFR. White cell casts (Option A) are pathognomonic for acute pyelonephritis which would present with a different profile of clinical symptoms, including dysuria, frequent urination, fever, and CVA tenderness. Protein (Option C) suggests a nephrotic syndrome such as membranous glomerulonephritis. The case would have some mention of periorbital and peripheral edema and lab tests would reveal hypoalbuminemia and hyperlipidemia. Glucose (Option D) would suggest poorly controlled diabetes mellitus where the body's filtered glucose load exceeds the kidney's reabsorption ability resulting in glucosuria.

24. **Answer: C (Case 50).** This patient presents with Reye syndrome. Given the patient's symptoms for the past 5 days, he most likely had influenza for which his mother gave him aspirin (Option C). This resulted in hepatoencephalopathy with microvesicular fatty change, hypoglycemia, and coma. The best alternative in this case would have been acetaminophen, which does not cause Reye syndrome in children. Moreover, if a patient overdoses on acetaminophen, it can be reversed with N-acetylcysteine. Reye syndrome is usually a fatal, irreversible condition. Chloramphenicol (Option A) is often associated with the "gray baby syndrome" which is common in premature infants because they lack liver UDP-glucuronyl transferase. Chloramphenicol is used to treat meningitis, not influenza. Trimethoprim-sulfamethoxazole (TMP-SMX) (Option B) may have precipitated a hypersensitivity reaction since TMP-SMX is a sulfa drug with potential for allergy to its chemical composition. The combination is used to treat recurrent UTIs, *Salmonella, Pneumocystis carinii* pneumonia, and *Shigella.* Ciprofloxacin (Option D) can cause headache, dizziness, and GI irritation. It is associated with damage to cartilage and is used to treat bacterial infections of the urinary and GI tracts. It most likely is not the cause of this patient's condition.

25. **Answer: A (Case 49).** This patient most likely has acute pancreatitis. Alcohol abuse (Option A) and gallstones are the most common causes. Gallstones specifically block the flow of bile into the intestine causing a backup into the pancreatic duct, irritating and inflaming pancreatic tissue. Hypercalcemia (Option B) and hypertriglyceridemia (Option C) are less common, but well-established causes of acute pancreatitis. Cystic fibrosis (Option D) causes chronic pancreatitis as thickened pancreatic secretions block the pancreatic duct owing to genetically defective chloride channels. Patients with cystic fibrosis present as early as a few days after birth with failure to thrive and meconium ileus. Additional findings include malabsorption of fats (especially fat-soluble vitamins A, D, E, and K) and steatorrhea. A key diagnostic test for cystic fibrosis is an increased concentration of chloride ions in a sweat test.

26. **Answer: C (Case 48).** This patient presents with the classic findings of systemic lupus erythematosus (SLE). Procainamide, quinidine, and hydralazine are well known for causing a lupus-like syndrome. Procainamide and quinidine are class IA antiarrhythmics whereas hydralazine is an arterial vasodilator used in the treatment of hypertension. Procainamide can cause a reversible lupus-like syndrome. Quinidine (Option C) can cause the same along with cinchonism (tinnitus, headache, dizziness). Spironolactone (Option A) is one of several K$^+$-sparing diuretics (others include triamterene and amiloride) used to treat potassium depletion, CHF, and hyperaldosteronism. Side effects include hyperkalemia and gynecomastia. Lithium (Option B) is used to treat bipolar disorder and is associated with tremor and polyuria as lithium acts as an ADH antagonist causing nephrogenic diabetes insipidus. Amiodarone (Option D) is also a class IA antiarrhythmic not associated with lupus. Instead, it is commonly cited for its multiple adverse effects including pulmonary fibrosis, hepatotoxicity, and hyper- and hypothyroidism.

27. Answer: A (Case 17). This patient most likely suffered a saddle pulmonary thromboembolus with sudden death from acute cor pulmonale resulting in right heart failure (Option A). Emphysema (Option B) can be a cause of his long-term smoking but would not cause sudden death as in this patient. Asthma (Option C) would also not cause sudden death. Both emphysema & asthma are obstructive lung diseases with respiratory acidosis and a decreased FEV_1/FVC. Bronchoconstriction (Option D) would be incorrect since the airways are not obstructed. Hence, the lungs do not collapse and there is no bronchoconstriction.

28. Answer: D (Case 1). Given this patient's age and gender, the diagnosis is most likely X-linked muscular dystrophy. An immunohistochemical stain for dystrophin (Option D) would probably reveal the absence of dystrophin, as shown in the figure below. This would confirm the diagnosis of Duchenne muscular dystrophy. Becker muscular dystrophy is similar to Duchenne muscular dystrophy in that it also is inherited in an X-linked pattern with a mutation to the dystrophin gene. However, in Becker muscular dystrophy, dystrophin is abnormal, *not* completely absent, resulting in a less severe muscle disease with middle-age presentation in males.

A blood eosinophil count (Option A) would confirm an allergic or parasitic disorder, such as trichinosis. An acetylcholinesterase antibody titer (Option B) would be elevated in myasthenia gravis which would present with muscle weakness after repetitive use.

Oligoclonal immunoglobulin bands in cerebrospinal fluid (Option C) would be present in multiple sclerosis, an idiopathic demyelinating disorder with intermittent remissions and exacerbations.

Dystrophin analysis in Duchenne and Becker muscular dystrophies

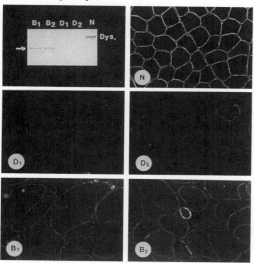

(Image from Rubin E, Farber JL. Pathology, 3rd Ed. Philadelphia: Lippincott Williams & Wilkins, 1999.)

29. Answer: A (Case 2). This patient most likely has trichomoniasis, a common STD caused by the parasite *Trichomonas vaginalis* (Option A). Symptoms are similar to this patient's with vaginal pruritus and a yellow, frothy discharge. The epithelium of the vulva and vagina are inflamed giving it the classic "strawberry cervix" appearance. This patient and all of her sexual partners should be treated with metronidazole and tested for other potential STDs.

Candida albicans (Option B) would be identified in a KOH preparation of a swab sample with a finding similar to Color Plate 2-1A. Moreover, the discharge is usually scant white with vulvar pruritus. *Gardnerella vaginalis* (Option C) presents with a malodorous white-gray discharge and *no* vaginal pruritus. Upon mixing KOH with the discharge, the "Whiff" test should be positive. Finally, herpes simplex virus (HSV) (Option D) is more likely in the perineal region because HSV-2 is latent in the sacral and lumbar regions while HSV-1 remains latent in the trigeminal nerve with oral infection upon activation.

30. **Answer: B. (Case 4).** Parathyroid adenomas (Option B) result in excessive secretion of parathyroid hormone (PTH) and cause primary hyperparathyroidism. This results in osteoclastic reabsorption of bone with microfractures that can give rise to hemorrhages. This results in an influx of macrophages and a reactive fibrosis. Giant cell tumor of the bone (Option A) would be in the epiphyseal region of the bone. On radiograph, the classic finding is a "soap bubble" appearance. Chronic osteomyelitis (Option C) would not have resulted in such a discrete lesion. Causes of osteomyelitis are summarized below:

    Overall: *Staphylococcus aureus*
    Neonates: *Streptococcus agalactiae*
    Sickle cell disease patients: *Salmonella*
    Drug users: *Pseudomonas aeruginosa*
    Sexually active: *Neisseria gonorrhoeae*

    Secondary parathyroidism (Option D) is more common in patients with chronic renal failure. The associated physiology is as follows:

Physiology of Chronic Renal Failure

↓ 1,25 dihydroxycholecalciferol and ↓ phosphate excretion (caused by ↓ GFR)

↓ serum calcium because of ↓ 1,25 dihydroxycholecalciferol

↑ PTH (2°)

Renal osteodystrophy (↑ bone resorption caused by ↑ PTH) and osteomalacia
(↓ 1,25 dihydroxycholecalciferol)

31. **Answer: D (Case 41).** Osteoarthritis (Option D) is a common problem among the elderly with a variety of joint types involved, from large, weight-bearing joints to small distal and proximal interphalangeal joints. Gouty arthritis (Option A) would have resulted in elevated serum levels of uric acid. The most common location is the MTP joint of the big toe (podagra). Multiple myeloma (Option B) produces lytic lesions in bones but does not typically involve the joints. Rheumatoid arthritis (Option C) can involve large and small joints with symmetric involvement of the small joints of the hands and feet. The following table summarizes the key differences between osteoarthritis (Option D) and rheumatoid arthritis (Option C).

	Osteoarthritis	**Rheumatoid Arthritis**
Etiology	Mechanical injury ("wear-and-tear")	Autoimmune (HLA-DR4)
Incidence	Older patients and women more commonly affected	Women ages 20–50
Joint involvement	Weight-bearing joints, Heberden nodes (DIP), and Bouchard nodes (PIP)	Symmetric joints of hands, knees, and feet; proximal interphalangeal and metacarpophalangeal joints
Notable features	Osteophytes, destruction of articular cartilage, and eburnation; no systemic symptoms	Subcutaneous nodules, pannus formation in MCP and PIP joints, rheumatoid factor (anti-IgG), ulnar deviation, and subluxation; systemic symptoms (fever, fatigue, pleuritis)

32. Answer: A (Case 10). The fact that this patient has no detectable C-peptide levels indicates no endogenous insulin production and hence, Type 1 diabetes in which there is no insulin production by the pancreas. In this case, the patient has experienced a hypoglycemic coma from either high levels of exogenous insulin (Option A) to treat her diabetes or a normal dose of insulin with a decreased appetite and hence, an inadequate glucose level. Nodular glomerulosclerosis (Option B) is a characteristic feature of renal involvement with advanced diabetes mellitus. Proteinuria and an elevated BUN level would have supported this diagnosis. A renal biopsy would have revealed Kimmelstiel-Wilson lesions. These are nodules of **pink hyaline material** that form in regions of glomerular capillary loops in the glomerulus. They are due to a marked increase in mesangial matrix as a result of nonenzymatic glycosylation of proteins. Type 2 diabetes (Option C) is characterized by peripheral insulin resistance, relatively decreased pancreatic insulin secretion, and increased hepatic glucose output. Ketoacidosis rarely occurs in Type 2 diabetes whereas it is very common in Type 1 diabetes. Biochemically, in Type 1 diabetes ketoacidosis results from a lack of insulin and increased release of glucagon. This leads to increased gluconeogenesis, release of fatty acids, and oxidation of fatty acids to form ketone bodies. Glucagon specifically accelerates fatty acid oxidation by increasing processing through the carnitine shuttle into the mitochondria, where oxidation occurs. Type 1 diabetes has weak genetic predisposition, but more than 90% of Caucasians with Type 1 diabetes have HLA-DR3, HLA-DR4, or both. Type 2 diabetes is strongly genetic with no association to the HLA system.

Zollinger-Ellison syndrome (Option D) is associated with one or more islet cell adenomas of the pancreas that secrete gastrin. This excessive secretion often results in peptic ulcer disease with gastric or duodenal ulcerations.

Kimmelstiel-Wilson disease.

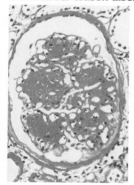

(From Rubin, E. and Farber, J.L. Pathology, 3rd Ed. Philadelphia: Lippincott Williams & Wilkins, 1999.)

33. Answer: B (Case 16). This patient most likely has developed staphylococcal acute mastitis (Option B) which produces localized abscesses. This is a common complication of lactation. Intraductal papilloma (Option A) is usually solitary and located within large lactiferous sinuses or ducts. Intraductal papillomas have a tendency to bleed. Fat necrosis (Option C) would have been high on the differential if there were some mention of trauma to the breast. The damaged, necrotic fat becomes phagocytosed by macrophages which become lipid laden. The lesion resolves in several weeks, leaving a collagenous scar. Fibroadenoma (Option D) is a neoplasm that is a discrete mass formed by a proliferation of fibrous stroma in ducts. Women often present with complaints of a lump in the breast that is discrete and freely movable. These neoplasms tend to enlarge in pregnancy and late in each menstrual cycle.

34. Answer: B (Case 31). During pregnancy, high levels of estrogen stimulate prolactin secretion which increases steadily throughout the three trimesters. Lactation, however, does not occur during pregnancy because increased estrogen and progesterone block the action of prolactin on the breast (Option B). Therefore, increased prolactin blood levels (opposite of Option C) and decreased estrogen and progesterone levels (after parturition) would result in lactation. Milk letdown is maintained by suckling which stimulates both prolactin and oxytocin secretion. During lactation, prolactin has three major inhibitory effects: 1) hypothalamic GnRH secretion (Option D), 2) GnRH's action on the anterior pituitary and hence, inhibition of LH and FSH secretion (Option A), and 3) LH and FSH on the ovaries. Therefore, ovulation is suppressed as long as lactation continues. The figure below summarizes lactation regulation.

Lactation regulation

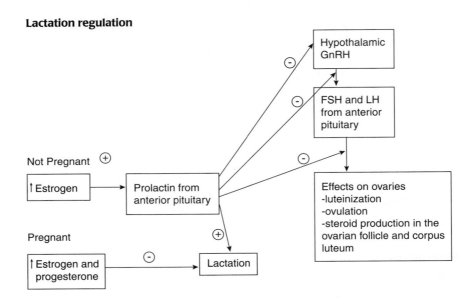

35. **Answer: C (Case 11).** This patient most likely has suffered an injury to his right axillary nerve, C5, 6 (Option C) which can be injured by a lesion near the shoulder joint. The nerve innervates the deltoid and teres minor muscles and hence, shoulder abduction is impaired. Sensory loss to the upper arm and shoulder is also common. The radial nerve, C5, 6, 7, 8 (Option A) innervates the triceps brachii, brachioradialis, extensor carpi radialis longus (wrist), and thenar extensors. Injury most often occurs near the spinal groove of the shaft of the humerus. Clinical features include paralysis of wrist extensors (wrist drop) and paralysis of the thenar extensors. "Saturday night palsy" can occur when the radial nerve is compressed after a person falls asleep with their arm over the back of a chair. The radial nerve provides sensory innervation to the dorsal aspect of the radial side of the hand, lower part of the thenar eminence, and all fingers except the hypothenar eminence and one half of the 4th finger. The long thoracic nerve, C5, 6, 7, 8, T1 (Option B), innervates the serratus anterior muscle, causing "winging of the scapula" leading to a protrusion of the scapula when a person pushes against a wall. There are usually no sensory deficits. The ulnar nerve (Option D), C7, 8, T1, innervates the flexor carpi ulnaris, half of the flexor digitorum profundus, and most of the intrinsic muscles of the hand. Injury can occur at the ulnar groove at the elbow, cubital tunnel, or the base of the palm. Clinical features would include impairment of wrist flexion, adduction, and impaired adduction of the thumb and 4th and 5th fingers. There may also be sensory loss or "tingling" of the medial proximal forearm and half of the 4th and all of the 5th fingers.

36. **Answer: C (Case 15).** This patient has a malignant melanoma with irregular borders and variability in pigmentation. Dysplastic nevi are often precursors of melanoma. There is significant risk of metastasis with the depth of the tumor correlating with the risk of spread. These lesions are associated with sunlight exposure, so option C would be likely because beach lifeguards often have prolonged exposure to the sun.

37. Answer: B (Case 24). This patient most likely has infectious mononucleosis which is a systemic viral infection caused by the Epstein-Barr virus (Option B). It is transmitted through respiratory droplets and saliva and is most common among teenagers and young adults ("kissing disease"). Epstein-Barr virus is also associated with an increased risk of Burkitt lymphoma, Hodgkin disease, and nasopharyngeal carcinoma. *Staphylococcus aureus* (Option A) is a catalase- and coagulase-positive, β-hemolytic, Gram-positive bacteria. It is associated with inflammatory diseases such as skin infections, pneumonia, and organ abscesses. It is also associated with toxin-mediated diseases such as toxic shock syndrome and rapid-onset food poisoning. *Chlamydia trachomatis* (Option C) is a Gram-negative obligate intracellular parasite that causes mucosal infections, specifically pneumonia, nongonococcal urethritis, conjunctivitis, and arthritis. Finally *Streptococcus pneumoniae* (Option D) is a Gram-positive, β-hemolytic, optochin-sensitive bacteria. It can be detected with a positive Quellung reaction and lancet-shaped, Gram-positive diplococci on Gram staining. It is the most common cause of community-acquired pneumonia. Clinical presentation would include a high-grade fever, pleuritic chest pain, and a productive, blood-tinged cough.

38. Answer: A (Case 26). This patient most likely suffers with hemophilia A, which is caused by a factor VIII (Option A) defect or deficiency. The transmission is X-linked given the family history of males who have a similar condition. The PTT is prolonged because factor VIII is required for the intrinsic pathway while the PT is normal because the extrinsic pathway does not depend on the function of factor VIII. β-globin chain (Option B) suggests either β-thalassemia minor (heterozygote) with underproduced β chains or β-thalassemia major (homozygote) with completely absent β chains. In both cases, fetal hemoglobin production increases to compensate but is still inadequate. α-globin chain (Option C) suggests α-thalassemia in which α-globin genes are lacking. There is no compensatory increase in other chains. Hb Barts lacks all four α-globin genes resulting in hydrops fetalis and intrauterine fetal death. Glucose-6-phosphate dehydrogenase (Option D) is also an X-linked disorder and results in hemolytic anemia RBCs susceptible to damage by oxidants. Patients often present with hemoglobinuria and there may be some mention of a new drug regimen because G6PD deficiency can be clinically triggered with drugs such as primaquine, sulfonamides, phenacetin, high doses of aspirin, and nitrofurantoin.

39. Answer: C (Case 32). Endometrial carcinoma is considered to be the most common gynecologic malignancy with a common clinical presentation of vaginal bleeding. Key risk factors are obesity, diabetes, hypertension, nulliparity (Option C) and prolonged estrogen stimulation from anovulatory cycles. All factors can cause endometrial hyperplasia that can progress to endometrial carcinoma. Adenomyosis (Option A) is not a risk factor for endometrial carcinoma and would have resulted in an increased uterine size. HPV infection (Option B) is associated with squamous epithelial dysplasias and carcinoma in situ of the cervix. Smoking (Option D) is a not a risk factor in endometrial carcinoma but can increase chances of atherosclerosis, which is a disease of elastic and muscular arteries. The general progression is from fatty streaks to plaques to atheromas. Body mass index (BMI) is a more accurate measure of body fat than weight alone. It is calculated by weight (kg) divided by height (meters) squared. An overweight person has a BMI greater than 25 while an obese person has a BMI greater than 30. This patient would qualify as obese.

40. Answer: D (Case 3). This patient has multiple sclerosis with a relapsing-remitting course. CSF electrophoresis reveals multiple oligoclonal bands and elevation in protein (IgG). The medial longitudinal fasciculus (MLF) syndrome (Option D), also known as internuclear ophthalmoplegia, is associated with multiple sclerosis. In this condition, patients have decreased ability for either eye to look medially but both eyes can converge because the pathway for convergence and vertical gaze (MLF) is different from the path for lateral conjugate gaze (paramedian pontine reticular formation). Therefore, a patient with MLF syndrome will have the following response to directions for eye movements:

Eye pattern.

Right	Left	
		"Look left"
		"Look right"
		"Converge"

Berry aneurysms (Option A) are associated with adult polycystic kidney disease, Marfan syndrome, and Ehlers-Danlos syndrome. Rupture of a berry aneurysm leads to subarachnoid hemorrhage and is classically described as the "worst headache of my life." Bronchogenic cancer (Option B) is often associated with excessive smoking and asbestosis, which presents with pulmonary findings. Horner syndrome (Option C) is associated with a Pancoast tumor in the apex of the lung that may affect the cervical sympathetic plexus resulting in ptosis, miosis, and anhidrosis—the classic triad for Horner syndrome.

41. **Answer: C (Case 7).** The aortic valve reveals large vegetations typical for infective endocarditis caused by highly virulent organisms like *S. aureus* (Option C). Positive antineutrophil cytoplasmic autoantibody (Option A) would indicate a vasculitis that does not involve the cardiac valves. Increased creatine kinase MB fraction (Option B) would suggest a myocardial, not endocardial, injury. Smaller, verrucous vegetations would suggest rheumatic fever and would be associated with an elevated antistreptolysin O titer (Option D).

42. **Answer: A (Case 8).** Given this patient's findings and the ferruginous bodies on microscopy, this patient most likely died of asbestosis, which is a diffuse pulmonary fibrosis caused by inhaled asbestos fibers, common in shipyard workers and plumbers. With asbestosis, there is an increased risk of mesothelioma and bronchogenic carcinoma (Option A). Esophageal adenocarcinoma (Option B) is associated with Barrett esophagus which results from chronic GI reflux. Hepatocellular carcinoma (Option C) is common with cirrhosis from alcoholism or hepatitis. Finally, there is increased risk of developing colonic adenocarcinoma (Option D) in patients with ulcerative colitis as opposed to patients with Crohn disease.

43. **Answer: D (Case 9).** The pulmonary function tests indicate that this patient has a restrictive lung disease. The progressive interstitial fibrosis associated with restrictive lung diseases such as pneumoconiosis can lead to dilation of remaining airspaces with a "honeycomb" appearance. Uniform dilation of air spaces (Option A) suggests emphysema with loss of lung tissue but no alveolar wall fibrogenesis. Edematous, congested lungs and prominent hyaline membranes (Option B) suggest diffuse alveolar damage such as in adult respiratory distress syndrome. Inflammation of the bronchial walls with eosinophilia (Option C) is common in asthma, which is not associated with fibrogenesis.

44. **Answer: B (Case 13).** This patient presents with atypical symptoms for angina and her vagal symptoms of nausea, vomiting, and bradycardia imply an inferior myocardial infarction. Additional clues to the diagnosis for right heart failure (Option B) include a jugular venous

distention (JVD) without pulmonary congestion on the X-ray or on chest exam. Aortic dissection (Option A) is unlikely because features of a dissection include some combination of pain radiating to the back, unequal blood pressures, and severe hypertension. Pericardial tamponade (Option C) would also present with dyspnea and JVD. However, it would not explain these ECG findings. Anterior myocardial infarction (Option D) would present with ST elevations in anterior leads.

45. **Answer: D (Case 19).** The clinical and histologic features in this patient are consistent with Crohn's disease. It is marked by segmental bowel involvement with transmural inflammation. This predisposes to fistulas (Option D). Inflammation limited to the mucosa (Option A) and continuous lesions (Option B) are typical of ulcerative colitis with diffuse mucosal involvement that is continuous. Hypertrophy of Brunner glands (Option C) is common with duodenal ulcers with increased gastric acid secretion or decreased mucosal protection. There is almost always an associated *Helicobacter pylori* infection with pain that decreases with meals. With gastric ulcers, pain is greater with meals, resulting in weight loss.

46. **Answer: D (Case 6).** This patient is presenting with occupational exposure to lead with subsequent lead toxicity. The peripheral smear reveals basophilic stippling, which is not specific for lead toxicity but is often seen in peripheral smears. The concentration of zinc protoporphyrin is elevated (Option D) in chronic lead poisoning, anemia of chronic disease, and iron deficiency anemia. High levels of lead in the blood interfere with heme synthesis, inhibiting the incorporation of iron into heme, and zinc is used instead. Elevated blood creatine kinase (Option A) would suggest muscle damage. Although neuropathy can occur, as in this patient who is experiencing difficulty grasping his tools, muscle enzyme creatine kinase would not be elevated. Elevated ALT and AST levels (Option B) suggest hepatic damage with elevation of liver enzymes ALT and AST. This is not associated with lead poisoning. Lead toxicity can also result in damage of renal tubules and even cause renal failure. However, alterations in electrolytes are not specific for lead-induced renal failure.

47. **Answer: A (Case 44).** This patient is presenting with acute pancreatitis. His symptoms of epigastric pain radiating to the back suggest this diagnosis with the elevated amylase and lipase levels confirming our suspicion. Didanosine (Option A), a reverse transcriptase nucleoside inhibitor, is used in HIV therapy but is also associated with acute, and sometimes fatal, pancreatitis. Fluconazole (Option B) is an antifungal agent that inhibits fungal steroid (ergosterol) synthesis. It can be associated with hormone synthesis inhibition which in males translates to testosterone inhibition and hence gynecomastia. Liver dysfunction can also occur with inhibition of cytochrome p-450. Isoniazid (Option C) is an antimicrobial that decreases the synthesis of mycolic acids. Toxicity includes hemolysis if a patient is G6PD deficient, neurotoxicity, and hepatoxicity. It is recommended that patients taking isoniazid also take pyridoxine (vitamin B_6) to prevent neurotoxicity. Rifampin (Option D) is also an antimicrobial that inhibits DNA-dependent RNA polymerase. It is associated with hepatoxicity and increases cytochrome p-450 interactions. Patients sometimes complain of reddish-orange urine when taking rifampin.

48. **Answer: B (Case 21).** This patient has Wilson disease with characteristic Kayser-Fleischer rings on slit lamp examination. Symptoms are a result of accumulation of toxic levels of copper, particularly in the eyes, liver, and brain. With a decrease in ceruloplasmin (Option B), copper cannot be secreted into the plasma. Increased serum ferritin (Option A) suggests hereditary hemochromatosis which is associated with pancreatic fibrosis, pigmentation of the skin, and micronodular cirrhosis. Ferritin is a measure of storage iron which is elevated in hemochromatosis. Positive antimitochondrial antibody (Option C) is common in primary biliary cirrhosis. Chronic liver disease or panlobular emphysema occurs with α_1-antitrypsin deficiency (Option D).

49. **Answer: A (Case 29).** Exophthalmos with pretibial myxedema suggests Graves disease with a hyperfunctioning thyroid gland leading to increased T4 levels and, via positive feedback on the pituitary, decreased TSH secretion (Option A). Decreased calcium levels (Option B) may be associated with hypoparathyroidism resulting in hypocalcemia. Clinical presentation includes neuromuscular irritability, carpopedal spasm, and, in advanced cases, seizures. Increased urinary

homovanillic acid (HVA) levels (Option C) are elevated in neuroblastoma, a pediatric tumor that produces high levels of catecholamines, and their metabolites, HVA. Increased urinary 5-HIAA levels (Option D) suggest a carcinoid syndrome which results in secretion of high levels of serotonin. Patients present with recurrent diarrhea, asthmatic wheezing, valvular disease localized to the right heart, and cutaneous flushing. Carcinoid tumors are derived from the neuroendocrine cells of the GI tract.

50. **Answer: A (Case 39).** This patient has developed central diabetes insipidus (DI) with a lack of ADH (Option A), most likely owing to his recent fall resulting in head trauma. In central DI, free water is not reabsorbed in the renal collecting tubules, diluting the urine. Deficiencies in prolactin (Option B) and melatonin (Option D) have no specific clinical effects in males. TSH (Option C) would suggest hypothyroidism with decreased TSH levels from feedback inhibition of elevated T_4 levels. Clinical presentation would have included some combination of proptosis, extraocular muscle edema, pretibial myxedema, or a diffuse goiter.

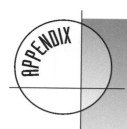

Complete blood count (CBC)	Reference value	Differential
Erythrocyte sedimentation rate	0–30 mm/hr	
Hematocrit		
Male	40.7–50.3%	
Female	36.1–44.3%	
Hemoglobin		
Male	13.8–17.2 g/dL	
Female	12.1–15.1 g/dL	
Leukocytes	$4–10 \times 10^3/\mu L$	
Neutrophils	$1.8–6.6 \times 10^3/\mu L$	38.7–74.5%
Lymphocytes	$1.2–3.3 \times 10^3/\mu L$	20.0–54.3%
Monocytes	$0.2–0.7 \times 10^3/\mu L$	2.7–9.8%
Eosinophils	$0.0–0.5 \times 10^3/\mu L$	0–6%
Basophils	$0.0–0.2 \times 10^3/\mu L$	0–3%
Mean corpuscular volume	$80.0–97.6 \ \mu m^3$	
Platelet count	$190–405 \times 10^3/\mu L$	
Reticulocyte count	0.5–1.5%	
Coagulation profile		
Activated partial thromboplastin time	25–36 sec	
Bleeding time	2.5–9.5 min	
Fibrinogen	150–360 mg/dL	
Fibrin degradation products	<8 mg/mL	
Prothrombin time	11–14 sec	
Thrombin time	11.3–18.5 sec	
Basic metabolic panel		
Carbon dioxide	–	
Chloride	97–110 mmol/L	
Creatinine	0.7–1.4 mg/dL	
Glucose	65–110 mg/dL	
Potassium	3.3–4.9 mmol/L	
Sodium	135–145 mmol/L	
Urea nitrogen	8–25 mg/dL	
Complete metabolic panel		
Albumin	3.6–5.0 g/dL	
Aspartate aminotransferase	11–47 IU/L	

(Doherty GM et: Barnes-Jewish Hospital Laboratory ReferenceValues. Department of Surgery, Washington University School of Medicine, St. Louis, Missouri: *The Washington Manual of Surgery*. Boston: Little, Brown, 1999, pp 642–46. Used by permission.)

313

Bilirubin, total	0.2–1.3 mg/dL
Calcium	8.9–10.3 mg/dL
Chloride	97–110 mmol/L
Creatinine	0.7–1.4 mg/dL
Glucose	65–110 mg/dL
Phosphatase, alkaline	38–126 IU/L
Potassium	3.3–4.9 mmol/L
Protein, total	6.2–8.2 mg/dL
Sodium	135–145 mmol/L
Urea nitrogen	8–25 mg/dL

Enzymatic activities and chemistries, other

Alanine aminotransferase	7–53 IU/L
Ammonia	19–43 μmol/L
Amylase	35–118 IU/L
Bilirubin, direct (conjugated)	0.0–0.2 mg/dL
Calcium, ionized	4.6–5.1 mg/dL
Carboxyhemoglobin	
Nonsmoker	0.0–1.5%
Moderate smoker	1–5%
Heavy smoker	5–9%
Ceruloplasmin	21–53 mg/dL
Cholesterol	
High	>240 mg/dL
Borderline	200–239 mg/dL
Desirable	<200 mg/dL
Copper	11.0–24.3 μmol/L
Creatine kinase	
Male	30–220 IU/L
Female	20–170 IU/L
MB fraction	0–12 IU/L
Ferritin	
Male	36–262 ng/mL
Female	10–155 ng/mL
Folate, plasma	3.9–28.6 nmol/L
Gamma-glutamyl transpeptidase	
Male	20–76 IU/L
Female	12–54 IU/L
Glycated hemoglobin	4.4–6.3%
Haptoglobin	44–303 mg/dL
High-density lipoprotein	27–98 mg/dL
Iron	50–175 g/dL
Binding capacity	250–450 μg/dL
Transferrin saturation	20–50%
Lactate, plasma	0.3–1.3 mmol/L
Lactate, dehydrogenase (LDH)	90–280 IU/L
Lipase	2.3–20.0 IU/L
Low-density lipoprotein	
High	>160 mg/dL
Borderline	130–159 mg/dL

Desirable	<130 mg/dL
Magnesium	1.3–2.2 mEq/L
5'-Nucleotidase	2–16 IU/L
Osmolality, serum	270–290 mOsm/L
Phosphatase, acid	0.0–0.7 IU/L
Phosphorus	2.3–4.3 mg/dL
Triglycerides, fasting	<255 mg/dL
Uric acid	4.0–8.0 mg/dL
Vitamin B_{12}	200–800 pg/mL

Selected serum hormones and tumor markers

Adrenocorticotropic hormone, fasting, a.m.	<60 pg/mL
Aldosterone	10–160 ng/mL
Alpha-fetoprotein	0.0–8.9 ng/mL
Beta-human chorionic gonadotropin	
Nonpregnant	0.0–5.0 mIU/mL
Pregnant	$5-200 \times 10^3$ mIU/mL
Carcinoembryonic antigen (CEA)	
Nonsmoker	0.0–3.0 ng/mL
Smoker	0.0–5.0 ng/mL
Cortisol, a.m.	8–25 µg/dL
Follicle stimulating hormone	
Male	2.4–19.9 IU/L
Female	
Follicular	3.1–19.7 IU/L
Luteal	1.7–11.2 IU/L
Midcycle	10.4–23.1 IU/L
Postmenopausal	18–126 IU/L
Gastrin, fasting	0–130 pg/mL
Growth hormone, fasting	<8 ng/mL
17-Hydroxyprogesterone	
Prepubertal	3–90 ng/dL
Male adult	27–90 ng/dL
Female adult	
Follicular	15–70 ng/dL
Luteal	35–290 ng/dL
Insulin, fasting	5–25 mU/L
Luteinizing hormone	
Male	0.0–8.9 IU/L
Female	
Follicular	1.4–11.5 IU/L
Luteal	0.1–16.1 IU/L
Midcycle	20.1–73.9 IU/L
Postmenopausal	8.4–46.5 IU/L
Parathyroid hormone	4.9 µEq/mL
Progesterone	
Male	<0.5 ng/mL
Female	
Follicular	0.1–1.5 ng/mL
Luteal	2.5–28 ng/mL

First trimester	9–47 ng/mL
Third trimester	55–255 ng/mL
Postmenopausal	<0.5 ng/mL
Prolactin	
Male	2–12 ng/mL
Female	2–20 ng/mL
Prostate-specific antigen	0.0–4.0 ng/mL
Renin activity, plasma	0.9–3.3 ng/mL/hr
Testosterone, free	
Male	52–280 pg/mL
Female	1.1–6.3 pg/mL
Testosterone, total	
Male	350–1,030 ng/dL
Female	10–55 ng/dL
Thyroid-stimulating hormone	0.45–6.20 μU/mL
Thyroxine, free	1.0–2.3 ng/dL
Thyroxine, total (T_4)	3.0–12.0 μg/dL
Triiodothyronine	80–200 ng/dL
T_4 index	0.85–3.50
Tumor uptake	20–40%
Vitamin D, 1,25-hydroxy	20–76 pg/mL
Vitamin D, 25-hydroxy	10–55 ng/mL

Immunology

Complement, total	118–226 U/mL
C3	77–156 mg/dL
C4	15–39 mg/dL
Immunoglobulin (Ig)	
IgA	91–518 mg/dL
IgG	805–1,830 mg/dL
IgM	61–355 mg/dL

Urinalysis

Macroscopic	
Bilirubin (qualitative)	Negative
Glucose (qualitative)	Negative
Ketones (qualitative)	Negative
Occult blood (qualitative)	Negative
pH	4.5–8.0 g/mL
Protein	0–150 mg/day
Specific gravity	1.003–1.040 g/mL
Urobilinogen	0.1–1.0 mg/dL
Microscopic	
Casts	None
Bacteria	0–1+
Red blood cells (RBCs)	0–3/high-power field
White blood cells (WBCs)	0–5/high-power field
Chemistries	
Amylase	0.04–0.30 IU/min
Calcium	0–250 mg/day

Copper	15–50 µg/day
Coproporphyrin	0–72 µg/day
Cortisol, free	20–90 µg/day
Creatinine	
Male	1.0–2.0 g/day
Female	0.6–1.5 g/day
Dopamine	100–440 µg/day
Delta-amino-levulinic acid	1.3–7.0 mg/day
Epinephrine	<15 µg/day
5-Hydroxyindoleacetic acid	<9 mg/day
Hydroxyproline, total	25–77 mg/day
Metanephrine	<0.9 mg/day
Norepinephrine	11–86 µg/day
Oxalate	
Male	7–44 mg/day
Female	4–31 mg/day
Protein	0–150 mg/day
Uroporphyrin	0–27 µg/day
Vanillylmandelic acid	2–10 mg/day

Therapeutic drug levels (serum)

Amikacin	
Trough	5–10 mg/L
Peak	20–30 mg/L
Amitriptyline	100–250 µg/L
Carbamazepine	4–10 mg/L
Clonazepam	10–80 µg/L
Cyclosporin A	125–300 ng/mL
Desipramine	100–300 µg/L
Digoxin	0.5–2.0 mg/L
Disopyramide	2–5 mg/L
Ethosuximide	40–100 mg/L
5-Fluorocytosine	
Trough	20–60 mg/L
Peak	50–100 mg/L
Gentamicin	
Trough	<2 mg/L
Peak	4–8 mg/L
Imipramine	150–300 µg/L
Ketoconazole	
Trough	≤1 g/L
Peak	1–4 mg/L
Lithium	0.6–1.2 mmol/L
N-Acetyl procainamide	6–20 mg/L
Nortriptyline	50–175 µg/L
Phenobarbital	10–40 mg/L
Phenytoin	10–20 mg/L
Primidone	5–15 mg/L
Procainamide	4–8 mg/L

Quinidine	1.7–6.1 mg/L	
Salicylate	20–290 mg/L	
Sulfamethoxazole		
Trough	75–120 mg/L	
Peak	100–150 mg/L	
Theophylline	10–20 mg/L	
Tobramycin		
Trough	0.5–1.5 mg/L	
Peak	6–8 mg/L	
Trimethoprim		
Trough	2–8 mg/L	
Peak	5–15 mg/L	
Valproic acid	50–100 mg/L	
Vancomycin		
Trough	5–10 mg/L	
Peak	20–35 mg/L	

Ascitic fluid	**Transudate**	**Exudate**
Amylase	–	Elevated
CEA	–	>10 ng/mL
CEA (ascites)/CEA (serum)	–	>2
Glucose	–	<60 mg/dL
Glucose (ascites)/glucose (serum)	<1	>1
LDH	–	Elevated
LDH (ascites)/LDH (serum)	–	>0.6
Lipase	–	Elevated
Protein	<3.0 g/dL	>3.0 g/dL
Protein (ascites)/protein (serum)	–	>0.5
RBCs	–	Elevated
Triglycerides	–	Elevated
WBCs	<300–500/μL	>500/μL

Cerebrospinal fluid	**Normal values**
Glucose	45–80 mg/dL
Pressure	70–180 mm H_2O
Protein	15–45 mg/dL
Total WBCs	0–10/μL

Pleural fluid	**Transudate**	**Exudate**
Amylase	–	Twice serum amylase
Glucose	–	0–60 mg/dL
LDH	<200 IU	>200 IU
LDH (pleural)/LDH (serum)	<0.6	>0.6
pH	7.4	<7.4
Protein	<3.0 g/dL	>3.0 g/dL
Protein (pleural)/protein (serum)	<0.5	>0.5
RBCs	<10,000/μL	>10,000/μL
Specific gravity	<1.016	>1.016
WBCs	<1,000/μL	>1,000/μL

Color Plates

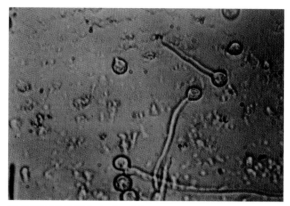

COLOR PLATE 2-1 C. albicans. [From Mahon CR, Manuselis G: Textbook of Diagnostic Microbiology, 2nd ed. Philadelphia, WB Saunders, 2000, p 751]

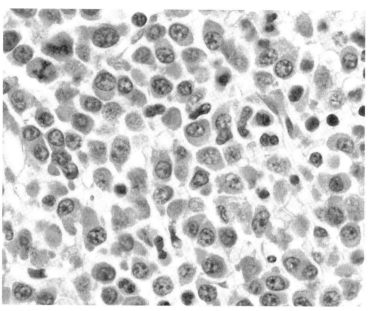

COLOR PLATE 4-4 Plasma cells and multiple myeloma. [From Burkitt HG, Stevens A, Lowe JS, Young B: Wheater's Basic Histopathology Color Atlas and Text, 3rd edition. Churchill Livingstone, 1996, p 193]

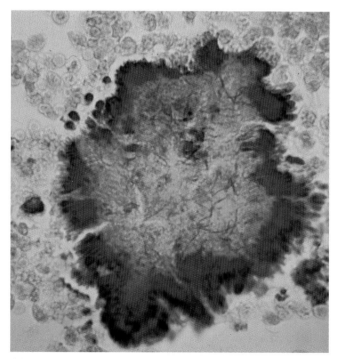

COLOR PLATE 8-1 Culture of exudate. Sulfur granules of Actinomyces israeli. [From Sweet, R.L. and Gibbs, R.S. Atlas of Infectious Diseases of the Female Genital Tract. Philadelphia: Lippincott Williams & Wilkins, 2005.

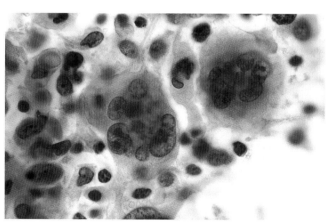

COLOR PLATE 9-1 Nasal swab and culture. Cytology of pleomorphic carcinoma with multinucleated giant cells. [From Cagle, P.T. Color Atlas and Text of Pulmonary Pathology. Philadelphia: Lippincott Williams & Wilkins, 2005.]

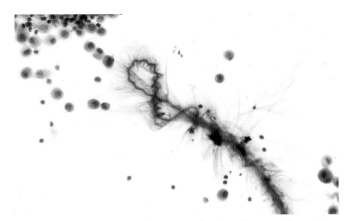

COLOR PLATE 9-2 Curschmann spiral. Corkscrew-shaped mucinous cast with radiating filaments in an exfoliative cytology specimen from a patient with asthma. [From Cagle, P.T. Color Atlas and Text of Pulmonary Pathology. Philadelphia: Lippincott Williams & Wilkins, 2005.]

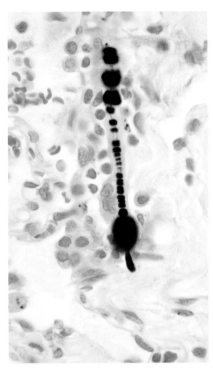

COLOR PLATE 13-4 Ferruginous bodies. Iron stains the beaded iron coat of an asbestos body bright blue around a clear asbestos fiber core, highlighting the asbestos body against a pale pink background. [From Cagle, P.T. Color Atlas and Text of Pulmonary Pathology. Philadelphia: Lippincott Williams & Wilkins, 2005.]

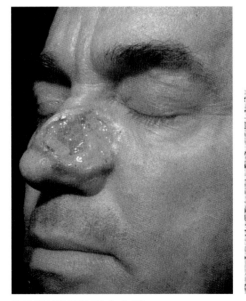
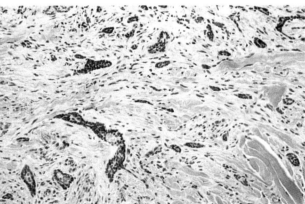

COLOR PLATE 15-1 A. The gross appearance of basal cell carcinoma. B. The microscopic appearance of basal cell carcinoma. (Reprinted with permission from Rubin E, Farber JL: Pathology, 3rd ed. Philadelphia, Lippincott-Raven Publishers, 1999, p 1292.)

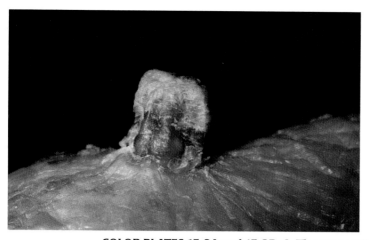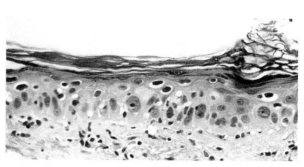

COLOR PLATES 15-2A and 15-2B **A. The gross appearance of actinic keratosis.** (Reprinted with permission from Fitzpatrick TB, Johnson RA, Wolff K, Suurmond D: Color Atlas and Synopsis of Clinical Dermatology, 4th ed. New York, McGraw-Hill, 2001, p 251.) **B. The microscopic appearance of actinic keratosis.** (Reprinted with permission from Rubin E, Farber JL: Pathology, 3rd ed. Philadelphia, Lippincott-Raven Publishers, 1999, p 1293.)

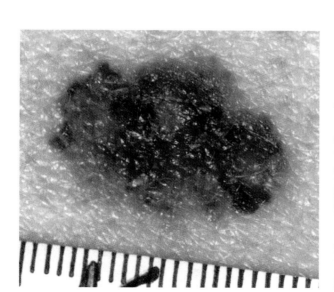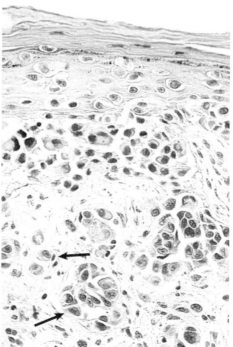

COLOR PLATES 15-3A and 15-3B **A. The gross appearance of malignant melanoma. B. The microscopic appearance of malignant melanoma.** (Reprinted with permission from Rubin E, Farber JL: Pathology, 3rd ed. Philadelphia, Lippincott-Raven Publishers, 1999, p 1281–1282.)

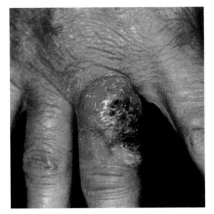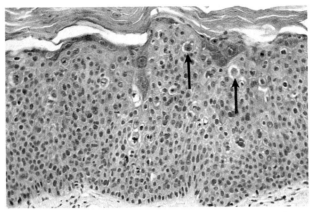

COLOR PLATES 15-4A and 15-4B A. The gross appearance of squamous cell carcinoma. B. The microscopic appearance of squamous cell carcinoma. (Reprinted with permission from Rubin E, Farber JL: Pathology, 3rd ed. Philadelphia, Lippincott-Raven Publishers, 1999, p 1293.)

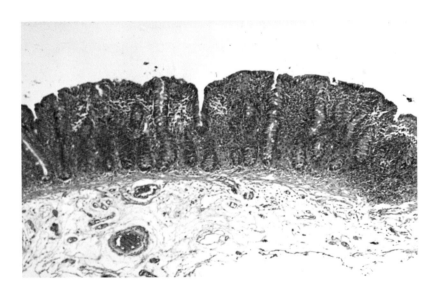

COLOR PLATE 19-1 Small intestinal biopsy (post). Villous atrophy with a flat surface, elongation of the crypts, and chronic inflammation of the lamina propria are characteristic of long-standing disease. [From Rubin, M.D. and Farber, J.L. Pathology, 3e. Philadelphia: Lippincott Williams & Wilkins, 1999.]

COLOR PLATE 19-2 Megaloblastic anemia. In this smear of peripheral blood, the erythrocytes are large, often with an oval shape, and are associated with poikilocytosis and teardrop shapes. The neutrophils are hypersegmented. [From Rubin, M.D. and Farber, J.L. Pathology, 3e. Philadelphia: Lippincott Williams & Wilkins, 1999.]

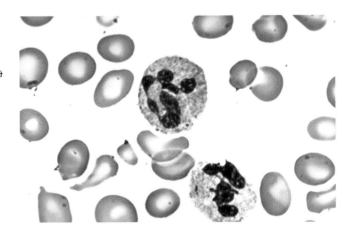

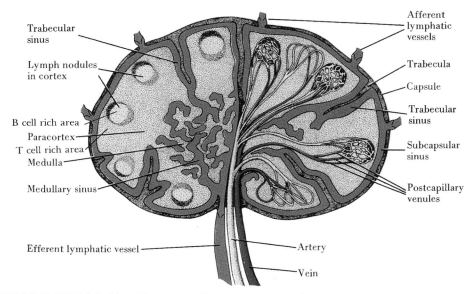

Trabecular sinus

Lymph nodules in cortex

B cell rich area

Paracortex

T cell rich area

Medulla

Medullary sinus

Afferent lymphatic vessels

Trabecula

Capsule

Trabecular sinus

Subcapsular sinus

Postcapillary venules

Efferent lymphatic vessel

Artery

Vein

COLOR PLATE 24-2 Blood from the afferent vessels are filtered through the lymph node before being recollected and exiting via the efferent vessel. [From Ross MH, Romrell LJ, Kaye GI: Histology: A Text and Atlas, 3rd ed. Philadelphia, Lippincott Williams & Wilkins, 1995, p 343. Based on Bloom W, Fawcett DW: A Textbook of Histology, 10th edition. Philadelphia, WB Saunders, 1975, p 473.]

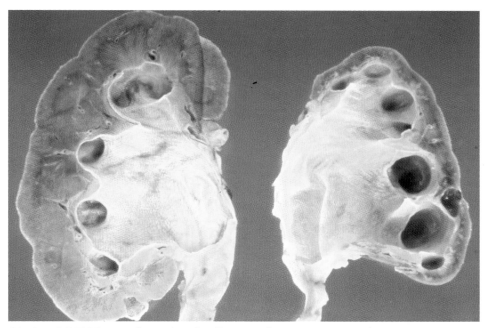

COLOR PLATE 25-1 Hydronephrosis. Bilateral urinary tract obstruction has led to conspicuous dilatation of the ureters, pelves, and calyces. The kidney on the right shows severe parenchymal atrophy. [From Rubin, E. and Farber, J.L. Pathology, 3e. Philadelphia, Lippincott Williams & Wilkins, 1999.]

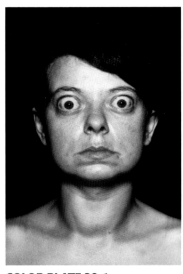

COLOR PLATE 29-1
Exophthalmos with proptosis and periorbital edema. [Reprinted with permission from Rubin, E. and Farber, J.L. Pathology, 3e. Philadelphia: Lippincott Williams & Wilkins, 1999.]

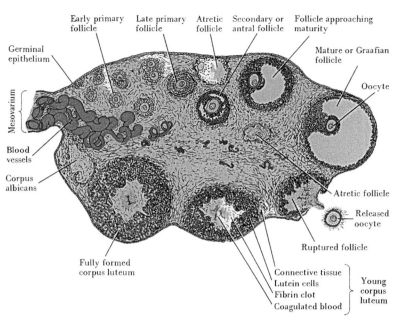

COLOR PLATE 32-2 Schematic drawing of a section through the ovary. Highly coiled blood vessels are present in the hilum and medullary regions. [From Ross MH, Romrell LJ, Kaye GI: Histology: A Text and Atlas, 3rd ed. Philadelphia, Lippincott Williams & Wilkins, 1995, p. 680 After C. E. Corliss.]

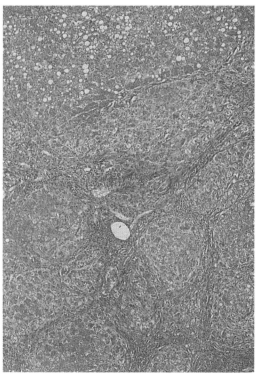

COLOR PLATE 33-1 Liver biopsy showing alcoholic cirrhosis. (From Damjanov I: A Color Atlas and Textbook of Histopathology. Philadelphia, Lippincott Williams & Wilkins, 1996, p 225.)

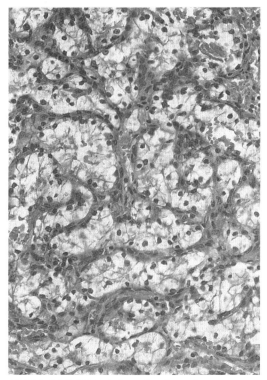

COLOR PLATE 37-1 Renal cell carcinoma. [From Damjanov I: Histopathology: A Color Atlas and Textbook. Philadelphia, Lippincott Williams & Wilkins, 1996, p 291]

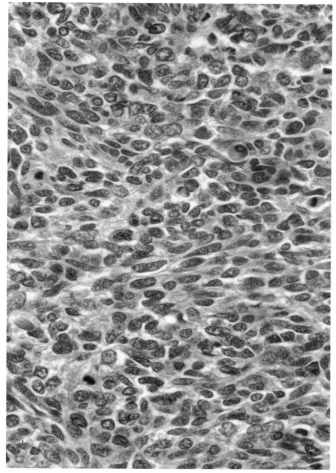

COLOR PLATE 39-5   No figure legend in case text provided.

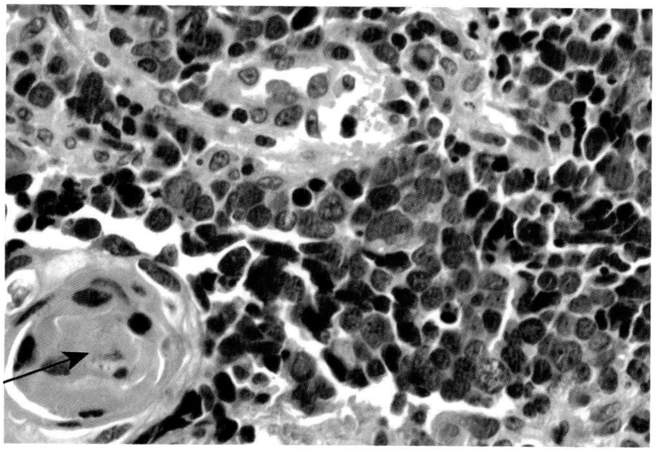

COLOR PLATE 39-6   No figure legend in case text provided.

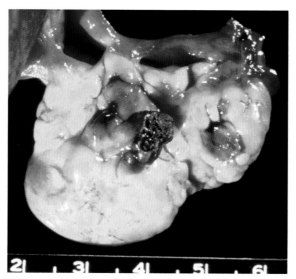

COLOR PLATE 45-1   Chocolate cysts.   [From Rubin, E. and Farber, J.L. Pathology, 3e. Philadelphia: Lippincott Williams & Wilkins, 1999.]

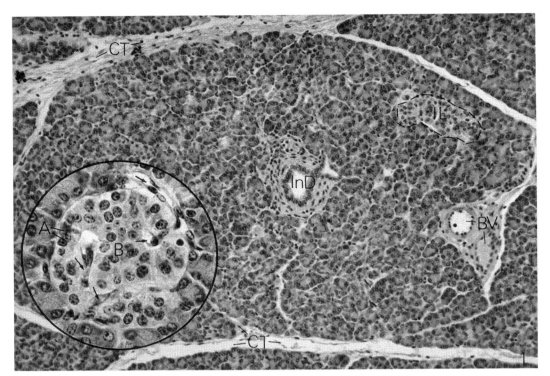

COLOR PLATE 49-1 Pancreatic histology [From Ross MH, Romrell LJ, Kaye GI: Histology: A Text and Atlas, 3rd ed. Philadelphia, Lippincott Williams & Wilkins, 1995, p 529]

Index

Page numbers followed by *f* refer to illustrations; page numbers followed by *t* refer to tables.